The American Geriatrics Society's

Complete

Guide to

Aging &

Health

The American Geriatrics Society's

COMPLETE GUIDE TO AGING & HEALTH

Mark E. Williams, M.D.

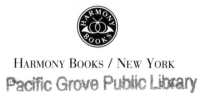

HARMONY BOOKS / NEW YORK

TO MY PATIENT FAMILY

Text copyright © 1995 by The American Geriatrics Society
Illustrations © copyright 1995 by Maureen Jones

Published by Harmony Books, a division of Crown Publishers, Inc., 201 East 50th Street, New York, New York 10022. Member of the Crown Publishing Group.

Random House, Inc. New York, Toronto, London, Sydney, Auckland

HARMONY and colophon are trademarks of Crown Publishers, Inc.

Manufactured in the United States of America

Design by Kay Schuckhart

Library of Congress Cataloging-in-Publication Data
Williams, Mark E.
    The American Geriatrics Society's book on aging / Mark E. Williams.
    —1st ed.
    Includes index.
    1. Aging. 2. Geriatrics. I. Title.   0'09
QP86.W53 1995
612.6'7—dc   94-32865
                                                              CIP

ISBN 0-517-59539-7

10 9 8 7 6 5 4 3 2 1

First Edition

Grow old along with me!
The best is yet to be,
The last of life, for which the first was made:
Our times are in his hand
Who saith, "A whole I planned,
Youth shows but half; trust God: see all, nor be afraid!"
—Robert Browning (1812–1889),
Rabbi Ben Ezra, stanza 1

CONTENTS

FOREWORD

The American Geriatrics Society (AGS) has a long history of affecting change in the provision of health care for older adults. Founded in 1942, the Society is an association of more than 6,000 health care professionals dedicated to improving the health, well-being, and independence of older adults and to promoting the provision of high-quality, comprehensive, and affordable long-term care to those chronically ill and/or functionally disabled. In the last decade, the AGS has become a pivotal force in shaping attitudes, policies, and practices in health care for older people, as greater attention is focused on the needs of our rapidly aging population. The AGS serves as a leader in and advocate for numerous and varied programs in patient care, aging research, professional and public education, and public policy.

The AGS receives thousands of calls and letters annually from the general public requesting information on a broad spectrum of aging-related issues. To address this demonstrated need for more information on aging and health, the AGS decided to develop a comprehensive resource for the general public, based on the Society's medical reference and self-assessment program for health care professionals entitled the *Geriatrics Review Syllabus: A Core Curriculum in Geriatric Medicine*. Dr. Mark Williams, the author of *The American Geriatrics Society's Complete Guide to Aging and Health*, was among the original editors of the *Geriatrics Review Syllabus*.

With the publication of this practical resource on aging and health for the public, the American Geriatrics Society hopes to bridge the gap between the expanding body of medical knowledge about geriatrics and a public in need of information about the aging process and geriatric health care. The Society envisions that this book will assist older adults and their caregivers in finding answers to their health care questions. The AGS also aims, through this book, to promote a positive, preventive approach to the health care of older adults.

The AGS hopes that *The American Geriatrics Society's Complete Guide to Aging and Health* proves an invaluable resource for readers who want to prepare themselves for a healthy old age, for dedicated caregivers of older friends and family members, and for people now in their fifties and sixties who are concerned about a particular disease, or who wonder what to expect as certain medical conditions advance with age.

The American Geriatrics Society extends sincere and heartfelt thanks to Dr. Mark Williams for his hard work and dedication in writing this book.

The American Geriatrics Society also expresses sincere appreciation to the following foundations for supporting the development of this book: The Robert Wood Johnson Foundation, The Josiah A. Macy, Jr. Foundation, The Pew Charitable Trusts, and The Retirement Research Foundation. Special appreciation is extended to Mr. Peter R. Seaver, corporate vice president, Worldwide Pharmaceutical Marketing, the Upjohn Company, for his early and ongoing support of clinical geriatrics.

—The American Geriatrics Society

ACKNOWLEDGMENTS

Although this volume is attributed to a single author, it is really a gift from numerous individuals. My thanks to them is hardly adequate. However, I am especially grateful to the contributing authors to the *Geriatrics Review Syllabus* published by the American Geriatrics Society. The combined clinical wisdom and skill of these leaders in geriatric care provided the core of the content for this book. Therefore, special thanks go to Richard Allman, Lodovico Balducci, Bruce Baum, Mark Beers, James Black, Ellen Brown, John Burkart, Ewald Busse, Anjan Chatterjee, Laura Chiodo, Seth Cohen, Leo Cooney, Jeffrey Cummings, Barry Cusack, Nancy Dubler, Craig Eisentrout, Roy Erickson, Bruce Ferrell, Joseph Fins, Joseph Francis, Susan Gaylord, Meghan Gerety, Tobin Gerhart, Barbara Gilchrest, Gail Greendale, Susan Greenspan, Ronald Hamdy, Peter Holt, Paul Katz, Susan Lehmann, David Lipschitz, Lewis Lipsitz, Bernard Lo, William McDonald, Graydon Meneilly, Susan Molchan, Stephen Montamat, Thomas Mulligan, Jane Murray, Gregory Pawlson, Paul Plattner, Peter Rabins, Neil Resnick, Charles Reynolds, Sheila Ryan, Carl Salzman, John Santinga, Jonathan Ship, Andrew Silver, Kenneth Solomon, Trey Sunderland, Marvin Swartz, Mary Tinetti, Roy Verdery, Thomas Walshe, Peter Whitehouse, and Thomas Yoshikawa.

A word of special thanks goes to John Beck, the editor of the *Geriatrics Review Syllabus* and to Bill Applegate, Dan Blazer, George Grossberg, David Reuben, and Gregg Warshaw, associate editors of the *Geriatrics Review Syllabus*, who devoted countless hours to refining and developing the syllabus.

The material that I contributed I learned from interacting with elderly people, teaching medical students, reading books and articles, regretting my own mistakes, and occasionally recognizing the mistakes of others. Because of this, I am deeply indebted to the innumerable students and patients I have encountered over the past two decades. I especially wish to acknowledge Nortin Hadler, my brilliant mentor, for his enduring impressions, provocative insights, and eternal patience. I also thank T. Franklin Williams, my fellowship director and friend, who devoted time and attention to show me firsthand the ways of the skilled and experienced geriatrician. His values and insights have had a considerable influence on my own geriatric practice. I owe a tremendous debt to the late Mack Lipkin, who shared his perspective and vast experience and who gave me the profound honor of having me as his personal physician. His wisdom is evident throughout these pages.

I also wish to acknowledge the support and assistance of Linda Hiddemen Barondess, AGS executive vice president, for her inspiration and insights regarding this project. This book was originally her vision, and I feel indebted to her for helping me to make this dream a reality. I wish to thank Bill Applegate, past president of the American Geriatrics Society, also for his strong friendship and support especially during the early phases of this project. The board of directors of the American Geriatrics Society deserves special recognition for allowing me to pursue this project in my own way.

A very special thanks goes to Madge Huntington, my remarkably helpful, perceptive, and meticulous managing editor, and to Laurel Coleman, my insightful and energetic junior editor. The illustrations are the handiwork of Maureen Jones, who has an obvious gift for artistic expression. Anne Flash, Robert Seymour, Florence Soltys, Dennis Jahnigen, Gregg Warshaw, Bill Applegate, John Burton, Joseph Fins, David Reuben, Laurence Rubenstein, Stephanie Studenski, Tom Yoshikawa, and Jane Williams read various portions of the text and offered numerous helpful suggestions. Janie Womble typed and reprocessed so many drafts of this book that I wondered if it would strain our friendship. Remarkably, she maintained her delightful sense of humor and extraordinary technical prowess. Betty Lineberry and Dorothy Jones also offered considerable technical assistance.

At Harmony Books, Valerie Kuscenko has been extremely helpful and Peter Guzzardi has been exceptionally encouraging and cooperative. Finally, my wife, Jane, and sons John and James have helped me in so many ways, supporting and sustaining me in the long hours of work. Their encouragement, patience, and love form the core of my life and clinical practice.

If I were to pick up a book on aging written by someone in his mid-forties I would want to know something about the credentials and qualifications of that individual.

I grew up in rural North Carolina, and frankly I never considered old people as any different from anyone else. My community was one where people spoke to each other on the street, took long walks after supper, and from whom no secrets were hidden. My family was not affluent but I was able to attend college on a scholarship. In medical school I began to sense an uneasiness that something was not right. Major scientific advances were elegant and held great promise to relieve suffering, but the application of this knowledge was often ineffective. I saw far too many instances where old people were not being treated as people.

About this time (the mid-1970s) leading medical journals were publishing articles on the "geriatric imperative," and Robert Butler had won a Pulitzer Prize for his book, *Why Survive? Being Old in America*. I completed my residency in internal medicine and was chosen to be a Robert Wood Johnson Clinical Scholar. This two-year program allowed my sense of social responsibility in aging to crystallize.

In the late 1970s I had decided on geriatric medicine as a career and I became one of the first group of physicians to receive formal training in the area. The problem was how to pursue instruction in this relatively new discipline. Fellowship programs were limited and none had a convincing track record. I set two strict criteria to guide my search: The program must have a director with substantial hands-on experience in caring for elderly people, and there must be a large facility to serve as a training site. In retrospect, the search was easier than it seemed at the time, and in 1980 my wife and I moved to Rochester, New York, for me to work with Dr. T. Franklin Williams at the Monroe Community Hospital. It was here that I spent almost five years learning the essential features of effective care to older people.

In the mid-1980s I was offered the best job in the country: developing geriatric programs and activities at my alma mater, the

University of North Carolina. An extraordinary stroke of good fortune placed my new office adjacent to Dr. Mack Lipkin, one of the true giants of medicine, who had retired to North Carolina to continue his teaching and writing. We established a close friendship, sharing numerous conversations and tuna fish sandwiches. One day I was stunned when Dr. Lipkin asked me to be his personal physician. This is one of the greatest compliments a physician can give a colleague. Our relationship deepened and I was honored to share the most personal insights and perceptions of a wise, sensible, and articulate physician. I felt the aging process from the inside out, witnessing it in Dr. Lipkin, my other older patients, and myself.

Again, I felt that sense that things were not quite right. I saw too many people who unnecessarily limited themselves because of their age. They were misinformed about aging and about the opportunities around them. The loss of human potential and productivity was staggering. My interest became focused on providing practical information to help older people live full and productive lives. This interest eventually led to the book that you now hold in your hands.

I set three strict principles to guide my writing.

1. The emphasis would be on facts and on connecting facts into a useful, practical framework.
2. The writing style would convey my sense that elderly people in general and you in particular should receive the best possible care.
3. Medical experts who care for elderly people would review the manuscript to ensure accuracy and balance in the presentation of the information.

I drew on a variety of sources: the *Geriatrics Review Syllabus* to abstract as much useful information as possible; current research in medical papers, journals, and periodicals for the latest data in geriatric studies; and standard medical texts for additional background material. Finally, because I am primarily a clinician, I have included much that comes from my own clinical experience and philosophy.

This book will not answer all your health concerns and it is not intended as a way for you to second-guess your doctor. Instead, I have offered some guidelines to help clarify what must sometimes seem like a confusing maze of medical information. I have stressed those things that seem of greatest importance in my clinical practice, and I have tried to address the concerns most frequently shared by my patients. It will not surprise me if my opinions are not uniformly shared by all doctors. This should not disturb you because medical practice changes rapidly and professionals should be expected to disagree. But the more complete your understanding of aging, the better prepared you will be to work with your doctor to develop an effective plan of care. Ultimately you will be the beneficiary of the health care network you establish for yourself. I believe you deserve the very best.

The technical (impersonal) aspects of medicine have advanced at a rate unparalleled in human history. However, the closer interpersonal qualities of the doctor-patient relationship have not seemed to keep pace. Of course, there are many reasons for this, and this book is not an attempt to be a substitute for an effective doctor-patient relationship. Nonetheless, the quality of that relationship may be improved if you and your doctor have a fuller understanding of the clinical conditions that affect older people and a more complete knowledge of how the body ages. Good health care does not happen by accident. You must be well informed and take an active role in care decisions.

This book is addressed primarily to you, the intelligent older person, your family, and others who care about someone who is old. It provides background information that can be useful in preparing for a visit to your physician or other health professional. It can also serve as a basic handbook to understand a symptom or a disease process, or simply as a way to learn more about how the aging process affects each of us.

The American Geriatrics Society's Complete Guide to Aging and Health is neither a textbook nor a how-to manual. It is intended to offer a fresh perspective on the medical conditions that affect you and to provide insights into their cause, symptoms, and treatment. Increasing clarity on health matters can empower each of us in our interactions with health professionals. The more informed you are, the more balanced and effective will be the health care you receive.

This book is organized into four sections.

Part I addresses how we age—the relevant differences between young and old people, how our minds and bodies change with the passage of time, and aspects of preventive care, particularly those aspects of aging that we can influence. Part II covers a number of issues related to health care decisions—the doctor-patient relationship, getting through a hospitalization, surgery in older people, the risk of surgery and complications following surgery, principles of rehabilitation, how our bodies handle drugs, and finally, the broad aspects of long-term care including home care and nursing home care. Part III covers ethical and legal issues and health care financing. Part IV, "Conditions That Affect Older People," contains fourteen chapters dealing with clusters of problems, concerns, and diseases. Each chapter in this section opens with a listing of its main headings. Hopefully, this will help you to find particular parts of these chapters more easily. Generally, chapter to chapter, information is organized in a sequence that starts with general information and moves to specific symptoms and conditions that a person might want to know more about. In some chapters, *symptoms* (the patient's complaint of pain or malfunction—chest pain, for instance) and *conditions* (the set of processes within the body causing the complaint— the pneumonia causing the chest pain, for instance) are distinguished from each other under these headings. In other chapters, symptoms and conditions did not fall into such clear groupings so these headings were not used. The last chapter addresses other important concerns and conditions that do not conveniently fit into the cluster format. However, these conditions are of vital importance to the care of older people and should not be overlooked.

This book is not intended to be read from cover to cover but rather to be a practical handbook covering a broad array of relevant health topics of concern to you. I have tried to make it comprehensive and yet easy to read so that you can quickly find the information you need.

PART I

HOW WE AGE

CHAPTER 1

IMPORTANT CONSIDERATIONS

Your health needs as an older person require a different perspective from when you were younger. Your range of problems is different; the signs of distress are more subtle and may have greater consequences; and improvements are sometimes less dramatic and slower to appear. You may face a wider array of diseases, and symptoms of illness may not point directly to the underlying disease. For example, changes in mental status, changes in behavior, walking problems, or weight loss are typical symptoms the physician may have difficulty interpreting. You are also now more likely to have a persistent condition. In such circumstances the goal for you and your doctor is to maintain your ability to function as comfortably as possible. Even when a total cure of a given problem is not available, any discomfort or disability can often be modified substantially.

Individual Variability

Although elderly people typically demonstrate some decline in organ function, there is a wide range of variation among individuals. These differences highlight the importance of your doctor developing an individualized approach to your care. In health care, one size does not fit all, and as we age our unique differences must become an integral part of health care decisions.

Having Multiple Illnesses

The likelihood of having one or more diseases increases as we age. Among people who are 65 and older, 85 percent have at least one chronic illness, and 30 percent have three or more chronic diseases. Having more than one disease complicates care in several ways. Sudden change or illness in one system may put stress on another system, making the interpretation of symptoms more complex. A common example is the difficulty in evaluating mental confusion when it occurs with fever caused by pneumonia. In addition, the symptoms of one disease may hide those of another. For example, a person with severe heart disease and arthritis may never express the symptoms of the heart disease because of limited physical activity caused by the arthritis. It can also happen that treatment for one illness will cause a problem with another illness. This occurs, for example, when treatment using an over-the-counter medication causes bladder problems in a person with previously normal bladder function. Because of this, it is important for you and your physician to recognize the extent to which multiple conditions may be present and be alert to possible effects that any treatment may have on other conditions.

Exposure to Many Medications

Because older people appear to be at a much greater risk of adverse drug reactions, you need to be alert to any medications that may aggravate other conditions. This issue is explored in more detail in Chapter 9. It is essential for you to reduce this risk by carefully reviewing your medication regimen with your doctor in order to determine its necessity, effectiveness, and any potential for harm. You need to examine both nonprescription and prescription medications to reduce your chance of experiencing an adverse event.

Reporting Your Illness

Older people often do not take full advantage of the health services available to them. This is due to many factors, ranging from personal attitudes to increased social isolation. Old age is not necessarily linked with disability, so you should not dismiss any changes by asking "What do you expect, at my age?" Although you may feel frustrated by an inaccessible or unresponsive system of health care, you must accept your responsibility in making your relationship with your doctor work. At times you may even experience depression, but instead of limiting yourself by asking "What do I have to gain?" you should know that depression is both common and treatable. You may also experience denial, resulting from fear of economic, social, or functional consequences—this is why you should know as much as possible in advance to alleviate any fears you may have. If you feel isolated, explore opportunities to increase your interactions with people and to discuss your state of health, attitudes, or ideas.

Some illnesses and disease, such as hip fractures or Parkinson's disease, are virtually confined to the later stages of life. Certain diseases, such as cardiovascular disease, malignancy, malnutrition, thyroid gland problems, and tuberculosis are more common in old age. You and your caregivers, therefore, should bear in mind such altered distributions of illness and disease when you notice symptoms.

Your changing response to illness is another important dimension of your health behavior. Personal attitudes, social factors, and changes in the sensory organ may affect how you perceive illness. The acute signs of some diseases diminish often as we age. For example, the chest pain due to a heart attack may be absent or less dramatic. And finally, symptoms in one organ may reflect abnormalities in another. For example, an older person with a urinary tract infection may also experience confusion and disorientation. Because of this nonspecific and possibly misleading presentation of significant problems, your physician must exercise very careful attention to evaluate any change in your health status.

How critical is it for your physician to determine the precise nature of the underlying *disease* (the abnormality in anatomy or physiology) when helping you with an *illness* (the manifestations or symptoms of distress)? Certainly, the quest to identify the disease causing your distress is important when the disease is reversible or remediable or both. Since the 17th century, a first principle of medical practice has been the mandate to define the one disease that underlies the person's distress. Treatment directed at this underlying disease represents the most direct and effective way to reduce the symptoms. Three arguments that favor precise determination of the underlying disease seem particularly compelling: The first is that identifying reversible or remediable disease is obviously rewarding to your welfare; the second is that your doctor's uncertainty is thereby reduced; and the third is that accurate prognosis may be possible.

Your Doctor's Response

Despite the overwhelming success of this disease-illness paradigm, its limitations must be remembered: Some symptoms are independent of the diseases; many diseases do not necessarily produce symptoms; and the quality of the distress may not be predictable from knowing that the disease is present. For example, knowing the extent of rheumatoid arthritis in a person does not allow a physician to predict the capacity of that person to work. Your doctor's search for reversible disease, while important, is secondary to the management of most of your conditions.

The discovery of a reversible disease when you are chronically ill remains an important medical responsibility, but a clinical relationship based solely on uncovering reversible disease can be detrimental if a search for remediable disease becomes the focus of your doctor's attention. It may undermine or distort the doctor-patient relationship when all reversible diseases have been excluded. Contrary to the situation in sudden illness, in which the expeditious discovery of remedies is an imperative, your doctor's search for reversible disease when you are chronically ill can be pursued in a more leisurely manner. Most experienced physicians readily define and treat remediable conditions in their elderly patients. Often these reversible problems are those produced by health care interventions, especially drug toxicities and abusive physical restraints.

A focus on disease deemphasizes the dominant issue in the management of chronic illness, which is the maximization of your productivity, creativity, well-being, and happiness. This goal of improving your function and satisfaction to the utmost is often achieved without curing the underlying problem.

The need to reduce clinical uncertainty, to leave no stone unturned, is another rationale for defining disease in the setting of a chronic illness. A common argument is that you may be spared unnecessary diagnostic procedures once any underlying condition is totally defined. The decision on how far to proceed with a diagnostic evaluation is ultimately between you and your physician. The benefit of a diagnostic procedure depends upon the likelihood that it will yield useful information, which in chronic illness is elusive. Diagnostic tests are often an exercise reflecting more the need to reduce your doctor's anxiety than to resolve clinical uncertainty, and testing is often counterproductive. If the relief of your distress is the primary concern of you and your doctor, many diagnostic tests become irrelevant.

As previously mentioned, the third argument for defining disease in chronically ill elderly people is to allow accurate prognosis, or prediction of a person's future health. Because prognosis generally involves estimating the remaining life span, its value is highest in diseases that markedly influence longevity. For such diseases, prognostic estimates help in making decisions regarding therapy. For example, treatment regimens that are especially toxic or risky are usually reserved for circumstances in which longevity is immediately threatened. Small reductions in life expectancy are a less important concern in the management of chronic disease and become nearly irrelevant for many elderly people. Even for some less chronic problems such as malignant disease, many people seem to prefer improved quality of life over extended life span.

Another factor that limits the utility and accuracy of prognostic estimates in older people relates to the constancy of the human life span. If the age at which people have their first infirmity continues to increase, then the overall period of infirmity must decrease, assuming that life span remains constant. In view of this compressed morbidity, delaying the onset or progression of the symptoms produced by chronic illness becomes as important as curing the disease. For example, if the progression of symptoms for Alzheimer's disease were delayed for ten years, the impact of dementing illness would be substantially reduced. Even limited prognostic inferences are unreliable because older people manifest such wide biologic variability.

The Importance of Function

The word *function*, as used in the health field, refers to your ability to manage your daily routine—a critical issue for all of us. Loss of this ability is invariably due to a serious illness and, in this country, often leads to long-term care. In some instances, the loss of independence results from organ dysfunction or failure, but that is the exception. Why should an older person with reasonably preserved organ, mental, and musculo-skeletal function be subject to the loss of independence?

Manual ability in particular appears to be intimately and principally associated with the ability to live independently. A person's manual ability, as measured by timing the performance of a few simple tasks that reflect the skills necessary to perform basic daily activities, is helpful in making decisions related to what type of assistance you may require. This means that an evaluation of your functional abilities can be more useful than a disease-oriented one in defining certain health needs. Because most older people have chronic disease, most assessments of an older person's well-being are based on measurements of functional ability.

When function rather than disease is the focus, your physician can be most helpful to you. Reliable care and your quality of life may be more important than thorough and efficient diagnosis of disease or prediction of life expectancy. In fact, your functioning can often be improved without even knowing what disease you may have; it is the knowledge of your disability that is necessary. For example, treatment of urinary incontinence focuses on determining how bladder control can be improved if not completely restored, as well as on improving the person's confidence and self-esteem. This treatment does not depend on knowing whether the bladder activity is due to brain injury, a stroke, dementia caused by Alzheimer's disease, or any other irreversible process. Knowledge of the disability rather than the underlying disease is what most enables your doctor to provide help. When your problems are treated in this way, both you and your doctor avoid the disappointment and frustration of not being able to define or cure the primary disease.

As we age, we experience different types of problems. We become more unique and notice more variability in our performance; our care must be individualized to address the chronic illnesses we will confront. And our doctors must be attentive to these changes. In our later years, care becomes more important than cure, and function becomes more important than diagnosis.

What Is Aging?

Aging is a progressive, predictable process that involves the evolution and maturation of living organisms. Aging is inevitable, but the rate of aging varies greatly among individuals. This chapter will address the aging process itself. We will explore current aging theories and review exactly what changes we can expect to take place in our bodies.

How Long Can We Realistically Expect to Live?

The maximum life span is the theoretical, species-specific, longest duration of life, excluding premature "unnatural" death. Life expectancy is defined as the average number of additional years of life that is expected for a member of a population. It can be a useful predictor of actual longevity for a given individual. Like most species, humans almost always die of disease or accident before they reach their biologic limit.

The percentage of a population that is alive at any one time is illustrated by the survival curves shown in Figure 1. Curve A, which might be representative of the human population 50,000 years ago in Africa, shows a population in which deaths occur randomly and for whom the probability of dying does not change with age. Curve B, which shows survival that is based on environmental

Figure 1. Survival Curves for Four Hypothetical Populations

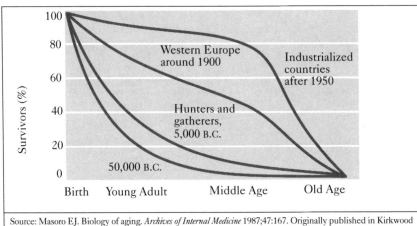

Source: Masoro EJ. Biology of aging. *Archives of Internal Medicine* 1987;47:167. Originally published in Kirkwood TBL, Holliday R. The evolution of aging and longevity. *Proceedings of the Royal Society of London.* 1979; B205:532. Reprinted with permission.

hazards, is the survival curve for animals that live in the wild and perhaps for prehistoric man. As environmental hazards are avoided, curves C and D result, representing the more dominant role that aging plays in mortality. The survival curve that has begun to be characteristic of the population in the United States in the past 50 years is represented by the rectangular shape of curve D.

While life expectancy at birth has increased significantly, life span, which is estimated at 85 to 100 years, has remained about the same. Eliminating the top ten causes of death would increase the life expectancy of people over the age of 65 by about 20 years, but the overall life span would not be affected.

The Influence of Genetics on Aging

The genetic basis of aging is clear. Even in the best of environmental conditions, various species of animals and plants mature, grow old, and die at widely differing rates. Identical twins, for instance, show much more closely correlated longevity than fraternal twins.

The strong genetic basis for aging is demonstrated by comparing normal aging to the premature aging process caused by the very rare disease of progeria. In this disease, the genetic mechanisms seem to involve just a single gene (or at most, a few genes). Further evidence for genetic influences on aging is provided by the selective breeding in animals for shorter or longer life spans and for various age-related traits. In almost all species, including the human species, females outlive males. This seems to be due to genetic factors, although the mechanism is not known.

Genetic influences seem to be more powerful than environmental factors in determining the enormous differences among species in aging and longevity. However, within a species a wide range of environmental conditions help shape the aging experience. Two groups of factors seem to be involved in determining longevity: those governing the rate of aging and those governing the age-dependent vulnerability to disease and death. The latter is much more susceptible to environmental factors.

Environmental Factors That Modify Aging

Random deaths have greatly decreased as a result of improvements in nutrition and sanitation and the decrease of such infectious diseases as tuberculosis, gastroenteritis, typhoid fever, and cholera. Preventive medicine has reduced the disability and mortality in infancy, childhood, and childbirth, and over the past 40 years the availability of antibiotics and other drugs has greatly reduced the death rate. These successes have added years to the lives of millions of people.

In addition to these environmental conditions, a person's lifestyle is an important factor in how we age. Health behaviors such as not smoking, moderation in alcohol use, adequate exercise and rest, a diet high in fiber content, effectively handling stress, and a positive outlook have all been suggested as a means to better health and longevity. Since our bodies are made up of cells, it is useful to explore how these cells age.

Aging of Cells

The aging of cells can be classified in three ways: cells that are continuously dividing, cells that are resting but can be stimulated to divide, and cells that are past the replicating phase altogether. Examples of continuously dividing cells include cells in the bone marrow that produce red and white blood cells and the cells that line the gastrointestinal tract. Cells in the liver, parts of the kidney, and the cells lining blood vessels are examples of the second type of cells, also called quiet cells, whose function is to respond to tissue injury.

Of the cells that do not reproduce, some have short life spans and others have long life spans. Those with short life spans (weeks to months) such as red blood cells and white cells, require continual replacement. Those with long life spans (years to decades) include nerves, muscles, heart cells, and reproductive cells.

The survival times of red blood cells are correlated with a species' life span. In humans, the survival of a red blood cell averages about four months. Changes in the membrane of these cells help identify the older cells and trigger a mechanism for their removal from the blood. This suggests that there may be a general mechanism for identifying and eliminating older body cells.

Little is known about aging and cell death in long-lived cells. Nerves, which have been extensively studied in humans, are lost at different rates in different parts of the brain. It is difficult to determine what changes are due to age and what changes are due to disease or environmental influences.

Although the cell's ability to reproduce typically declines with normal cellular aging, it is interesting to note that many age-associated processes seem, paradoxically, to involve increases in proliferation. For example, the prostate gland tends to increase its cells with age. One hypothesis is that aging may cause inappropriate cellular responses to signals to proliferate and to signals that tell cells to stop proliferating.

Theories of Aging

Cells are only one area that researchers examine in their search for how we age; they also focus on molecular, organic, and individual stages of organization. No single theory has accounted for how we age, but each seems to hold some interesting clues. According to the two main lines of thought, the aging process either results from genetically programmed changes or it occurs because of an accumulation of genetic errors due to environmental damage. Since programmed cell death appears to be a regular feature of human growth and development, it seems reasonable to use this as a model for the aging process. For example, we have to lose our baby teeth to make room for our permanent teeth. But aging could also be viewed as a phase in which the person, having passed his or her reproductive stage, no longer has a genetic program to follow and becomes increasingly vulnerable to random hazards. This process may be analogous to riding a ski lift. Genetics (the lift) gets you up the mountain, but the ride down is under your control, becoming more hazardous with steeper and longer runs.

One set of theories regarding programmed changes involved in aging suggests that the immune system is the regulator of aging decline and the thymus gland is akin to a biologic clock. The thymus gland is the site where special lymphocytes called T cells mature, and its hormones are important in the development of white blood cells. The thymus gland (located behind the breast bone) is large at birth and continues to grow until adolescence. It begins a rapid withering after adolescence, so that by the time a person is 45 years old, the gland has only 10 to 20 percent of its former cell mass. After people reach the age of 30, the level of thymic hormones goes down; by the time people are 60, thymic hormones can no longer be detected in the blood.

There are a number of theories that attribute aging to the accumulation of various errors in cell functioning and environmental exposures. According to this group of theories, aging results from changes in the information that is provided by the cell nucleus during normal cell function. Aging could result from changes in DNA (deoxyribonucleic acid—the molecule that carries the genetic code of a cell), errors in the synthesis of other nuclear proteins, or alterations in the structures that modify gene expression.

As part of normal metabolism, humans produce chemically reactive substances called free radicals. Free radicals are highly toxic and can damage delicate cellular elements, particularly membrane fats and genetic materials. These chemical-free radicals have been implicated in a number of age-related phenomena, including cancer and arthritis. However, the damage produced by free radicals is so general that the current assumption is that there are some yet undefined intermediates that may cause specific damage to genes and to DNA.

Although compelling evidence suggests that aging is genetically determined, the number of theories tells us that no one knows for sure how this happens. However, a number of environmental factors seem to influence the rate of aging with harsh exposures tending to accelerate the process. Many of these environmental factors have been controlled to such an extent that for the first time in human history people in nations like ours can expect to live into their seventies, eighties, or even older. Old age, once the privilege of the very few, has now become the shared destiny of humankind.

Body Changes with Aging

Normal aging in the absence of disease is a remarkably benign process. In terms of body systems, aging involves the steady decline of organ functioning and of the regulation of body systems. We may not even notice these changes except during periods of maximum exertion or stress. We may experience slower reactions to stimuli, wider variations in functioning, and slower returns to resting states. Some biological changes are predictable though. Following are some of the most common changes in our body systems.

Normal Aging and Disease

Aging is not the accumulation of disease, although aging and disease are related in subtle and complex ways. Several conditions once thought to be part of normal human aging have been shown to be due to disease. For example, heart and blood vessel diseases are less common in populations that eat no meat and little fat, and cataract formation in the eye is largely dependent on the degree of exposure to ultraviolet radiation in sunlight.

The range of individual response to aging deserves emphasis. Biologic and chronologic age are not the same, and body systems do not age at the same rate within any individual. You might have marked arthritis or severe loss of vision while enjoying excellent heart or kidney function. Even those aging changes that are considered usual or normal do not necessarily represent the optimum outcome for an aging individual or society.

Changes in the Regulation of Body Systems

The regulation of body systems changes as you age. Progressive changes in the heart and blood vessels impair your body's ability to control blood pressure. Because increases in blood pressure may also impair blood pressure control mechanisms, you have the greatest risk for sudden drops in your blood pressure if you have high blood pressure. Changes in the brain and kidney with aging can amplify these effects.

Your body cannot regulate its temperature as it could when you were younger. This can result in hypothermia if the ambient temperature is low or hyperthermia (heat stroke) if the temperature is high. There may also be aging-related changes in your body's ability to mount a fever in response to an infection. The regulation of the amount and composition of body fluids is diminished in healthy elderly people. Resting levels of the hormones that control fluid volume are unchanged, but abnormalities of fluid regulation frequently occur during illness or physiologic stress. Water regulation involves mechanisms in the central nervous system and the kidneys. The thirst response that follows water deprivation is decreased in elderly people.

What are the relevant implications of these age-related changes in our body systems? First, advancing age results in increasing differentiation and biologic diversity; we become less like each other, and health care must be individualized. Various strategies of diagnostic investigation and the allocation of resources are likely to be far less than optimal if they are based only on chronologic age criteria.

We also need to consider how our biologic systems that are minimally affected by age are often *profoundly influenced by lifestyle circumstances such as cigarette smoking, physical activity, nutritional intake, or economic advantage. Although the precise mechanisms by which these environmental and lifestyle factors induce changes in body systems are unknown, some exposures seem to accelerate the aging process.* The potential interactions of environmental and physiologic conditions are shown in Figure 2. The upper line represents the maximum potential performance for a given organ system such as the musculoskeletal or cardiovascular system. Ideally, this line is almost horizontal with minimal decrements in maximum function occurring over time. The position and slope of this line may be affected by various environmental factors. For example, cigarette smoking in youth may reduce optimal respiratory potential in later years. The lower line represents the rate of atrophy when the system is put at complete rest (never stressed); the system always functions at some point between these lines.

The third consequence of aging physiology is the prospect of living with diminishing resources with which to meet increasingly complicated environmental demands. The decline of functional capacity is often compounded by losses of social status, income, family support (for example, through death), and self-esteem. Diseases may

Figure 2. Effect of Conditioning and Age on the Organs

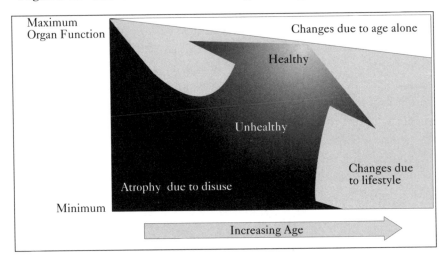

reduce physical and mental capabilities, which are magnified by rapidly changing social expectations, especially for people who have accepted a self-reliant lifestyle.

However, the capacity to learn and adjust continues throughout life, strongly influenced by interests, activity, motivation, health, and income. With years of rich experience and reflection, some of us can transcend our own circumstances. We call this wisdom. Old age, despite the physical limitations, can be a time of variety, creativity, and fulfillment.

Aging and Body Defenses

This section will review various age-related changes that influence our bodies' ability to resist and control infections.

The Barrier Defenses

The skin and mucous membranes that line body cavities are primary barriers to infection. Some of the barrier and antimicrobial properties of the skin may be impaired with age. In addition, certain skin conditions that predispose one to infection—pressure ulcers and trauma (wounds, lesions, bruises, etc.), for example—become common.

The lining surfaces of body tissues, the mucosal surfaces, help prevent infection by trapping organisms in secreted mucus and removing them by a process called ciliary transport. This transport system works like a tiny escalator conveying the trapped material toward a body opening such as the mouth. Aging may compromise this barrier function, which commonly occurs in the mouth, urethra, and vagina.

Disturbance in swallowing, a common and age-related change, predisposes individuals to aspiration (drawing substances into the lungs instead of swallowing them through the esophagus), which is a common cause of pneumonia in older people. (Aspiration and pneumonia are each addressed in Chapter 21.) Our cough mechanism decreases as we age, further reducing our ability to eliminate organisms. Changes in the lung, especially the collapse of small airways and the overall loss of lung elasticity, also increase the risks of infection.

Physical and Mechanical Defenses

In the gastrointestinal system, the stomach secretes reduced amounts of acid, the bowel's contractions can change, and outpouchings called diverticula often form in the bowel lining. (See Chapter 22 for a discussion of diverticula.) Each of these changes makes it easier for bacterial populations to increase in the stomach and intestines. Changes in the urinary tract lower resistance to infection: the chemistry of the urine; decreased prostatic fluid (with reduced ability to kill organisms); diminished flushing mechanism of the bladder; backward flow of bladder contents toward the kidney; and the potential obstruction of urine flow by prostate enlargement, bladder prolapse, narrowings in the urethra, or stones.

In general, white blood cells do not appear to change as we age. Their ability to attack organisms does not seem to be impaired, and they respond normally to signals that they are needed in order to combat infecting organisms. While you can probably develop fever with infections, reduced or absent fever responses are not rare.

Other Body Responses to Infection

Declines in immune responsiveness as we age may explain our increased likelihood of infections, cancer, and various immune diseases. Our body's production of antibodies is impaired in old age.

Specific Changes in the Immune System

The changes in the thymus (see page 13) play a crucial role in impairment of the immune system. An impaired response to a stimulus, a fundamental defect in immunity, appears to be due to reduced numbers and diminished responsiveness of certain lymphocytes and other cell lines. Older people show less vigorous skin test reactions, suggesting that the response to antigens is impaired.

Physical Activity and Aging

Decreases in physical activity and accompanying changes in body composition may cause some of the declines in body metabolism and cardiovascular function that occur with advancing age. In addition, aging produces several changes in the ability of our body to acquire and deliver oxygen to the tissues. These changes include increasing stiffness of the chest wall, impaired blood flow through the lungs, diminished strength of each contraction of the heart, and decreased muscle mass. It is not surprising that because of these changes the physical work capacity of the average 70-year-old person is about half that of a 20-year-old. Although the decrease over this 50-year age span is progressive, the rate of loss accelerates after our mid-fifties.

Total body metabolism declines slightly but steadily. The maximum oxygen consumption with exercise, a measurement of fitness, declines more rapidly because of the decrease in lean muscle mass and a fall in maximum heart rate. While there is considerable variability among older individuals, the maximum oxygen consumption tends to be higher in physically active people than in sedentary individuals. It may be higher still in older athletes who are in training. Even after correction for height, weight, and other differences, maximal oxygen consumption is higher in men than in women.

Regular physical exercise is the best antidote to many of the effects of aging. The major benefits from regular exercise include favorable effects on fats in the blood, better handling of blood sugar, increased maximal oxygen capacity, greater strength, denser bones, an improved sense of well-being, and better sleep. It has not yet been proven, however, that an exercise regimen reduces the chance of eventual disability or prolongs life expectancy. Nonetheless, these benefits are likely to be demonstrated in the next several years as a result of current studies.

We have just reviewed how aging affects our bodies' control systems and defense systems, and that regular physical exercise may well forestall some of these changes. Let us now consider some of the more visible manifestations of aging.

The Anatomy of Aging

Difficulties in making health care decisions result when normal aging changes are not appreciated or are misinterpreted. Because of this, a knowledge of the anatomy of aging is fundamental to our care. While the cause of most of the aging changes remains unknown, many changes are not inevitable.

Changes in Height

We all lose height as we age but with great variability both in the age of onset and the rate of loss. Generally, before the decline begins, our height increases until our late forties, then approximately two inches are lost by age 80. Changes in posture, changes in the growth of vertebrae, a forward bending of the spine, and the compression of the disks between the vertebrae cause a loss in trunk length. Increased curvature of our hips and knees, along with decreased joint space in our trunk and extremities, contribute to a loss of stature. The length of the bones in our legs shows little change. In our feet, joint changes and a flattening of the arches can also contribute to the loss of standing height.

Changes in Body Weight

In men, body weight increases until the mid-fifties; then it declines, with the rate of weight loss accelerating in the late sixties and seventies. In women, body weight increases until the late sixties; it declines thereafter at a rate slower than in men. People of less technologically developed societies do not show this sequence of weight change, which suggests that reduced physical activity and changes in eating patterns may be causes of the change in body weight rather than the aging process.

Changes in Body Composition

Total body fat as a proportion of the body's composition doubles between the ages of 25 and 75. Exercise programs may prevent or reverse much of the proportional decrease in lean muscle mass and the increase in total body fat. Because the fat just beneath the skin decreases with age, fat accumulation is presumed to occur in our muscles and body organs. These changes in body composition have important implications for nutritional planning and metabolic activity. They also strongly influence the distribution and disposition of various drugs. For example, because of this increase in our body fat, drugs that are dissolved in fatty tissues remain in our body much longer than in a younger person's body.

The loss of lean body mass is due to a decrease in arm and leg muscle mass, with some decrease in our bones and body organs. Hormone changes seem to influence these losses: In women the decrease of estrogens that occurs with menopause is proportionally much greater than the fall of total androgens in men. Other organs also show losses; our liver and kidneys, for example, lose about a third of their weight between the ages of 30 and 90. The prostate gland, however, doubles in weight between the ages of 20 and 90.

Changes in Body Systems

Skin and Hair Changes

The aging changes in normal human skin are shown in Figure 3. Little change occurs with aging in the outer layer of the skin called the stratum corneum. The contact area between the dermis and the epidermis decreases, and the number of deeper cells called basal cells and pigment-producing cells, called melanocytes, is reduced. With advancing age, the number of Langerhans' cells, cells that come from the bone marrow and provide assistance to the immune system, is also modestly reduced. The reduction of these cells is striking in skin that has been exposed to sunlight; this reduction is thought to contribute to the development of sun-related skin cancers. The graying of hair reflects the loss of pigmented cell (melanocyte) function.

The dermis thins by approximately 20 percent as we age, and the number of cells decreases. The blood supply is reduced. The collagen, a basic chemical building block of skin, decreases with age, which results in less skin elasticity. The collagen fibers in younger skin exhibit an orderly arrangement similar to fibers in a rope. These fibers become coarser and more random with aging, resembling a mass of unstirred spaghetti. Alterations in elastic tissue cause a loss of resiliency and produce wrinkles.

Skin changes caused by excessive sunlight exposure compound these changes. The main features of sun-damaged skin include irregularity in the cell membranes with loss of the organization of skin cells, damage to the lower levels of skin, a loss of collagen, and a modest infiltration of inflammatory cells. Generally speaking, normally aged skin shows thinning, a loss of elasticity, and the deepening of normal expression lines whereas sun-damaged skin is characterized by wrinkled, yellowed, rough, leathery, and spotted skin.

The tissues below the skin may undergo site-specific atrophy or enlargement. A well-recognized occurrence is the relative increase of fat along the waistline in men and the thighs in women. Locations that show atrophy include our face, the back of our hands, our shins, and the soles of our feet.

Hair changes play a prominent role in the perception of age. Hair graying results from a progressive loss of pigment cells from the hair bulbs. The loss of these pigment cells is more rapid in the hair than in the skin, possibly because of the rapid proliferation of cells during hair growth. The graying of hair in the armpit is thought to be one of the most reliable signs of aging. There is a decrease in the number of hair follicles of the scalp. Changes in the growth rate of hair depend upon the site. The growth rate of scalp, pubic, and armpit hair declines; however, possibly because of changes in hormones, an increased growth of facial hair is sometimes seen in elderly women. An increased growth of eyebrow and nostril hair occurs in elderly men.

Figure 3. Aging Changes in Normal Skin

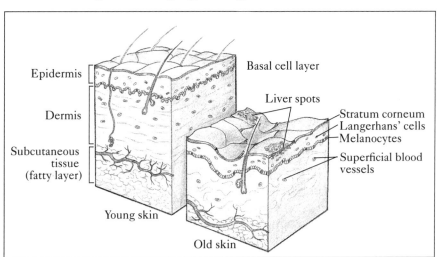

Changes in Muscles and Bones

Aging changes in our muscles include a decrease in muscle strength, endurance, size, and weight relative to total body weight. However, the late onset of these changes and their unpredictable rate of appearance suggest that they may not be due to aging but rather due to inactivity, nutritional deficiency, disease, or other long-standing conditions.

Older muscles appear to have a reduced blood supply, although the utilization of oxygen appears to be unchanged. Curiously, both the diaphragm and the heart, two muscles that work continuously, appear to be relatively unchanged by aging.

Age-related chemical changes occur in cartilage, the substance that provides the lubricating surface of most joints. Because cartilage contains no blood vessels, it depends upon the blood supply of the synovium (the tissue that produces joint fluid) for nutrients that pass through the joint fluid. The water content of cartilage decreases, and changes in the deeper structures such as the underlying bone may influence the cartilage and may reduce its ability to adapt to repetitive stress.

Bone loss is a universal aspect of aging that occurs at highly individual rates. (The section on osteoporosis and osteomalacia in Chapter 17 provides further information on bone loss.) Aging affects and reduces the bone cells that produce bone more severely than those cells that reabsorb bone. While bone-remodeling occurs throughout life, the balance between the amount of bone reabsorbed and the amount of bone formed is impaired with aging; the growth of bone slows and the bone begins to thin and become more porous. The internal latticework of bones loses its horizontal supports, which significantly compromises its strength. These changes mean that the smallest trauma may cause the bone to collapse.

Our skull appears to thicken with age. All of our skull dimensions increase, but greater increases are noted deep in the skull and in the frontal sinuses located just over the eyes. Bone growth has also been demonstrated well into advanced age in the ribs, the fingers, and the femur (the large bone in the hip and thigh). These changes in the hip may be important, because growth in the midportion of the bone results in a wider but weaker bone.

Conditioning, nutrition, vascular and neurologic abnormalities, and hormones influence the degeneration in our muscles and bones. Conditioning is the most significant because disuse or underuse produces marked declines in bone and muscle structures. Nutrition affects bone and mineral metabolism, and blood vessel and neurologic abnormalities accelerate muscle degeneration. In addition, a variety of hormones—growth hormone, estrogens, androgens, and many others—modifies our musculoskeletal integrity.

Changes in the Nervous System

The brain's weight declines with age, but this decline appears to be in a few specific places rather than overall. Atrophy of the outer surface of the brain, called the gray matter, is usually moderate in healthy older people, as compared with a more extensive loss of cells in older people with dementia. From ages 30 to 70, the blood flow to our brain decreases by 15 to 20 percent.

With aging there is a loss of neurons in the gray matter, the cerebellum, and the hippocampus, a structure deep in the brain resembling a seahorse (hence the name), that seems to be involved in some aspects of memory function. Less dramatic losses occur in deeper brain structures.

For some nerves, the density of their interconnections seems to be reduced with aging. However, there is slow and continued growth of the very end connections between nerves, which suggest a possible repatterning of the nervous system.

Brain proteins, including an impressive number of enzymes, generally decline, notably, those that involve glucose breakdown and a key enzyme in carbon dioxide detoxification. Not all proteins are reduced, however. Some abnormal proteins increase with age.

Brain Function

Aging changes in brain structure and biochemistry do not necessarily affect our thinking and behavior. (Chapter 3 has more information about thinking and behavioral changes.) Our basic language skills and sustained attention are not altered with aging, but some aspects of our cognitive ability do seem to change, the earliest being the ability to retain large amounts of information over a long period of time. Naming tasks and abstraction are altered late in life. However, none of these changes develops uniformly or inevitably, and many older people continue to perform

Figure 4. The Eye

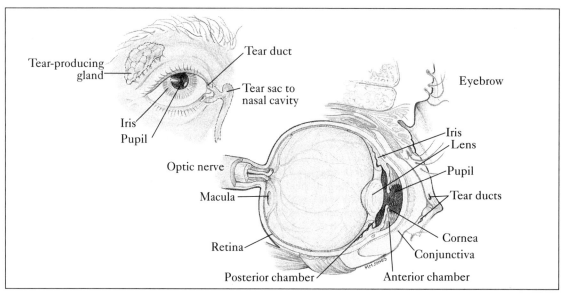

Tear-producing gland
Tear duct
Tear sac to nasal cavity
Eyebrow
Iris
Pupil
Iris
Lens
Optic nerve
Pupil
Tear ducts
Macula
Retina
Cornea
Conjunctiva
Posterior chamber
Anterior chamber

at levels that are comparable to, or even exceed, those of much younger people.

Changes in the Senses

Sight. The normal anatomy of the eye is shown in Figure 4. With age, the tissues around our eyes atrophy and fat around the eye is lost; this may result in the upper lid drooping and the lower lid turning inward or outward. The decreased production of tears combined with atrophy around the eye increases the chance of eye infection. Changes in the cornea can also occur, although they are usually related to disease and not aging. The iris, or the colored part of the eye, becomes more rigid, the pupil becomes smaller, and changes around the lens occur, predisposing us to glaucoma.

What changes in the lens? As newer lens fibers proliferate at the periphery, older fibers migrate to the center to form a denser central section. This process is like continually forming a ball of yarn. The lens progressively accumulates yellow substances, possibly from a chemical reaction involving sunlight with amino acids in the lens. These substances reduce the amount of light and color entering the eye, and this yellow filtering causes the lens to become less transparent to the blue part of the color spectrum. To older eyes, blue appears greenish blue.

The jellylike substance inside of the eye, called the vitreous body, tends to shrink, causing traction, or pulling, on the retina. It also becomes more liquid, and densities may form in it that produce visual images called floaters. Changes in the retina have not been clearly identified, although blood vessel disease involving the retina is common. Changes in the blood supply of the retina and possibly the pigmented layer of the retina can cause macular degeneration, one of the most common causes of vision loss in older people. (Macular degeneration is discussed in Chapter 18 in the section on vision problems.)

The most common change in our vision associated with aging is called presbyopia, a condition in which it becomes harder to focus on nearby objects. This is mainly due to decreased elasticity of the lens and atrophy of the muscle that controls the lens shape. It affects men and women equally and begins in our early twenties, although it is usually not noticeable until 20 or 30 years later. Eyeglasses usually correct the problem.

With age, the sharpness of our vision when looking at static objects, called static visual acuity, shows a gradual and steady decline. This decline is due to change in the diameter of the pupil, loss of the focusing power of the lens, and increased scattering of light. Much of this loss of vision is correctable by glasses. Dynamic visual acuity, or the ability to discriminate detail in a moving object, decreases more rapidly as we age than static acuity. This decline seems to be at least partially attributed to a loss of the cells along the visual pathway in the brain.

Changes in the shape of our eyes and the formation of cataracts reduce visual acuity, and both increase in likelihood as we age. Women are more likely than men to have cataracts. Unprotected exposure of the eyes to the sun is a major cause of cataracts. Chapter 18 contains additional information on cataracts.

As we age we adapt more slowly to an abrupt change from light to dark areas. So consistent is this correlation with age that a person's age may be predicted to within three years on the basis of this performance. These changes are not trivial: After two minutes of reduced illumination, young people's eyes are almost five times as sensitive as older people's eyes; after 40 minutes, there is a 240-fold difference.

The discrimination of objects in the presence of a source of glare declines so that older people require 50 to 70 percent more light than younger people to recognize an object near a source of glare. The increased effect of a glaring light is due to the scattering of peripheral light caused by the more opaque lens in the older eye. When the lens is removed because of a cataract, the amount of glare perceived is decreased.

Older people need greater contrasts between the object of focus and its background in order to identify it accurately, especially in dimmer light. Other changes in vision are discussed in Chapter 18.

Hearing. Changes in our ears also occur with aging. The ear canal atrophies, resulting in thin walls and decreased production of ear-wax. Our eardrum thickens, often appearing dull and white to the physician. Degenerative changes and even arthritis can develop in the small joints connecting the bones in the middle ear. Significant changes take place in the inner ear. Whether aging alone produces these changes or whether they are due to excessive noise exposure is unknown. Noise exposure apart from aging can clearly cause diminished hearing.

These changes in ear structure significantly affect hearing. Presbycusis is the name for hearing loss for pure tones, which increases with age in men and women. Higher frequencies become less audible than lower frequencies; overall the loss is slightly less severe in women than it is in men.

The decrements in our hearing occur not only in the absolute threshold of tones of varying frequency but also in the point at which a change in pitch is detectable. Between the ages of 25 and 55, our pitch discrimination decreases, but after age 55 the decline is steeper. This is especially true for very high and very low frequencies. Combined with this loss in sensitivity is a distortion of signals that makes the localizing and understanding of sounds more difficult.

Pitch discrimination plays an important role in our speech perception. As we age, speech discrimination declines, even when pure tone hearing loss is taken into account. From the ages of 6 to 59, our intelligibility declines less than 5 percent. Thereafter it deteriorates rapidly, dropping more than 25 percent from peak levels after the age of 80. When exposed to loud background noise or indistinct speech, older people hear less, but at the same time they may be very sensitive to loud sounds. Hearing impairments are discussed further in Chapter 18 on hearing disorders.

Taste. The evidence regarding taste sensitivity is inconclusive and varies both among individuals and the substance tested. The tongue atrophies with age, which may result in diminished taste sensation; however, the number of taste buds remains unchanged and the responsiveness of these taste buds appears to be unaltered.

Smell. Our sense of smell declines rapidly after the age of 50 for both men and women, and the parts of our brain that are involved in smell degenerate significantly. By age 80, the detection of smell is almost 50 percent poorer than it was at its peak. Taste and smell work together to make the discrimination and enjoyment of food possible. As we age we may have trouble recognizing a variety of blended foods by taste and smell.

Touch. In general, our response to painful stimuli is diminished with aging. Sensitivity of the cornea of the eye to light touch declines after the age of 50 (touch sensitivity to the nose declines by age 15). Pressure touch thresholds on the index finger and the big toe decline more in men than in women.

Changes in the Cardiovascular System

Our cardiovascular system changes in ways that affect its overall function. With aging, our hearts tend to show disease in the heart muscle, heart valves, and coronary arteries. It is unclear whether any age-related changes of the heart occur in the absence of disease. The cells responsible for producing heartbeats become infiltrated with connective tissue and fat. Similar but less dramatic changes occur in other parts of the heart's electrical system. Poor blood supply does not seem to be an underlying cause.

Age-related declines in the ability of the heart to contract include a prolonged contraction time, decreased response to various medications that ordinarily stimulate the heart, and increased resistance to electrical stimulation (normally these changes do not result in disease). The elastic properties of the heart muscle are altered.

Changes in the blood vessels also occur as we age (see Figure

Figure 5. Aging Changes in Arteries

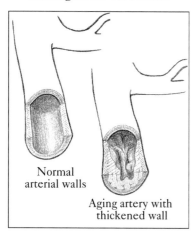

Normal arterial walls

Aging artery with thickened wall

5). Irregularities in size and shape develop in the cells that line blood vessels, and the layers in the blood vessel wall become thickened with connective tissue. Our large arteries increase in size and thickness.

The cardiovascular system responds less efficiently to various stresses with age. The maximum heart rate changes in a linear fashion and may be estimated by subtracting our age from 220. The resting heart rate and the amount of blood pumped by the heart over time (cardiac output) do not change. The cardiac output with work may increase, even though there is a decrease in the maximum heart rate. This increase in cardiac output occurs because the amount of blood pumped with each beat increases to compensate for the decreased heart rate with age. The extent of blood flow within various organs varies: In the kidney it may decrease by 50 percent, and in the brain by 15 to 20 percent. Following stress, it takes longer for our heart rate and our blood pressure to return to resting levels.

Whether blood pressure increases as an inevitable consequence of aging is unknown. Several studies have shown that aging is associated with an increase in the blood pressure. Stiffness within the blood vessels is thought to be the reason for these increases; however, an age-associated increase in blood pressure is not found in individuals who live in isolated, less technologically developed societies or in people who grow old in a special environment such as a mental institution.

Changes in the Respiratory System

The trachea (windpipe) and large airways increase in diameter as we age. Enlargement of the very end units of the airway results in a decreased surface area of the lung.

Decreased lung elasticity contributes to the increase in lung volumes and to the reduced amount of surface area. The decreased elasticity causes the chest to expand and the diaphragm to descend. The end of our ribs calcifies to our breastbone producing stiffening of the chest wall, which increases the workload of the respiratory muscles.

The consequences of these aging changes are an increased likelihood that we will have lung disease and progressive declines in measurements of lung function. From the ages of 20 to 80, our vital capacity declines linearly. The amount of residual air left in our lungs after each breath increases from about 20 percent of the total lung capacity when we are 20 to 35 percent at age 60.

The amount of oxygen dissolved in the blood decreases, largely as the result of impaired matching of blood flow with the parts of the lung that contain air. Aging does not cause any problems in our ability to get rid of carbon dioxide.

Well-conditioned older people may reach levels of lung function that exceed those of much younger people. Endurance training can produce a striking increase in the lung capacity of sedentary older persons. Of all the factors that influence lung function, smoking continues to produce the greatest amount of disability. Because smoking seems to accelerate aging changes, older smokers should stop smoking—now.

Changes in the Gastrointestinal System

On the whole, the gastrointestinal tract shows less age-associated change in function than other systems. The lining of the gut maintains an extraordinary capacity for replacing itself.

Age-related dental changes do not necessarily lead to the loss of teeth. Poor dental hygiene is a more important factor than age in this dental loss. Usually the losses have been caused by cavities or periodontal (gum) disease, both of which can be prevented by good care. With age, the location of cavities changes, and an increasing amount of root cavities and cavities around existing sites of previous dental work are seen. Tooth loss leads to changes in diet and can increase the likelihood of malnutrition. False teeth reduce taste sensation and do not completely restore normal chewing ability. Alterations in swallowing are more common in older people without any teeth. As we age we do not chew as efficiently as younger people and tend to swallow larger pieces of food. Swallowing takes us 50 to 100 percent longer, probably because of subtle changes in the swallowing mechanism.

The word *presbyesophagus* refers to normal aging changes in the muscle contractions of the esophagus. The principal abnormality is in the size of the contraction during swallowing. All other measures of esophageal contraction do not differ as a result of age. Moreover, the decreased size of the these contractions does not appear to cause any symptoms. Because of this, disorders of the esophagus are not due to aging but rather to diabetes mellitus, central nervous disorders, malignancy, or other diseases.

Continuing down our aging gastrointestinal system, stomach contractions appear to be normal, although according to some reports, we may need more time to empty liquids from our stomach. The amount of stomach acid secreted declines, probably as a result of a loss of the cells that produce gastric acid.

The small intestine shows a modest amount of atrophy of the lining. Changes in the large intestine include atrophy of the lining, changes within the muscle layer, and blood vessel abnormalities. Approximately one in every three people who are 60 years or older has diverticula, or outpouchings, in the lining of the large intestine, the likelihood increasing with age. The condition results from increased pressure inside the intestine, which is caused by a disorder of intestinal muscle function. Weakness in the bowel wall is another contributing factor. (For more information on diverticula, see page 371.)

Direct measurements of the speed with which substances are transported through the small intestine have not shown any age-related changes when people are not eating. However, upon eating, elderly people show reduced intestinal muscle contractions. Since the food transport in the large intestine slows down, constipation is common. Subtle changes occur in the coordination of large intestinal muscle contractions. The number of certain narcotic (opiate) receptors increases as we age, and this increase may lead to significant constipation when we ingest narcotics. Our intestines' ability to absorb foods as well as drugs generally does not change significantly. Changes can occur in the metabolism and absorption of some sugars, calcium, and iron. Highly fat-soluble compounds such as vitamin A appear to be absorbed faster as we get older. The activity of some enzymes such as lactase, which helps us digest some sugars (particularly those found in dairy products), appears to decline, but the levels of other enzymes remain normal. The absorption of fat may change, but this may relate more to changes in the pancreas and the digestive enzymes it produces rather than the ability of the intestine to absorb fat.

With age, the liver decreases in size and blood flow declines. There is reduced capacity to regenerate damaged liver cells. The shape of the liver adjusts to the contours of the adjacent organs, and the common bile duct that drains into the intestine enlarges. However, the portion of the bile duct just at the opening to the intestine narrows somewhat.

The pancreas commonly drops a little in the abdomen and the pancreatic ducts gradually increase in size. Atrophy is common in the pancreas as is scar tissue and fat. The liver and pancreas maintain adequate function throughout life, and, thankfully, age-related failure in the liver or pancreas does not occur. The metabolism of specific compounds, including numerous drugs, can be significantly prolonged in elderly people. (See Chapter 9 on how our body handles drugs.)

Changes in Kidney Function

With aging, there is a 25 to 30 percent decrease in kidney mass. There is probably a steady age-related decline in our kidney function; nevertheless, absolutely no fall in kidney function was observed in some older people who were studied for as long as 18 years; a few even showed an increase.

The reduced kidney function leads to decreased clearance of some drugs. The kidneys' hormonal response to dehydration is reduced, as is the ability to retain salt under conditions when it should be conserved. The ability of our kidneys to modify vitamin D to a more active form may also decline.

Bone Marrow Changes

Like the cells lining our intestines, the bone marrow cells have remarkable restorative capacity. The normal values for red blood cells in terms of number, size, and hemoglobin concentration remain essentially unchanged throughout life. The average life span of red blood cells remains constant at about 120 days, although these cells may be more fragile. The blood volume is also usually well maintained throughout old age.

Despite the continuing production of bone marrow cells, the amount of active bone marrow diminishes whereas marrow fat increases. While anemia is commonly seen in older people, it is not a normal consequence of aging and is always caused by something other than age, most frequently malnutrition, blood loss, or a malignancy. In some situations, however, the cause of the anemia is never found. (See the section on anemia in Chapter 20 for more details.)

The number of white blood cells and platelets remain unchanged, and the white blood cells continue to be effective in fighting off bacteria.

Changes in Reproductive Function

While women lose the capacity to reproduce well before they reach the average life span, men maintain this ability in extreme old age. In women, the rapid decline in eggs produced by the ovary is precisely and quantitatively age related. After menopause very few, if any, eggs can be seen in the ovary, which becomes scarred and withered.

At menopause, the production of ovarian estrogen is markedly reduced. This is responsible for the "hot flashes" felt by some women and changes in the uterus and the vagina. The lining of the uterus (endometrium) thins and the connective tissue increases. This thinning of the vaginal lining and reduced secretions can cause pain with sexual intercourse and can contribute to urinary incontinence. Changes in breast tissue are attributed to hormonal changes, and cysts may appear. The stretching of ligaments and the loss of muscular tone alter the contour of the breast.

In men, the decline in reproductive ability is a gradual process since sperm cells continue to be formed. The prostate tissue is replaced by scar tissue. The gland enlarges, particularly around the urethra. Changes in the concentration of testosterone, particularly its conversion to dihydrotestosterone, appear to cause the enlargement. (For more on this, see the section on prostate disease in Chapter 25.) Changes in the penis include progressive decline in blood flow and the formation of scar tissue in the inner compartments.

The frequency of sexual activity generally declines with age, but how much this is due to aging and how much to circumstance is not known. The most important factor may be the presence of a willing and able partner. Social and cultural circumstances tend to reinforce the decline in sexual activity, especially for older women.

Biologic changes that affect reproductive function, such as reduced responsiveness to erotic stimuli, may also influence sexual activity. It is not possible to predict how menopause will influence a woman's sexuality, although vaginal lubrication diminishes. In men, the ability to develop and maintain an erection can be impaired. Older men may also notice a decreased sensitivity of the penis, thus requiring more stimulation.

To sum up, bodily changes associated with aging generally increase our vulnerability to environmental conditions, to side effects of medical treatment, and the complications of medical procedures.

CHAPTER 3

HOW OUR MIND CHANGES WITH AGING

For young people time seems to span infinitely to the future. Years pass and suddenly we realize that the number of years remaining is limited. This realization that one is now old can be traumatic. The attitude we take about aging will be very important in affecting the success with which we age.

This section provides a brief overview of the psychology of aging and includes such topics as information processing, cognition, intelligence, personality, and life satisfaction. (Specific issues in mental health such as dementia and depression are addressed in Chapters 13 and 15.)

Psychologic characteristics of aging have a strong genetic component. A longitudinal study of aging human twins shows that identical twins have a greater similarity in cognitive performance than do nonidentical twins.

Men and women differ biologically in both obvious and subtle ways that affect their physical, psychologic, and social experience of aging. From the time of birth, differing sexual characteristics, such as men's generally greater physical strength and women's ability to bear offspring, have a profound influence on roles and behavior.

One obvious difference between the sexes is the greater longevity of the female, which is characteristic of most species. For us, this trait has psychologic and social implications since reduced numbers and proportions of aging men mean that aging is predominantly the experience of women. Women in our society usually marry men who are older than they are and, consequently, widowhood is common. Older women are most often called upon to make the psychologic adjustments to greater independence at a time that is often marked by less functional capabilities and consequent dependence on others for daily functioning and support.

Changes in Learning and Memory as We Age

Changes in mental function are perhaps the most feared aspect of aging. Significant mental impairment threatens our lives and our independence since we use our brains to perceive and act on risks in the environment. For most of us this fear of becoming mentally incompetent is groundless. Much harm results from the mistaken assumption that all mental functions decline with age. We begin to believe the stereotype, which encourages us to withdraw and lose our self-esteem. Mental function does not have to decline; the capacity to learn continues through life.

There are three phases of information processing—getting information into the system, keeping it in, and getting it out again. These may be referred to as encoding, storage, and retrieval.

Encoding New Information

As we age, we require more time and effort than younger people to encode an equivalent amount of new information. The reason for this is not known. However, it seems likely that changes in our vision, hearing, and other senses place barriers that reduce our memory efficiency. Optimal learning for us involves reading or following instructions on how to organize information, finding tasks meaningful and rewarding, and being able to link the visual information with auditory information. At best, sensory memory lasts much less than a second, and because of sensory changes that occur with aging, we are at a disadvantage at this first stage of information processing. Short-term memory only lasts a few seconds and declines with increasing age.

Storage and Retrieval

Recall and recognition are two types of memory tasks. Recall involves search and retrieval of information from storage. Recognition involves matching information in storage with information in the environment. Several studies have shown that for all ages recognition is superior to recall and that recall worsens over time. Little decline is noted in recognition.

Long-term memory (what most of us mean by the word *memory*) is said to decline as we age but perhaps only as a result of poorer encoding (getting information into the memory system). Very long-term memory, spanning months or years, is defined as information that is relatively permanent, acquired during a lifetime of education and day-to-day experience. This type of memory increases from the age of 20 to about the age of 50 and then remains relatively constant until well after we turn 70.

Most of us learn to adapt to changes, often by such compensatory behaviors as slowing down movements, increasing the rehearsal of elements to be committed to memory, or avoiding unfamiliar environments. As a result, a particular deficit may not even be noticed until a new challenge occurs, such as a move out of familiar surroundings or the death of a spouse.

Intelligence   Whether intelligence declines as we age remains a hotly debated topic. We may do less well than younger people on standard intelligence tests; however, when an individual is studied over a long time, little decline is seen. The results of verbal tests, such as measuring information retention, vocabulary, and comprehension, remain fairly steady. Tests of performance, in which, for example, the speed of copying a picture is measured, show decline with increasing age.

Traditional intelligence tests are probably not appropriate to measure intellectual functioning in older adults. First, the fact that speed of response is usually given great weight in these tests puts older people at a disadvantage. As we age we tend to be more cautious and more unwilling than younger people to make a mistake in judgment. In real-life situations, such caution has survival value, but in experimental settings it may bias psychological-test results in favor of younger people, making us appear slower and apparently unable to respond to test items. This makes it difficult to interpret studies examining psychological aspects of aging.

The times needed by healthy adults to react to a physical stimulus, particularly with respect to cardiovascular function, are faster than those of less healthy adults of similar age. Furthermore, our reaction times are quicker when we engage in regular physical activity. In fact, there are many healthy, physically fit elderly adults whose response times do not differ from those of less healthy, inactive younger adults.

The Speed of Processing Information

As we age we tend to process sensory information at a slower pace than when we were younger. Slowing outside the brain accounts for about 5 percent of this loss; 95 percent is due to changes in our nervous system. In addition, it takes longer to perceive a stimulus.

While we tend to be slower in performing simple cognitive tasks, we are even slower when the responses are more complicated. When an event is a surprise, we are particularly slow to respond. In addition, as we age we value accuracy, and therefore tend to be slower but more accurate in our responses.

Another criticism of most intelligence tests is how relevant are the tests in our daily lives. For example, on a test dealing with practical information items, including the use of a telephone directory, elderly adults score better than younger adults, even when they had scored less well on conventional tests.

Most of us continue to gain rather than decline in our ability to manage our daily affairs; it is usually only in time of stress or loss that our mechanisms may be pushed beyond their limits. At that point, social support represents an important external compensatory mechanism. In the ideal, we receive support, care, respect, and status and a sense of purpose by interacting with younger people. In turn we can provide cultural meaning, stability, and a continuity with the past. Meaningful participation in family and community activities is a major source of personal satisfaction and is the product of cultural attitudes and decisions made earlier in life.

Life satisfaction relates to subjective well-being, which in turn is strongly associated with health, socioeconomic factors such as income, and the degree of social interaction. When these variables are factored out, there is no correlation between the level of well-being and age or gender. Moreover, life satisfaction may be a

Life Satisfaction

relatively stable personality characteristic that is most associated with our previous sense of life satisfaction. Predictors of life satisfaction in older age may be different for men than they are for women. In one study, older men and women who had been interviewed about psychosocial issues 40 to 50 years earlier, when they were young parents, were reinterviewed. For the men in the study, the strongest predictors of life satisfaction were their wives' emotional characteristics as well as their own emotional and physical well-being. For the women, life satisfaction was most strongly associated with the amount of income and leisure time they enjoyed rather than with their husbands' personality.

Overall, except for extremely old people, life satisfaction does not seem to decrease with aging, despite age-associated events such as poorer health, reduced financial resources, widowhood, loss of friends, and reduced activity.

People tend to adapt to changing situations—pleasant or unpleasant—if the situations themselves cannot be changed. Since aging is a normal part of our developmental process, it is not surprising that we adapt to most of the physical, mental, and social changes. Role shifts that occur when we expect them to are less stressful than those that happen unexpectedly. For example, women who are widowed during old age experience less stress than those who are widowed during midlife. Many people, not taking this mechanism of adaptation into account, have mistakenly viewed the conditions of old age from the perspective of a youth-oriented society.

Stress is the body's response to a demand, and inordinate stress is associated with a variety of psychological and physical states, including anxiety, headaches, and ulcers among others. Causes of stress have been found to vary depending on one's age group. Elderly people have generally reported that they experience less stress than younger people. The comparative lack of stress in the older age group seems to be due to the lesser importance that older people attach to particular stimuli. For example, in one study both older and younger women expressed low satisfaction with social relationships but for the younger women these social relationships were very important whereas they were considered much less important by the older women. Thus, the younger women had higher expectations that were often not satisfactorily met, and the older women had either achieved their valued expectations or had placed less importance on attaining them.

As most of us are aware, there are healthy coping responses to stress, such as exercise or meditation, and there are unhealthy ones, such as overeating or substance abuse. However, coping responses also vary with age. In one study it was found that younger women relied on talking, rest and relaxation, and isolation to relieve stress, whereas elderly women used work, religion, and ignoring the problem.

Our ability to manipulate aspects of our environment represents personal control. Loss of this control can result in helplessness. Depression, or lack of motivation and even some cognitive deficits, may be manifestations of learned helplessness. In addition, passiveness and helplessness are the effects of repeated failures to control, escape, or avoid events. Even positive events that cannot be controlled may result in feelings of helplessness and depression. The explanation people give for an uncontrollable bad event may indicate the extent of their sense of helplessness or depression. For example, if they explain events in global terms such as "This always happens to me," "I can't do anything right," and "It's all my fault," then they are more likely to experience hopelessness and depression than if they explain events in event-specific terms.

Personal Control

Loss of perceived control often accompanies our aging experience, particularly in situations of disability. Feelings of helplessness, which are commonly experienced as we age, can produce adverse reactions and may contribute to early death. Our ability to predict events may be a form of control in that it allows us to adapt to the situation. In a study that involved nursing-home residents, members of the experimental nursing home were encouraged to take responsibility for themselves, were given the opportunity to care for a plant, and were also invited to participate in a residents' council. Patients in the control nursing home received no such interventions. The consequences of the intervention were significant reductions in hopelessness, increases in activity, and positive changes in behavior for the experimental group.

The acceptance of limits and a finite future is a quality of maturity, not a matter of resignation or defeat. With years of rich experience and reflection, some of us can transcend our own circumstances. We call this ability to see the truth in the light of the moment, wisdom. So as we age in creativity, in deepening wisdom and sensibility we become *more*, not less. And we realize that aging confronts us with the tension between ourselves now and ourselves in the future. We have an enormous amount of choice regarding our own aging. What are we sowing, and what is it we wish to reap?

CHAPTER 4
PREVENTIVE CARE

What Aspects of Aging Can We Influence?

Since we are apt to be active and functional in old age, we should expect to benefit from programs to promote health just as younger people do. It is important for us to remember that on average a person who is 65 can expect to live another 16 years. People 75 and 85 can expect to live another 10 and 6 years, respectively, and can expect to be functionally independent for at least half of that period. Because of this, the goal of promoting our health care shifts from maximizing longevity to postponing dependency. Health promotion emphasizes prevention of decline in function while supporting those abilities we need to remain independent.

In order to make optimal use of our health care resources, all of us—old and young—need to understand the overall organization of health care institutions. This is just as important in preventing illness and disease as it is in getting help once a health problem occurs. Prevention of illness and disability has been traditionally considered in terms of primary, secondary, and tertiary prevention. Primary prevention refers to interventions that are designed to reduce the risk of getting a disease. The methods of intervention include counseling to encourage a change in behavior (regarding diet, exercise, alcohol or nicotine use, etc.), and immunization.

Secondary prevention refers to efforts to improve outcomes in people who already have a given disease. This type of prevention is most effective when routine screening during a medical checkup allows the early detection of the disease. Tertiary prevention refers to efforts to prevent the progression of disability through systematic identification, treatment, and rehabilitation. Tertiary prevention is particularly applicable to older persons who often do not seek care for common sources of disability.

It is clear that the goals of prevention change in late life. In younger people, the goals target disease-specific disability and death, but in view of the multiple chronic conditions that commonly occur as we age, this focus loses its value. Our focus is on vitality, function, and quality of life, rather than on survival alone.

Primary Prevention

Exercise is an important means of preventing a wide range of health problems, including cardiovascular disease, falls, and depression. Older adults probably receive more health benefits from regular physical activity than adults who are younger and more fit. One long-term study of health-related behavior that started in the middle 1950s identified seven good health practices: seven to eight hours of sleep at night, weight control, exercise, limited alcohol consumption, not smoking, eating breakfast, and seldom snacking. Walking, which is available in all settings at a low cost, is recommended to all persons who are physically able. Activity should be habitual and not unduly strenuous. People who engage in light to moderate exercise daily, equivalent to sustained walking for about 30 minutes a day, can achieve health gains. Evidence suggests that even small increases in exercise by those who are least active produces benefits.

When older smokers quit, they can increase their life expectancy, reduce their risk of heart disease, and improve the function of their lungs and circulation. Cigarette smoking remains the single most preventable cause of death in the United States for both men and women. Those who have stopped smoking have found it helpful to set a quit date, to have scheduled reinforcement visits, to use self-help packages that are available from several voluntary organizations, and to make visits to community-based smoking-cessation programs. Some physicians prescribe nicotine gum or the nicotine patch to help, but smokers should have completely stopped smoking before they begin using these products. They should use them for at least three months—the time during which the risk of relapse is highest—but for no more than six months.

Dietary excesses are important causes of disease as we age, and therefore a regular review of dietary intake of calories, fluid, cholesterol, fiber, sodium, and minerals is useful. Caloric intake should be balanced against the expenditure of energy. Saturated fats should be reduced to less than 10 percent of the total calories. This can be done by eating fish, chicken without skin, low-fat dairy products, and lean meats. Whole grains, fruits, and vegetables are also highly recommended. Salt use should be modestly restricted by limiting the salt that is added at the table and by reducing the use of prepared (canned) foods. Women generally need to increase their calcium intake. In addition, if you have specific health problems and dietary needs, you should receive individualized counseling from a nutritionist, dietitian, or physician.

Approximately 5 percent of people who are over the age of 65 have an alcohol problem. Excessive alcohol use not only increases injuries, gastrointestinal illness, and liver disease, but it may also be a cause of potentially reversible dementing illness. (Alcohol and drug abuse are considered in Chapter 15.)

Motor-vehicle accidents are the leading cause of fatal injuries in adults up to age 75. Although the number of crashes sustained by older drivers as a group is no higher than that of the driving population in general, their crash rate adjusted for the actual miles that they drive is higher than for any other age group except for people under the age of 25. All drivers, of course, should wear seat belts and avoid using alcohol before driving. More specifically, as older drivers we must be aware of adjustments in driving techniques and habits to accommodate the changes of aging. Driving schools are often able to provide an assessment of the person who has experienced a recent decline in driving skills. Driver education or retraining is offered through the American Association of Retired Persons (AARP) and the American Automobile Association (AAA). It's sensible to take a refresher course to improve your knowledge and skills. Drivers with severe visual or hearing loss, dementing illness, or various neurologic diseases should seriously consider not driving.

Unintentional injury is the sixth leading cause of death among people who are 65 years and older. While a third of these injuries are related to falls and motor vehicle accidents, choking, burns, and drowning are also relatively common causes of death. Again, alcohol use contributes significantly to injuries due to falls, burns, and drownings.

Regular dental checkups are important as we age. Both daily brushing with fluoride-containing toothpaste and flossing are crucial to good dental health.

Although cholesterol remains a risk factor for coronary heart disease as we age, it is less important and less powerful a risk factor than smoking, hypertension, or lack of exercise. In fact, our risk in old age is not completely known. All of the studies evaluating cholesterol-lowering drugs have excluded or contained very few older people. Encouraging a balanced low-fat diet is beneficial not only for preventing heart disease but also for preventing cancer and other forms of disease. Specific high-risk groups, such as those with heart disease, may benefit from more aggressive cholesterol-lowering programs.

In spite of the availability of an effective vaccine, pneumococcal infections continue to be the leading cause of pneumonia and are a significant contributor to disability and mortality. The Centers for Disease Control and Prevention estimate that more than 40,000 deaths are due to these infections each year—80 percent occurring in people over age 65. While the vaccine, commonly known as the flu shot, has been available since 1977, it is greatly underutilized; less than 20 percent of the targeted population has ever received any vaccination. A number of expert panels recommend that all people 65 years and older receive the pneumococcal vaccine. The limiting factor in demonstrating the true benefit of the vaccine is the failure to deliver it to those of us at highest risk.

Yearly vaccination for influenza continues to be necessary because of the changes that occur in the influenza virus itself, a factor that explains the failure of protective antibodies in our blood to develop in spite of previous infection. If you have allergies to eggs or egg products you should not receive the vaccine nor should anyone who has any history of sensitivity to any part of the vaccine. Additionally, you should postpone immunization if you have a sudden respiratory infection or any illness that produces fever. During influenza epidemics, older people may be hospitalized at two- to fivefold increased rates, which poses significant health and economic problems.

While diphtheria and tetanus are rare (in 1987 they occurred in only 25 people over the age of 60) they are associated with a high rate of fatalities. Because of this, a tetanus-diphtheria booster every ten years is recommended.

To prevent coronary heart disease, the leading cause of death in the United States, low-dose aspirin therapy (325 milligrams of aspirin every other day) is recommended if you have two or more of the following risk factors: diabetes mellitus, a low HDL cholesterol, high blood pressure, a high LDL cholesterol, male gender, severe obesity, strong family history, or smoking. However, you should not take aspirin if you have uncontrolled high blood pressure, severe liver disease, ulcer disease, or any other condition that increases the risk of bleeding.

An estimated 25 percent of women who are 65 and older have spinal compression fractures, and about 15 percent will have a hip fracture during their lifetime. Estrogen therapy is often recommended for women who are at increased risk for osteoporosis. (This issue is further discussed in Chapter 17.)

By adopting preventive health behaviors, we can gain control over some factors that influence the nature and rate of our own aging. Smoking hastens the aging of the cardiovascular system; protein in the diet affects the aging of the kidney; excessive sunlight accelerates aging in the skin and the eye; exercise prolongs muscle function.

Secondary Prevention

Screening to detect early disease and initiate treatment is the chief element of secondary prevention. Table 1, compiled from a review of recent recommendations on prevention, lists the diseases, conditions, and risks that are associated with older people, along with the most commonly suggested screening intervals. Routine screening for diabetes mellitus is not recommended. Only if you have such risk factors as obesity, a family history of diabetes, or diabetes mellitus occurring during pregnancy should you be screened.

An electrocardiogram is not an effective screening test; however,

Table 1. Prevention in Older People

SCREENING RECOMMENDED FOR EVERYONE	INTERVAL
Alcohol, drug, and tobacco abuse	Yearly
Breast cancer	Yearly
Decline in function	Yearly
Deconditioning	Yearly
Dental problems	Yearly
Hearing problems	Yearly
High blood pressure	Yearly
Malnutrition	Yearly
Risk of falls	Yearly
Thyroid disease	Yearly
Vision problems	Yearly

SCREENING RECOMMENDED FOR PEOPLE AT HIGH RISK		
Cervical cancer	(women who have not had previous normal exams)	Every 3 years
Colon cancer	(family history, previous polyps or inflammatory bowel disease, previous breast, ovarian, endometrial, or colon cancer)	Every 3 years
Coronary heart disease	(two or more coronary risk factors, sedentary males beginning an exercise program)	Every 3 to 5 years
Diabetes mellitus	(obesity, family history, diabetes during pregnancy)	Yearly
Oral cancer	(excessive tobacco or alcohol use)	Yearly
Skin cancer	(previous history of skin cancer, significant sunlight exposure, precancerous changes)	Yearly
Tuberculosis	(residents of nursing homes, homeless people, immigrants from endemic countries, people with impaired immune function)	Every 10 years

NOT RECOMMENDED FOR SCREENING BUT WORTH WATCHING FOR
Abuse or neglect
Dementing illness
Depression
Obesity
Prostate cancer
Transient ischemic attack

cardiac stress testing may be useful before you begin an exercise program. If you have had a heart attack, the aggressive control of risk factors such as cigarette smoking, high cholesterol, and high blood pressure is important to prevent another. In addition, treatment with beta-adrenergic-blocking drugs in the first three years following a heart attack seems to reduce mortality. These are important concerns to discuss with your doctor.

Over the past 40 years cervical cancer in the United States has decreased by approximately 80 percent. There are significant racial differences in the pattern of the disease. As black women age, they experience a much higher incidence in mortality from cervical cancer than do white women. The National Health Interview Survey estimates that up to 40 percent of black women and 15 to 20 percent of older white women have never had a Pap smear. Pap smears can be stopped at age 65 if a woman has had several (at least three) previously documented normal exams.

Breast cancer screening by means of an annual examination and mammography every one to two years is recommended by the U.S. Preventive Services Task Force. Unfortunately, there is no reliable information for deciding whether there should be an upper age limit to screening. On average, breast cancer takes about ten years to grow to about the size of a large pea (1 centimeter in diameter). In older women, breast cancers are generally slower growing and less aggressive than they are in younger women. The U.S. Preventive Services Task Force registered uncertainty as to the benefits of screening in low-risk women 75 and older whose prior mammograms had been normal. Its ultimate recommendation was that screening be discontinued at age 75, but reliable data to support this directive are unavailable. Since years of remaining life constitutes a major issue in determining the benefit of early detection, recommendations regarding screening mammography could be made on the basis of anticipated survival rather than chronologic age.

There is not enough evidence to make a judgment about screening for colon or rectal cancer. As we get older, the potential benefit of screening is heightened by the increased likelihood of the disease, but is reduced by our diminished tolerance of the various aggressive curative and investigative procedures. Screening for

Table 2. Areas of Priority for
Health Promotion in Older People

Cancer screening

Depression

Falls

Hypertension

Infectious diseases

Misuse of medications

Nutrition

Oral health

Osteoporosis

Physical inactivity

Sensory loss

Smoking

Social isolation

Source: Berg R, Cassells J, eds. *The Second Fifty Years: Promoting Health and Preventing Disability.* Washington, DC: National Academy Press; 1990. © 1990, National Academy of Sciences. Published by the National Academy Press, Washington, DC. Reprinted with permission.

colon cancer is recommended if you have the following risk factors for the disease: (1) a first-degree relative with colon cancer, (2) a personal history of endometrial, ovarian, or breast cancer, or (3) a previous history of an inflammatory bowel condition, polyps, or previous colon or rectal cancer.

Screening for prostate cancer is controversial because of the usually slow progression of the disease. Only 1 in 380 men with prostate cancer will die of the disease. In addition, there is a lack of evidence supporting the benefit of treatment of early disease.

It is also not recommended that bone density in asymptomatic women be routinely measured. However, as mentioned, women who are at increased risk for osteoporosis and who are being considered for estrogen therapy might consider this measurement to help them decide whether therapy is appropriate.

Usually the areas of health care priorities for older people as outlined in Table 2 are identified when we become symptomatic. Osteoporosis, sensory deprivation, depression, malnutrition, unintentional injury, oral disease, taking too many medicines, urinary incontinence, and arthritis are all major health problems in elderly people that deserve to be given priority in preventive care.

The comprehensive geriatric assessment is one way to determine current medical problems, sources of disability, and priorities for future care. It includes screening to identify problems, including the targets of tertiary prevention, and usually involves the contributions of a multidisciplinary team. This assessment is particularly important for us when rapid changes are occurring in our health status or when a change in living arrangements appears necessary. (Chapter 8 on principles of rehabilitation has more information regarding the restoration of function if you are already disabled.) Checklists that outline health promotion strategies have been shown to improve the involvement and compliance of older persons and their physicians with the current recommendations. Properly timed and effectively delivered, preventive care can be expected both to extend our life and to postpone the period of functional disability. We have a considerable amount of control over the quality of our health in old age.

Tertiary Prevention

PART II

MAKING HEALTH CARE DECISIONS

CHAPTER 5

CHOOSING A DOCTOR

If a sudden illness occurs, your life can be thrown into a state of disarray requiring immediate decision making. Moreover, decisions such as whether to have surgery or to undergo a potentially life-threatening treatment can have significant consequences. Our views and values about these consequences will strongly influence our decision. In order to avoid making some of the most important decisions of our lives at a time we might feel the most helpless and out of control, we need to take as many steps as we can in advance. Of these steps, the most important by far is the selection of a physician whose expertise and judgment you trust. In this chapter we will examine the importance of the doctor-patient relationship, discuss how to find a doctor if you do not already have one, and how to make the most of your doctor visits.

Your relationship with your doctor can have a tremendous impact on your response to care and treatment. If you have confidence in your physician, you may experience a healing power that goes far beyond a comforting feeling of security or peace of mind. Your body can be significantly affected by stress, and every doctor has seen a situation improve dramatically by reassurance. Your doctor is an essential part of your treatment—you should have the best you can find.

Your regular doctor should be someone who understands you in particular and the needs of elderly people in general. An appropriate choice of physician might be a family practitioner, a general internist, or a geriatrician. In order to receive a medical license, all physicians must have graduated from an accredited medical school and have at least one year of training after medical school. However, for your care, this minimal level of training is far from adequate. Physicians must complete additional training, usually called a residency, to become eligible for certification by the board of the given medical specialty. Residency programs vary from two to six years of rigorous, supervised experience. Physicians must then pass a certifying exam to demonstrate that they have at least the minimal knowledge in the specialty. At this level of training, the name of the physician's medical school is not as important as whether the physician is board certified in a medical specialty. You will want a physician certified in a primary medical care discipline such as family medicine or internal medicine.

Geriatric care is a relatively new specialty; geriatricians specialize in the care of the older adult. A specialist in geriatric medicine has first been certified in either internal medicine or family practice and has had additional experience in caring for elderly people, either by completing two additional years of intensive hands-on training called a fellowship, or by having extensive clinical experience. Generally, physicians specializing in geriatrics focus their skills on very frail elderly people who have extremely complicated medical and social problems. You are probably too healthy to need the specialized services that can be performed by a geriatrician.

If you do not have a regular doctor, you should select a physician before you get sick. If you wait, you may be forced to take the first available doctor regardless of quality. Good medical care does not happen by accident and it is very risky not to have one personal physician in charge of the process. Your personal doctor can keep things coordinated so that you are not on too many medicines, you do not have unnecessary medical or surgical procedures, and so that recommendations from consultants are carefully considered to advise what is best for you. Someone needs to have the full picture of what is going on, to make sure that all the information has been gathered appropriately, and to see that nothing is missing.

You want your physician to have character and be competent and you want to be compatible. Character implies honesty, humility, an awareness of strengths and limitations, and a sense of responsibility. Compatibility is ultimately the physician's ability to gain your confidence, which depends upon an agreement of personalities.

Medical competence is also difficult to evaluate. You should not rely on a layman's testimony alone because people can be easily misled about a doctor's competence, and many people feel grateful to anyone who makes them feel comfortable. As a rough guide, doctors use the medical school, residency training, hospital privileges, and any specialty certifications when considering the competence of another physician.

Many personal preferences are involved in choosing a new doctor. The attributes you want, however, generally center around someone who is concerned about you, who can communicate with you, and who can anticipate your problems. A good physician will listen carefully to you and explain things clearly and completely, leaving time for questions and discussion. In addition, a good doctor must be available to you when you need his or her services. At the very least, alternatives to office visits with your doctor need to be provided, whether this means having another doctor on call if your doctor is unavailable or being able to reach your doctor for consultation over the telephone, or receiving visits at home. Other considerations in choosing a new doctor are more personal. Some women may feel more comfortable with female doctors, and some men may feel more comfortable with male doctors.

What to Look for in a Doctor

You already have a doctor whom you see for checkups, minor problems, or for medical conditions that have occurred in the past. However, you may need to find a new doctor if you move, if your regular doctor retires or dies, or if you become dissatisfied with your current doctor's services. If you live in a small community, your choice may be limited. If not, your search may be challenging. Your best source of information is a level-headed, responsible physician. A medical school's chairman of internal medicine or family practice can provide recommendations. The chief of medicine at the best hospital in your area can also give you some names.

How to Look for a Doctor

If you have moved, your previous physician might be able to recommend someone in your new location.

Giving a New Doctor a Checkup

Doctors play such an important role in our lives that you should be prepared to spend whatever time, money, effort, and energy you need to find the best possible physician. Therefore, once you have identified a person as a potential physician, schedule a visit to find out in advance whether this particular physician will suit your needs. To do this, when you make your telephone call to a new doctor's office, notice how the assistants respond to you. Are they abrupt or courteous, helpful or aloof? Ask if the doctor is accepting new patients and how soon you can have an initial examination. An appointment within a month is acceptable; any longer may imply that the doctor is overworked.

Getting the Most from Your Doctor Visit

You and your physician will need to work together to develop a comprehensive plan for your health. Your responsibilities are to be prepared to ask the right questions and to be a good listener. This book can help you in two of these three areas. You should gather all your relevant past medical information, including any old records from past physicians. You can send a written request to your previous physicians to have copies of your records sent to your new physician. You should also compile a brief family history, which includes any illnesses or causes of death within your immediate family. It is also important to bring all your current medications with you, including any medicines you may have purchased without a prescription. Because you will probably need to undress for the physical exam, it is important to wear clothing that you can remove easily.

Allow time for traffic and parking when you reach the doctor's office and try to get there a few minutes early. Your first impressions of the office are important. Are things organized? Someone will probably first check your blood pressure and weight and then either have you wait in the waiting room or direct you to an examining room. It is not unusual that doctors become a little behind their scheduled appointments. If, however, you have to wait for more than 20 minutes, ask someone about the reason for the delay. You may wish to reschedule the visit if the delay is going to be excessively long and, in any case, just knowing the reason for the delay can be reassuring.

When the doctor arrives, you will want to make every second count. To use the time efficiently, have a list of your concerns with you. The first time your doctor sees you, there will probably be an extensive interview and physical examination, which may take up to an hour or even longer. The conversation should be balanced with neither you nor the physician doing all the talking. Ask plenty of questions and make sure that you understand the physician's answers. You do not want to be confused or uncertain when you leave the office and certainly not when you arrive home. If your doctor has used medical terms that you do not understand, ask for simple definitions. An example of a list of questions related to an illness would be: Exactly what is wrong with me? Is this a common problem? What other conditions could possibly cause this and how likely are they? What do I need to do now? Is there anything that I shouldn't do or that would cause me difficulty? What are the options and alternatives for treatments? You will very likely have additional questions, based on the specific problems and concerns you may have, but the point is for you to leave the office with a clear understanding of what is going on and a basic understanding of the treatment.

After the office visit, think clearly about what has happened and always remember that you have an active role in making the decisions about your own health. Your doctor's advice is certainly important, but you are free to accept or reject this advice. You are the one who must consent to various medical or surgical treatments, and your decisions must be made on the basis of your personal beliefs along with the doctor's advice, but remember, *nothing can be done without your consent.* If you have continuing concerns about the visit, go to the next person on your list. You must have trust and confidence in your physician.

Every significant relationship requires careful maintenance to allow it to grow. Once you have chosen your doctor, understanding a few basic principles can help make the most of the relationship. Having an up-to-date list of your medical problems or health concerns is important. You should know what to do in the case of an emergency. Should you call the physician first, go to the emergency room first, or have the doctor call the emergency room in advance? Find out the hospitals for which your doctor has admitting privileges. If you go to the emergency room of a hospital where your doctor does *not* have admitting privileges, you will consult and be examined by one of the doctors who are associates, with privileges, to that particular hospital.

It is important to let your doctor know if there are any aspects of your care that you are unwilling or unable to do. Discuss all tests with your doctor before they are ordered to find out why they are being performed, what the risks are, and how much they cost. Keep track of the test results and review them periodically with your doctor to understand how the evaluation is progressing. Obviously, if medications are prescribed, you will need to understand the reasons for their use, any side effects that may be expected, if any less expensive or dangerous alternatives exist, and how long you will need to be on the medications.

Information that you give your doctor is strictly confidential and therefore honesty between you and your doctor is very important. Although some information may be very embarrassing for you to share, it is essential for your doctor to know everything.

Deciding on a personal physician is one of the most important decisions you will ever make: One day your life may depend on your choice.

Chapter 6

Going into the Hospital

Hospitalization may be necessary for a specialized medical procedure, for an elective surgical procedure, or because your illness has become so severe that it cannot be managed elsewhere. Ideally, there should be time to schedule a hospitalization without the pressure of an emergency. Very often, however, this is not the case, and when you need immediate medical attention, you go to a hospital emergency room. The physicians who are on call will evaluate your condition and decide or recommend whether you need to be admitted. *State and federal laws prohibit hospitals and emergency rooms from refusing care to anyone who needs it.* When you are seen in the emergency room, your personal physician will be notified. Your doctor, if available, may come into the emergency room if he or she has privileges to practice in that hospital.

Before you agree to be admitted into a hospital there are several important questions you should ask: Is being admitted the best of any alternatives? What procedures or treatments are likely to be done during the hospitalization? How long will the stay be? What would happen if you were not admitted?

When you are hospitalized for elective surgery, a number of additional health care personnel become involved: the surgeon, the anesthesiologist, the radiologist, as well as others. You will experience a number of different hospital environments that may well be unfamiliar and confusing: the operating room, the recovery room, and, possibly, the critical care unit. (Surgery is discussed in more detail in the next chapter.)

Before you go to the hospital, try to do some planning.

- Make a list of questions or concerns to discuss with your doctor prior to your hospitalization
- Ask your doctor how to reach him/her while you are in the hospital
- Carry with you a list of your medical conditions and current medications, any drug or food allergies you have, your insurance information, names and phone numbers of family and friends
- Label personal items (hearing aids, dentures, eyeglasses) with your name and address to avoid loss
- Leave jewelry and other valuables at home
- Take to the hospital a personal belonging (not a valuable one) such as a photograph of a loved one, to provide comfort and reassurance

There are other aspects of hospitalization that may dismay or bewilder you aside from the discomfort of being ill or undergoing uncomfortable medical or surgical procedures. Knowing about them ahead of time may help dispel these frustrations. Hospital admission usually requires filling out a number of forms and making a number of complicated decisions. There will be significant changes in your daily routine and you will likely be put through a number of tests in unfamiliar settings. Your normal familiar clothing will generally be replaced with unflattering and rather revealing hospital gowns. The food is not always appetizing and may be served at unusual times of day. And you will probably experience some lack of privacy. Medical staff and hospital personnel will be going in and out of your room continually to ask you important, but fairly demanding questions or to take your temperature, give you medication, change your linens, adjust your bandages, and so on. Most people will knock on your door and then barge on in before you can respond. Although you may feel intimidated or dependent in the face of all of this authority, remember that your health is your first concern in such circumstances and, ultimately, your responsibility. In the end, you—not the hospital staff—are the person in control of your well-being.

It is important that throughout your hospitalization you look out for yourself regarding your care. After all, mistakes and accidents can happen in the hospital, and the best way to avoid these is to ask plenty of questions. Ask about medications, ask about procedures, ask about when or how things are supposed to occur, and so on. Some of the anxiety of a hospital stay can be relieved if a family member, a friend, or other interested person can be there to help look after you and be your advocate.

When you're admitted, you need to consider what type of room to get, how much it will cost, whether a telephone or television is or can be provided in the room, and whether special dietary concerns can be handled. Generally, you will have to sign a form agreeing to the type of care that is being provided: This is not a consent form for specific kinds of treatment. Other forms involving the method of payment give the hospital permission to share information concerning your circumstances with various organizations, such as insurance companies that may be involved in paying for your hospitalization and any procedures. Once you have completed filling out forms, which may be time-consuming, you are generally taken either to your room or to other sites within the hospital where you will receive various tests (blood tests, X rays, electrocardiogram, etc.) that may be required as part of your hospitalization.

While you are in the hospital, you should expect your doctor to visit you daily and sometimes more than once a day, depending on your situation. Besides talking with you during these visits, your doctor will evaluate your condition and write various orders and progress notes in your chart so that nurses and other staff members are kept up-to-date on your care. You should feel free to talk with your doctor about these orders so that you will understand what is being asked of other staff members while you are a patient. Also, you should know how to reach your doctor while you are in the hospital.

While in the hospital, you have a number of rights:

- The right to be free of restraints and abuse
- The right to leave the hospital, even against the advice or wishes of your doctor
- The right to refuse medical care, even if life prolonging
- The right to know the truth about your condition
- The right to keep your condition a secret from your family or anyone, unless you have a contagious disease

You also have the right to know the truth about your condition, including an honest description or statement. You also have the right to keep your condition a secret from family members or anyone else. The exception to this is when you have a contagious disease.

As soon as possible after being admitted to the hospital, you, a family member, or a close friend should speak to a hospital discharge planner. Preparing for your discharge can take anywhere from a few hours to several days, depending on the nature of your condition and your personal situation. It's best when family members and others who will care for you after hospitalization are involved in the planning. The main issues are the ease or difficulty you will have in performing daily activities after discharge from the hospital and who will assist you on a day-to-day basis. Once this has been settled, it is important to determine the date of discharge. You should receive written notice of the discharge date, after which you have until noon of the following day to decide whether this date seems appropriate. If you decide that the discharge date is inappropriate, you should discuss this as soon as possible with both your doctor and the discharge planner. If you have good reasons for objecting to the date of discharge, it can often be changed without any lengthy process. The main objective is to remain in the hospital only as long as you need the care that can be obtained only in the hospital.

We have acknowledged that a hospitalization can be a trying process that is made even more challenging because it happens when you are not always feeling your best. Although you may feel a loss of control and a sense of intimidation, the key to overcoming these feelings is to look out for yourself and ask plenty of questions. Having another person with you is also very reassuring.

CHAPTER 7

UNDERGOING SURGERY

The current annual rate for surgery on people over age 65 is 15 percent and rising. Twenty percent of all open-heart procedures are on people over the age of 70. Improved evaluation and management techniques for older people undergoing surgery are being introduced. In the following pages we will discuss the key issues concerning surgery: determining whether the operation is necessary, agreeing to the surgeons, minimizing your risks, and trying to reduce complications. (More detailed discussion of specific conditions mentioned here can be found in Part IV.)

You should be aware of your responsibility in selecting a surgeon. Sometimes your personal physician helps by recommending the surgeon, but you are ultimately in charge of this decision. Approximately one-quarter to one-third of all surgical procedures currently performed in the United States are unnecessary. You should always obtain a second opinion before deciding to have any kind of elective surgery. If your physician recommends surgery, find out as much as possible about what will happen during surgery. Also, determine the surgeon's experience in performing the operation, and what the surgeon considers acceptable as quality of life for a person before and after the surgery. If you want to know who will perform the anesthesia during the surgery, ask the surgeon. What matters most concerning an anesthesiologist is that the surgeon feels comfortable with the anesthesiologist's work, reputation, and expertise. Also, you should not assume that the surgeon you have chosen will be the person who actually performs the operation. Ask the surgeon who will perform the operation. Some hospitals are teaching hospitals, and the actual surgical procedure may be done by a surgical resident who is learning the technique. You have every right to know who will be performing the surgery on you.

Aging and Surgical Risk

Although the risk associated with many operations increases as we age, the overall risk for older people has been steadily declining over the past 30 years. In fact, elective surgery on people who are over 80 years old is safer in the 1990s than the same procedures were when performed on younger people in the 1960s. Coexisting medical diseases and the urgency of the procedure are more important factors than age in predicting possible complications. Moreover, people over the age of 80 can undergo major surgery without excessive mortality.

Complications involving the heart are the most life-threatening. In surgical cases involving elderly individuals, mortalities due to heart disease are about 3 to 5 percent. The average risk of a heart attack after surgery is 1 to 4 percent and that of congestive heart failure is between 4 and 10 percent.

Complications involving the lungs, the most common cause of postoperative complications in the older age group, affect 15 to 45 percent of older people who undergo surgery. Pneumonia is more than twice as common as other respiratory causes of death. Cancer is the next most common condition that is associated with postoperative death in older people. Kidney failure, stroke, and bleeding are less common causes.

Three issues are most often considered in the evaluation for surgery: What medical conditions could adversely affect the surgical risk? What is the overall level of risk associated with the conditions identified? How should these conditions be managed to control the risk?

Because problems with your heart and lungs comprise the majority of serious postoperative complications, the assessment of your surgical risk involves determining your cardiovascular risk and your pulmonary risk. Reduced blood flow to your heart, heart attacks, congestive heart failure, and disturbances of the heart rhythms are serious problems. Interestingly, stable angina pectoris, compensated congestive heart failure, and well-controlled high blood pressure do not seem to contribute to your risk of cardiac complications.

Determining Your Risk of Surgery

Assessing your heart function is particularly important, since the effects of age are first seen as a reduction in heart function with physical stress. The preoperative assessment often includes an electrocardiogram if major surgery is expected. If you have a known heart disease or if multiple risk factors are present, you may be asked to take a stress test of your heart. If you cannot complete the stress test or raise the heart rate above 100 beats per minute, you may be vulnerable to increased risk after surgery.

In order to avoid the risk of postoperative lung complications, most notably pneumonia, you must be able to generate enough airflow to expel the mucus that can accumulate in your lungs during surgery. The progressive, age-associated loss of lung function and common nonlung conditions such as obesity, malnutrition, skeletal abnormalities, and general muscular weakness may place you at risk for these lung complications after surgery.

Cigarette smoking is a major risk factor for complications after surgery. Smokers are most likely to have significant lung disease, increased amounts of airway secretions, bacterial contamination of the airways, and diminished ability to clear up secretions. All smokers should stop smoking eight weeks prior to surgery. (If you smoke, stop smoking now.)

Detectable clots (thromboses) in the deep veins of the leg develop in about half of all elderly surgical patients. Orthopedic surgery (especially hip surgery) and surgery in people with cancer also produce an increased risk of clots in the large veins in the leg. Additional risk factors include obesity, heart disease, a history of prior blood clots, and immobility. Other factors that cause concern include additional chronic diseases, malnutrition, a diminished will to live, kidney disease, dementing illness, and active infection.

Complications Following Surgery

Your risk of a heart attack extends through the first week after surgery, with the greatest risk on the fourth postoperative day; in over half of these heart attacks there is no chest pain, so many physicians perform an electrocardiogram on the day of surgery and on the first two or three postoperative days. Others suggest continual monitoring of the heart during this time. Nonetheless, you should have at least one electrocardiogram after surgery.

Congestive heart failure after surgery is most likely to occur in people with heart failure before surgery, although half of the people who develop heart failure after surgery have had no prior evidence of it. Other reported risk factors for heart failure after surgery are an abnormal preoperative electrocardiogram, surgery in the chest or abdomen, and advanced age.

Collapse of the small airways in the lungs and increased secretions in the lungs are responsible for pneumonia after surgery. The development of airway collapse is associated with lying on the back, incisions near the diaphragm, obesity, pain on breathing, sedation, and an excess of sticky secretions that cause plugging. Before surgery, stopping smoking for eight weeks or more and the treatment of lung disease may significantly reduce your risk of having pneumonia after an operation.

You may receive heparin, a blood thinner sometimes given to prevent blood clots from forming in the deep veins in the legs. Heparin is often given as an injection twice a day. If you are undergoing hip surgery or surgery for cancer, the anticoagulant warfarin is often given instead because heparin does not seem to be adequate.

If you have diabetes, you should receive glucose and insulin before and after surgery. You should also avoid having low blood sugar by discontinuing oral medications used to lower blood sugar one or two days before surgery.

The death rates after surgery in people with dementia may be as high as 20 percent one month after the operation and 50 percent at six months. In addition, delirium after surgery is much more commonly seen in people who have dementia before surgery. Depression, which is common in older people, may limit their interest in recovery. Depression should be treated prior to having any elective surgical procedures.

The overall likelihood of delirium in older people who have

general surgery is between 10 and 15 percent. The factors that would precipitate delirium include medications, infection, low oxygen, heart problems, changes in body chemistry such as low sodium in the blood or a low blood sugar, fecal impaction, and urinary retention. Sleep deprivation, sensory deprivation, immobility, and being in an unusual place are also contributing factors. Because of this, the first priority in the management of a person with delirium after surgery is to recognize and correct any of these factors. Obviously, you will not be able to recognize delirium in yourself, so close observation and orientation by family members, hospital staff, or paid sitters may help reduce your risk of injury until you recover.

We have seen in this chapter that surgery presents you with a number of responsibilities: agreeing to a surgeon, determining the necessity of the operation (since one in three operations performed is not necessary), finding out who will actually perform the operation, minimizing your risks, and trying to reduce complications. Heart and lung complications and blood clots cause the most serious problems; delirium after surgery is common, and you must be prepared for postoperative confusion.

CHAPTER 8

PRINCIPLES OF REHABILITATION

The primary focus of rehabilitation is function. The goal may be to restore a function that you have lost, or it may involve maintaining function that you need to modify and strengthen.

Rehabilitation can then be characterized as either a restorative or a maintenance process. Restorative rehabilitation aims to reverse a new disability and improve function and is often funded by Medicare or other payers. Examples include the short-term rehabilitation that follows a stroke or a hip fracture. Maintenance rehabilitation is less intense, with continued outpatient physical therapy or occupational therapy three times a week. This continual therapy offers the possibility of a person making further gains in function or preventing further functional loss.

The maintenance of function is a central aspect of your general care, particularly when you experience a sudden illness or become immobilize. In these situations you would benefit from maintenance therapy that consists of exercises designed to prevent joint contractures, maintain your muscle tone, and avoid significant decline in function. Begin rehabilitation early—it will help you preserve and maintain function and can increase your chances of returning to your previous level of function.

Usually, rehabilitation means working with a team of trained professionals. The members of the rehabilitation team will vary significantly according to the setting. The disciplines represented may include medicine, rehabilitation medicine (physiatry), nursing, physical therapy, occupational therapy, speech therapy, social work, nutrition, psychology or psychiatry (or both), and recreation therapy (see Table 3).

Rehabilitation settings include special units in acute care hospitals, rehabilitation hospitals, nursing facilities, outpatient centers, homes, or private offices. If you have a sudden onset of a new disability and are an appropriate candidate for 4 to 12 weeks of restorative rehabilitation, you may benefit from an intensive rehabilitation program with a team effort. Such programs are usually carried out in a rehabilitation unit, whether in an acute hospital, a freestanding rehabilitation hospital, or a nursing facility with a designated rehabilitation program. If you cannot tolerate or do not need an intense therapy program, you may receive services at the nursing facility level, in your home, or as an outpatient. These programs may also be more appropriate when ongoing maintenance therapy follows the inpatient restorative rehabilitation program.

Techniques used in rehabilitation may not be limited to specific programs such as stroke rehabilitation or hip fracture rehabilitation. People can often be evaluated when they are having difficulty performing various activities of daily living (ADL). These activities include mobility, transferring (from wheelchair to bed, toilet, chair, etc.), eating, bathing, dressing, and communication.

Assistive Devices

Assistive devices can be used to help people with difficulties performing such activities of daily living as feeding, bathing, and dressing. Most people benefit from an evaluation by an occupational therapist to ensure that the assistive device is the appropriate one for improving the impaired capability. Several important principles need to be considered.

1. A person must be physically and cognitively capable of using the device effectively.
2. People tend to use aids that are not conspicuous, complicated, cumbersome, or cosmetically unappealing.

Table 3. Members of the Rehabilitation Team

DISCIPLINE	ACTIVITY
Medicine	Manages acute and chronic medical illnesses.
Nursing	Assists in coping and adaptation to illness; integrates medical and nursing care plan with rehabilitation treatment plan.
Nutrition	Assesses and improves nutritional status.
Occupational therapy	Assesses and improves upper-extremity function; improves performance of activities of daily living; helps compensate for visual and other perceptual deficits; assists in evaluation and treatment of swallowing disorders.
Orthotics	Makes and fits orthopedic appliances.
Physiatry	Develops the plan for continued physical, occupational, and speech therapy.
Physical therapy	Assesses and improves lower-extremity function; improves range of motion, strength, balance, and endurance; teaches use of assistive devices and provides gait training.
Psychiatry	Provides psychiatric evaluation and treatment for patient; provides support for family.
Psychology	Provides psychologic support and assistance to rehabilitation team.
Social work	Assists in discharge planning, helps families cope with illness and disability; does financial and personal counseling.
Speech therapy	Evaluates and treats communication, speech, and swallowing disorders.
Therapeutic recreation	Helps plan leisure-time activities and hobbies; develops realistic goals and motivation.

3. A person with perceptual problems may have difficulty using a device effectively.

4. Assistive devices may be a significant out-of-pocket expense since they are usually not funded by insurance or other payers.

5. An evaluation of a person's home or other living situation may be necessary to determine the most appropriate and effective use of assistive devices in improving function and ensuring safety.

Older people with upper-extremity weakness, deformity, uncoordination, and limited range of arm motion frequently find assistive devices for eating very helpful. A rocker knife and fork, for example, may allow a person with paralysis on one side of the body (hemiplegia) to cut and pick up food with one hand (see Figure 6). Similar assistive devices can be used for spoons, bowls, and plates. Eating utensils can also be modified for people who have limited motion or poor grasp. For example, silverware handles can be enlarged with foam padding or other materials, and a cuff that straps around the hand to hold eating utensils in place can be used to help a person with a weak hand to hold the device.

Because fatigue frequently aggravates uncoordination, energy-saving techniques are often helpful. Foods that eliminate the need for extensive cutting, chopping, or mixing are generally recommended along with easy-to-open packages and containers. You can hold food steady by using a board with spikes, a rubber mat, or sponges. The use of blenders, coffee urns, Crock-Pots, microwave ovens, and electronic skillets all reduce the need to use the stove or oven. These need to be placed at the appropriate

Figure 6. Eating Aids

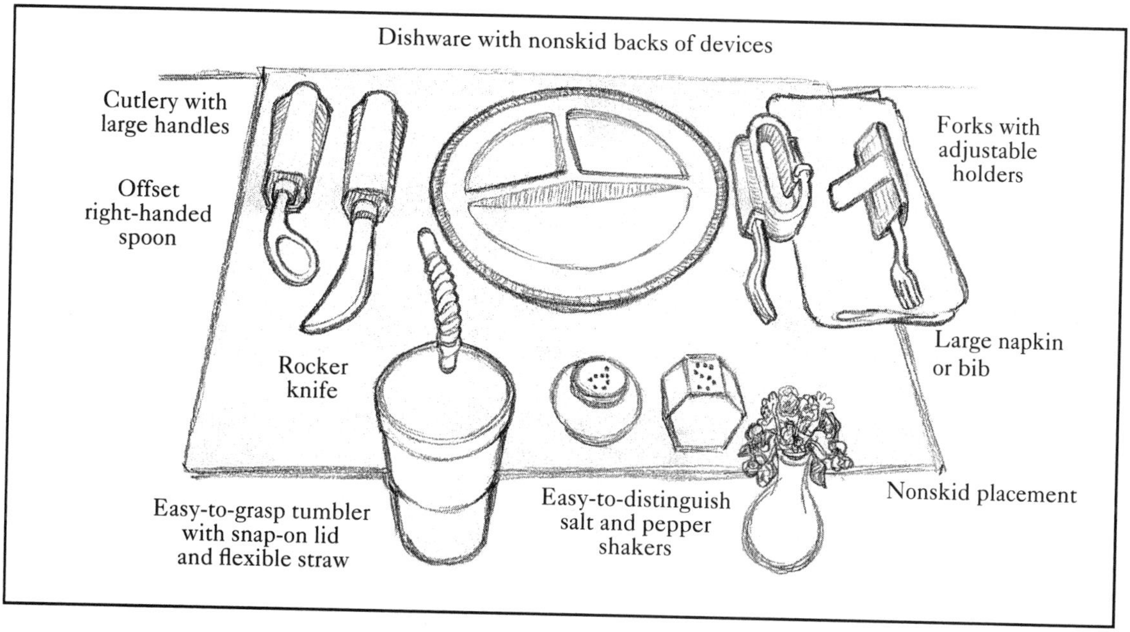

Dishware with nonskid backs of devices

Cutlery with large handles

Offset right-handed spoon

Rocker knife

Easy-to-grasp tumbler with snap-on lid and flexible straw

Easy-to-distinguish salt and pepper shakers

Forks with adjustable holders

Large napkin or bib

Nonskid placement

Figure 7. Dressing Aids

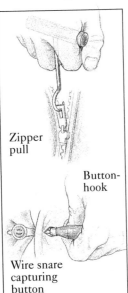

Zipper pull

Button-hook

Wire snare capturing button

heights on a stationary work surface. Pizza cutters can sometimes replace knives. Oversized bowls, plate guards, and soup dishes with high rims can be used to avoid spills during the extra movements or for people with tremors. For people who have loss of manual dexterity, electric can openers and jar openers can be extremely helpful.

In addition to raised toilet seats and tub transfer benches (see Figure 11), a variety of other devices can help with bathing and maintaining personal hygiene. Long-handled bath sponges, "soap-on-a-rope," and wash mitts can be helpful bathing aids for people who have limited motion, weakness, or difficulty with coordination. As an aid in grooming, the handles of combs and brushes can be enlarged by foam padding to help compensate for limited grasping ability. A wall mirror may be tilted downward to permit better visibility from a wheelchair.

Assistive devices are also available to help with dressing (see Figure 7). For example, the use of a buttonhook or zipper pull can make dressing much easier, and Velcro attachments are excellent substitutes for buttons or shoelaces. A dressing stick can aid older persons to dress as they sit, allowing them to hook or pull the cuff or sleeve of a shirt or pants into position. A stocking-donning device or slip-on dressing aid can also assist in dressing the legs. This can permit older people to pull up their stockings themselves even though they cannot reach their feet. For people with limited motion of the arms or shoulders, various reaching aids (see Figure 8) can help in pulling hats off a shelf as well as paper off a floor.

Other Rehabilitation Techniques

People who are receiving either restorative or maintenance rehabilitation may benefit from electrical stimulation and thermal approaches.

Electrical Stimulation

Two kinds of electrical stimulation are generally available: (1) functional electrical stimulation and (2) transcutaneous electrical nerve stimulation (TENS). In functional electrical stimulation, an electrical current is used to produce a muscle contraction. It not only prevents atrophy in muscles that have not been used for a while but also increases the range of muscle motion and strength, helps increase the voluntary function of a previously paralyzed muscle, and reduces muscle spasticity. For older people who have severe weakness of the upper arm, functional electrical stimulation can help prevent a dislocation of the shoulder and the development of a "frozen" shoulder. (Shoulder problems are found on page 243.) Electrical stimulation has also been used to improve the strength of pelvic muscles in older women who suffer certain forms of incontinence. (See page 389 for a complete discussion of urinary incontinence.)

Transcutaneous electrical nerve stimulation, in addition to improving muscle strength and bulk, may have a pain-relieving effect. It has been used to treat the pain that is associated with various conditions, such as rheumatoid arthritis, poor circulation, and nerve diseases. In addition, this technique may reduce the amount of pain medicine that a person may need. TENS involves the direct electrical stimulation of the spinal cord. It has been used to treat older people with shingles (herpes zoster), to reduce the spasticity of a limb after a stroke, and to relieve the nerve pain sometimes associated with diabetes or poor circulation. While TENS is

Figure 8. Reaching Aids

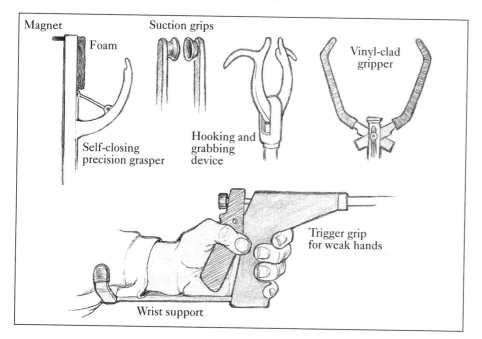

Magnet

Suction grips

Foam

Vinyl-clad gripper

Self-closing precision grasper

Hooking and grabbing device

Trigger grip for weak hands

Wrist support

sometimes used for long-standing low back pain, evidence of its efficacy is lacking.

Thermal Approaches

Various thermal approaches are used primarily to treat pain, reduce inflammation, and increase muscle tone. Heat can be applied either superficially with a heating agent such as a hot pack, or with deep-heating devices such as ultrasound or diathermy. Locally applied heat can promote muscle relaxation and pain relief, help with tissue healing, and prepare stiff joints and tight muscles for exercise. Hot packs can be applied to most body surfaces, while baths of liquid paraffin are most often used for the application of heat to the hands or feet. For example, hot packs may reduce muscle spasm in older people who have arthritis involving the neck, muscular low back pain, or muscle contractions. Heated paraffin may be particularly helpful to reduce the hand stiffness and pain in people with rheumatoid or osteoarthritis.

Ultrasound is a deep-heating technique that is capable of elevating the temperatures deep in the tissues. This can be used to relieve joint tightness and loosen scar tissue, as well as to reduce pain and muscle spasm. It has been used to treat bursitis, tendinitis, and low back pain.

Hydrotherapy in the form of a whirlpool or other pool therapy may be helpful. It has been used to treat arthritis, joint injuries or replacements, and to promote pain relief, wound healing, and to help with various neurologic disorders. Cold treatments or cold packs have been commonly used to treat people with sudden muscle or bone injuries. They can sometimes reduce pain and muscle spasms, especially those caused by brain injury.

Who Benefits from Rehabilitation?

When evaluating a person with a disability, the health care provider concentrates on understanding the history of the progressive loss of function, its severity, and the potential for recovery. These factors are vital to determine whether a person can regain function. The present level of functioning can be evaluated both in terms of activities and of daily living.

Knowledge of your level of functioning before a disability is essential when evaluating your potential for rehabilitation. For example, it may be very realistic for a previously healthy older person who could walk without the use of an assistive device before suffering a hip fracture to be able to walk again within several months after a program of rehabilitation. However, the same goal may be less attainable for a person of the same age whose walking ability was previously poor, limited perhaps by arthritis or poor circulation.

Generally, a person is evaluated for coexisting medical conditions, such as heart disease, lung disease, and joint diseases, that might limit participation in an intense rehabilitation program. Although moderate to severe heart and lung disease may reduce the possibility of intensive rehabilitation, many people can improve their exercise tolerance gradually.

Another essential factor is your commitment to ongoing rehabilitation along with the commitment to your family—or caregiver—when you return home after the rehabilitation program. The severity and type of disability often influence the decision of all involved as to whether the affected person is best off returning home. From a standpoint of function, the minimum prerequisite for people living at home is that they be able to transfer safely from a bed to a chair, and from a wheelchair to the toilet. For people who have cognitive impairment or perceptual problems, 24-hour supervision may be necessary. Often the critical factor for discharge from a rehabilitation unit is whether the person has this type of 24-hour support at home.

Settings for Rehabilitation Programs

Rehabilitation programs within hospitals or special rehabilitation hospitals utilize a multidisciplinary team approach. For a person to qualify for insurance coverage of comprehensive rehabilitation at the hospital level, Medicare and most other insurance carriers stipulate that the person must need (1) close medical supervision and care by a rehabilitation physician; (2) rehabilitation nursing on a 24-hour basis; (3) participation in more than one therapeutic discipline, such as physical therapy, occupational therapy, or speech therapy; (4) a multidisciplinary team approach to therapy, with a coordinated rehabilitation program; and (5) clear, realistic, attainable goals in rehabilitation, with the expectation and documentation of significant functional improvement during the rehabilitation program.

In general, rehabilitation programs in these settings are short-term. Depending upon the person's needs and anticipated gains from therapy, inpatient hospital-based rehabilitations on average require six to eight weeks for the person who has had a stroke, a longer time for those who have had a major injury, and a shorter time for those who have less complicated problems.

Nursing facilities frequently provide rehabilitation services for older people, particularly those who have recently had a hip fracture, as well as those who have had an amputation. In contrast to the Medicare requirements for the hospital level of rehabilitation, the requirements for insurance coverage at the nursing facility level of rehabilitation do not include occupational therapy, a multidisciplinary approach, or the services of a rehabilitation physician. However, the requirements do specify that a person must need daily physical therapy and skilled nursing care and that continued, significant functional improvement be documented. Under these guidelines, a person with a hip fracture who has minimal impairment of arm function and is medically stable would be covered for rehabilitation at a nursing facility rather than at a hospital.

Outpatient rehabilitation services, also quite varied in scope, range from private practitioners' offices that offer fee-for-service care to outpatient rehabilitation facilities that provide the same comprehensive, multidisciplinary team efforts as hospital rehabilitation units. Generally, these outpatient units are appropriate for people with short-term, self-limited syndromes or illnesses, such as low back pain or minor trauma. Other services may be appropriate for people who require follow-up services after being discharged from a rehabilitation hospital or for whom an inpatient rehabilitation program is not feasible, suitable, or acceptable. Often, the availability of transportation is what determines whether the person can participate in an outpatient rehabilitation program.

For a number of older people, home care rehabilitation programs can be an important component of follow-up care for people who have been discharged from either a hospital-based or nursing facility–based inpatient rehabilitation program. In addition, home rehabilitation services can help with the evaluation and provision of maintenance therapy or for short-term therapy for self-limiting illnesses. The Medicare criteria for in-home rehabilitation services are similar to those for outpatient or inpatient programs, with one notable addition: The person must be completely home-bound. This requirement often restricts the number of people who might benefit from therapy services at home and limits opportunities for developing a comprehensive, multidisciplinary approach to therapy in this setting.

For most of us, walking difficulties frequently occur as a result of an abnormality of our nervous system, or problems with our muscles and joints. There are various assistive devices for walking, such as canes, walkers, orthotics (braces), and prostheses, designed to improve balance and support during standing and ambulation.

Rehabilitation of Walking Problems

Canes, the simplest assistive devices for walking, provide the least amount of support and balance. While they support up to 25 percent of the body weight, they are best reserved for people whose ability to walk is limited by weakness or pain on one side. The use of canes is governed by the following principles: (1) Single-prong canes provide the least degree of support but are lighter and less conspicuous. (2) A pistol-shaped grip allows for greater comfort, better weight bearing, and more secure handling than the evenly rounded handle of the standard wooden canes. If necessary, the handle of the cane can be modified to adapt to physical impairments or deformities of the hand. (3) Quadripod canes provide greater support than the single-point cane and are usually better for people who have significant walking problems. The wider base for these canes provides greater support. (4) In general, you should hold the cane in the hand of your *unaffected* side. This allows you to form an arch between the affected side and the cane to help support the weight. This also permits a shorter "stance phase" of walking and a decreased period of weight bearing on the affected side when you walk. (5) The length of the cane is important for ensuring stability and comfort. When the cane is properly positioned on the ground and your hand is resting on the handle, your elbow should be flexed upward at a 20- to 30-degree angle. Another measuring method is to let the arm dangle beside the cane: A correctly sized cane will come to the crease of your wrist.

Canes

Walkers   Walkers, another common assistive device, surround you with four broadly spaced posts. Walkers can support up to 50 percent of your body weight, so you should consider them if you have problems on both sides or if you have general weakness. Among the several types of walkers in use are the standard pick-up walkers, which have four, often adjustable, posts covered by rubber tips. To use one of these walkers effectively, you must have sufficient upper-arm strength, a reasonable amount of standing balance, and the cognitive ability to walk in sequence with the walker. A person with Parkinson's disease will often have a tendency to fall backward, and would not do well with this kind of walker. People who have trouble with standing balance or who don't have enough upper-body strength can use rolling or wheeled walkers, which have either two or four wheels in place of the posts. Walkers with two wheels on the front are relatively easy to control, and can help a person maintain a forward gait—a useful feature for the person with Parkinson's disease. The four-wheeled walkers are of limited use and are probably best reserved for people with significant arm weakness who are building up enough strength to use a two-wheeled walker. Walkers can also be modified to benefit people who have significant upper-arm dysfunction or weakness. For example, if you have deformed upper extremities caused by rheumatoid arthritis, you can use a modified platform walker with arm rests. These platform walkers permit you to walk as well as to participate in active physical therapy of your lower legs despite significant upper-arm disability. Rolling walkers can be made into "auto-stop" walkers, so that when the person presses down on the front wheels the walker stops rolling.

If you are considering using a walker, your home situation needs to be evaluated carefully. If you functioned well with a walker in a rehabilitation unit, you may find new challenges at home, including thresholds, throw rugs, narrow passages, and short stair treads.

Orthotics or Braces   Orthotics (from the Greek, meaning "straight") are another category of assistive devices. They are braces that are designed to modify the support and functional characteristics of the musculoskeletal system. The goals of these braces include (1) relieving pain by limiting motion or weight bearing; (2) immobilization and protection of weak, painful, or healing body parts; (3) reduction of weight on that body part; (4) prevention and correction of deformity; and (5) improvement of function.

Orthotics can be applied to the arms, legs, and spine. Orthotics are usually referred to by an acronym formed from the first letter of the joints braced by the device or an orthosis. For example, WHO signifies wrist-hand orthosis, and AFO signifies ankle-foot orthosis.

Common reasons for using an orthosis on your legs include weakness, deformity, increased muscle tone (spasticity), ankle or knee instability, or pain on weight bearing such as that which sometimes occurs after surgery or with inflammatory arthritis. These orthotics not only help with your walking but also encourage more energy-efficient walking. An ankle-foot orthosis can improve the efficiency and speed of walking as well as decrease your body sway.

A foot orthosis can be as simple as a modified shoe in which a wedge, lift, bar, or other device has been inserted. These are sometimes used for people whose legs are different lengths, a condition called leg length discrepancy. Foot orthoses outside the shoe sometimes provide additional rigidity to align a malformity of the foot caused by severe joint deformity, reconstruction after surgery, or severe muscle contraction.

Ankle-foot orthoses, which are normally used for limited weight bearing or to preserve joint alignment, are commonly used in older people with mild to moderate leg weakness due to a stroke or some process affecting the nerves. These devices are designed to provide support for unstable joints, particularly the ankle. Some are as simple as a plastic shell that fits into your shoe and extends up the back of your calf to prevent the foot from dropping. This device can offer short-term benefit for the person whose foot drop is caused by a stroke or a nerve problem.

Knee-ankle-foot orthoses (KAFOs) are essentially ankle-foot orthoses with additional support surrounding the knee. These are sometimes used to provide knee support during weight bearing in cases of severe weakness of the lower leg, such as severe paralysis of one side of the body (hemiplegia) following a stroke. These devices can be made more sophisticated by the addition of a knee joint hinge.

Orthoses are not appropriate for everyone who has a leg disability. For example, if you have poor balance, strength, or coordination, a lower-extremity orthosis may aggravate rather than improve your walking. In addition, if you have considerable loss of sensation as well as muscle control of the leg, you may be vulnerable to skin breakdown because of the direct pressure and force produced by the orthotic device. The presence of a poorly fitting device, underlying skin disease, impaired circulation, or swelling increases the likelihood of skin breakdown.

Spinal braces are sometimes worn by people who have compression fractures of the spine or disk disease in the neck. For the majority of people with mild compression fractures, the most important principles of treatment are adequate pain relief and temporary limitation of movement. Abdominal binders or corsets are not routinely recommended for rib or spinal fractures.

Rigid braces can be valuable for people who have significant spinal injuries resulting in a need for stability of the spine. The use of rigid metal supports, however, makes it important to monitor carefully the areas where pressure ulcers and skin breakdown might develop.

If you have neck problems, whether caused by muscle strain, a narrowing of the spinal canal, or arthritis, you can sometimes benefit from the use of a cervical collar. Soft, foam collars or molded plastic collars are often used but various collars all provide similar levels of support to the neck, spine, and muscles. Keep the following important principles in mind when using neck supports: (1) As with most spinal devices, you should only use neck braces for a very short time to avoid psychological dependency. (2) The prolonged use of these collars may actually reduce your neck muscle strength and result in atrophy of the neck muscles. Therefore, use them very conservatively.

The principles that apply to the use of orthoses for the arms are similar to those that apply to the legs. Arm braces may be appropriate for neurologic problems, severe arthritis, or burns. Like other devices, arm braces provide immobilization, improve alignment, and assist or restore function. For stroke victims, a hand or forearm splint helps maintain the optimal position and can improve the function of the weak limb. In people with lower nerve problems, such as carpal tunnel syndrome where a nerve may be pinched, a special splint can reduce nerve entrapment. In people whose arthritis involves the joints of the hand and wrist, a wrist-hand splint may help prevent joint deformity.

Seventy-five percent of all amputations occur in people older than 65. The leg is the site of 90 percent of amputations, with two-thirds of these occurring below the knee. Fortunately, fewer than 15 percent of people with below-the-knee amputations eventually need above-the-knee amputations. However, 30 percent of people who require amputation because of poor circulation require an amputation on the other side within five years. For people whose poor circulation has been worsened by diabetes mellitus, the amputation rate affecting the opposite side is about 30 percent within two years and about 50 percent within five years. While this information suggests significant potential disability, 70 to 80 percent of older people can regain their ability to walk with or without assistive devices if they undergo the proper rehabilitation program before and after they acquire a prosthesis.

Amputations and Prostheses

The energy expenditure required for walking is related to the length of the residual limb. An amputation just above the ankle requires only a 10 to 15 percent additional energy expenditure. The standard below-the-knee amputation, however, requires expenditures of 25 percent of additional energy. Below-the-knee amputation of both legs requires a 40 to 45 percent increased energy expenditure, and an above-the-knee amputation of one leg requires 65 percent more energy.

The use of prostheses is governed by the following principles: Age alone is never a reason to avoid use of a prosthesis. In general, the weight of the prosthesis should be minimized, and the attachment chosen should be the one that is easiest and most appropriate. You should be trained to perform simple transfer movements without the prosthesis. For example, transferring from a bed to a wheelchair or to the toilet in the middle of the night should not necessarily be delayed for the attachment of a prosthesis. People expecting amputation should be reassured of the fact that 70 to 80 percent of older people who have had an amputation are able to walk with a prosthesis and that many below-the-knee amputations result in the ability to walk independently without an assistive device such as a cane or walker. Often, meeting with a person who has successfully completed a rehabilitation program and who walks independently can be informative and can improve your motivation if you are faced with a choice of amputation. Depression after an amputation is common. Emotional support, treatment of severe depression with antidepressants, and the involvement of caregivers and families are critical in reversing the depression. Often, your functional state before the amputation is one of the most reliable predictors of your success. This occurs both in short- and long-term prosthetic training.

The Use of Wheelchairs

Wheelchairs become an easy and frequently used (if not overused) way to move about for some older people. However, there are important factors to be considered in wheelchair use, whether it is used during the rehabilitation process or on a long-term basis.

You must be properly fitted and measured to your wheelchair, because if this is not done correctly, a wheelchair might actually impair rather than aid your mobility. Ideally, your weight, strength, skin condition, heart function, mental capacity, and vision should all be evaluated. In the process, you need to balance your concerns about seating comfort with those for mobility and your general functional needs.

For most people, a chair with the large rear wheel is adequate (see Figure 9). While sitting in the chair with your feet on the floor, you should be able to raise your feet off the floor, if necessary. The chair should be as narrow as possible, with a clearance of at least two inches on each side for entering doorways. A seat that is too narrow can hinder transferring and can increase your risk of pressure ulcers. If the seat is too wide, you may become unsteady while sitting and have difficulty in propelling the wheelchair and overcoming various architectural barriers, such as narrow doors. Armrest height is also important, because if the armrests are too high, your shoulder muscles can become fatigued. If the armrest height is too low you may develop poor posture as a result of leaning forward, and your balance within the wheelchair may become impaired. Homes may need to be modified to accommodate a ramp for an entrance. Doorways, for example, need to be 30 to 36 inches wide,

Figure 9. Basics of a Good Wheelchair

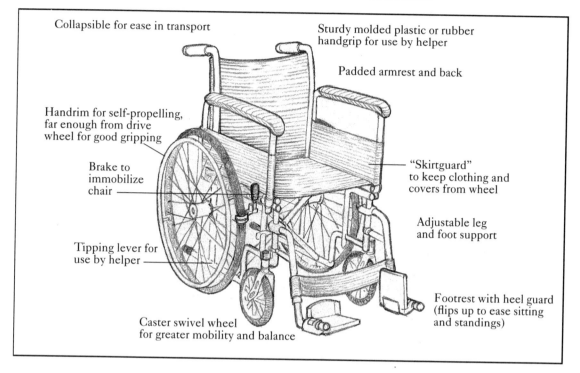

Collapsible for ease in transport

Sturdy molded plastic or rubber handgrip for use by helper

Padded armrest and back

Handrim for self-propelling, far enough from drive wheel for good gripping

Brake to immobilize chair

"Skirtguard" to keep clothing and covers from wheel

Adjustable leg and foot support

Tipping lever for use by helper

Footrest with heel guard (flips up to ease sitting and standings)

Caster swivel wheel for greater mobility and balance

and bathrooms at least 5 to 6 feet wide to permit the turning of the wheelchair.

Footrests need to be properly positioned, because if they are too low, they may increase the pressure under the thigh and may allow the foot to drag. If the footrest is too high, this can create greater pressure on both the foot and calf, thus increasing the risk of pressure ulcers and blood clots in the legs.

The seating can be modified to reduce the risk of pressure ulcers by using low-pressure cushions made of foam or gel, which transmit the body weight over a broader surface. A wheelchair can adjust to accommodate a person who can only use one limb and can be modified so that the arms can be raised up, down, or folded back on each other to facilitate transferring.

Powered or motorized wheelchairs are generally reserved for people who have been unable to achieve sufficient functional mobility with a manual wheelchair. In general, these people suffer from increasing disability as a result of a progressive disease.

Powered wheelchairs are made in three-wheeled and four-wheeled versions. They vary substantially in terms of their quality, adjustability, and durability. Powered wheelchairs are very expensive and should be used for people who have seen a physiatrist in collaboration with a physical therapist.

Transferring from One Place to Another

A transfer refers to a pattern of movement that involves shifting from one surface to another. It can occur in the sitting, standing, or lying positions, and may be accomplished with or without the help of another person, or an adaptive device (see Figure 10).

Safe and efficient transfers require a combination of physical and perceptual capacities, proper equipment, and training and techniques that are tailored to your special abilities. The achievement of sitting balance is a prerequisite for safe and comfortable

Figure 10. Bed Aids to Assist Changing Position, Doing Exercise, and Getting in and out of Bed

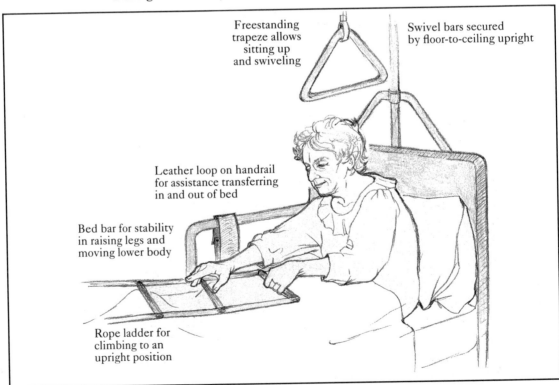

Freestanding trapeze allows sitting up and swiveling

Swivel bars secured by floor-to-ceiling upright

Leather loop on handrail for assistance transferring in and out of bed

Bed bar for stability in raising legs and moving lower body

Rope ladder for climbing to an upright position

transfers. To perform standing transfers, you must have good sitting balance and be able to stand evenly without assistance. In addition to lower-leg stability, you also need a reasonable degree of upper-arm strength to accomplish a transfer safely in the standing position.

A bed-to-wheelchair transfer can be initiated from a sitting position. The person locks the brakes on both sides of the wheelchair, grasps the side rails of the bed to come to a sitting position, and then while grasping the front arm of the wheelchair with the unaffected arm (in the case of a person who is paralyzed on one body side—the hemiplegic person) sits down in the wheelchair. This type of transfer is also known as a stand-pivot transfer. Early in the course of therapy, or if the person cannot stand, a board can be used to bridge the space between the bed and the wheelchair.

Wheelchair-to-toilet transferring is similar to the bed-to-chair transfer. However, you must be able to manage clothing and undergarments for this maneuver. Special adaptive equipment may be used to help make these transfers more independent (see Figure 11). For example, toilet seats should be approximately 20 inches from the floor. If necessary, raised toilet seats can be attached to the standard height toilet bowl. Handrails can be attached to the wall if it is close enough, or they can be freestanding. They should be placed on your unaffected side if you have a paralysis or on both sides of the toilet if you have weakness on both sides.

Transfers in and out of the bathtub (see Figure 11) are especially

Figure 11. Bathroom Aids

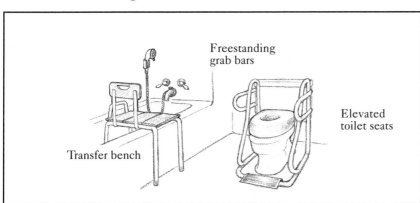

Freestanding grab bars

Elevated toilet seats

Transfer bench

important because this is a potentially dangerous procedure. Unlike most transfers, which should be made normally from your strongest side, a tub transfer usually makes use of your weaker side, depending on which is easier for you. Adaptive equipment, such as a tub transfer bench, which bridges the tub side by having one leg in the tub and one leg on the other side of the tub, can be helpful to move you safely along the bench to the tub. In doing this, a person with hemiplegia may first move the affected leg into the tub and then the unaffected leg. To help with bathing, a hand-held shower hose can be attached to the faucet. Safety-tread tape will secure a bath mat to the tub surface. There are also a number of bed aids that are useful for the transferring of positions and for exercising.

Stroke Rehabilitation

Most stroke therapy programs take place in a rehabilitation hospital, a rehabilitation unit in an acute hospital, or a nursing facility. The physical therapy plan in these programs is targeted at obtaining safe ambulation, usually with the use of an assistive device. Generally, occupational therapists address problems with upper-extremity function in terms of upper-muscle weakness and coordination, as well as perceptual and cognitive difficulties. For people with speaking or language problems, speech therapists develop specific treatment programs, both to try to restore some language and, if necessary, to develop alternative communication systems.

Since swallowing difficulty is a common but frequently under-recognized complication of strokes, an evaluation of swallowing function by a speech or occupational therapist should be done. The involvement and education of family or caregivers during the stroke rehabilitation program is crucial to the entire rehabilitation process. This is important in establishing the appropriate goals for rehabilitation and in planning for discharge. Before discharge, physical and occupational therapists generally visit the home to evaluate it for safety and the need for any adaptive equipment. Depression after a stroke is common and may also seriously affect rehabilitation. (Depression is covered on page 192.)

Hip Fracture Rehabilitation

The goal of rehabilitation for people who have had a hip fracture is the return to full ambulation. The focus is physical therapy that strengthens the leg muscles. This approach is intended to prepare the person for walking and to prevent any displacement of a hip prosthesis or the destabilization of a hip fracture that has been fixed by a pin or screw. Arm muscles are strengthened to help people in using assistive devices such as walkers. Arm strength and function are also important for bathing and dressing, which may be affected by the lower-extremity disability. Generally, people progress from using a walker to using a wide-based four-prong cane, to walking with a handheld single-point cane.

Several factors influence both the course and outcome of hip-fracture rehabilitation. For example, the person's weight-bearing status depends upon the type and severity of the fracture and the resulting repair. The capacity for early full weight bearing increases the intensity and shortens the duration of therapy services that are needed. Not surprisingly, the risk of institutionalization for people with a hip fracture increases in the presence of dementia and with significant functional impairment.

Ordinarily, the rehabilitation process takes longer for an amputation than for either a stroke or hip fracture. The program begins before surgery and involves not only the evaluation of the site for the amputation but also a comprehensive evaluation of your medical condition and an evaluation of your motivation to participate in the program. Whenever possible, the preoperative management should include stabilization of any medical problems, especially heart and lung disease. The surgeon, primary care physician, physiatrist, and you and your family should discuss the care plan for postoperative management as well as preprosthetic conditioning and training, and to prepare you for the phenomenon of "phantom limb" sensation, in which you feel as if the amputated limb were still present.

Rehabilitation if You Need an Amputation

The initial postoperative efforts are directed to proper care of the stump to promote healing, the initiation of an exercise program to strengthen the muscles above the site of the amputation, and the maintenance of proper positioning as well as exercise to prevent contractures of the knee or hip. Shrinking of the stump to accommodate the socket of a temporary prosthesis is usually accomplished by either using tight elastic cuffs or by frequent wraps with tight elastic bandages. Usually, people are measured for a temporary prosthesis 4 to 8 weeks after surgery and for a permanent prosthesis 8 to 12 weeks after surgery.

In preparation for an amputation, the therapy program initially involves training in transfer techniques, such as from bed to wheelchair or from chair to toilet. After amputation, you will progress to practicing weight bearing on a temporary prosthesis, first on parallel bars and eventually using a walker, then crutches, then a cane for assistance. By the time you complete the rehabilitation program, you will probably be capable of walking without any assistance. People with amputation of both limbs may progress to needing, at most, a walker for ambulation.

Common Medical Problems During Rehabilitation

During the course of rehabilitation, you may need ongoing medical evaluation and intervention to treat or prevent significant illness and disability. If you have had a stroke or have suffered a hip fracture, you are at increased risk for blood clots and the complication of pulmonary embolus. This refers to the situation where a blood clot breaks away from its origin in the veins in the legs and travels up to the lungs. Generally, people are given blood thinners during the rehabilitation process to keep blood clots from forming.

Most physical therapy programs do not require a high level of physical activity. It may come as a surprise that occupational therapy results in greater cardiovascular stress than physical therapy. This is because exercise of the arms causes a greater increase in blood pressure and pulse rate than does leg exercise. Therapy activities for people with known heart disease are generally modified, especially if they induce chest pain, shortness of breath, light-headedness, or fatigue. The blood pressure and pulse rate are frequently monitored to avoid undue stress. Sometimes a physician will recommend that other tests be performed to assess cardiac risk.

People with preexisting arthritis may experience a worsening of their disease during rehabilitation as a result of progressive weight bearing and stress during therapy. Other people may develop bursitis around the shoulder, or especially around the hip. Some of this is due to the increased physical activity in their rehabilitation program. Treatment approaches for these individuals, however, are generally the same as those for people with arthritis who are not in a rehabilitation program.

For people who have moderately severe lung disease and who become short of breath while participating in a physical therapy or occupational therapy program, a reevaluation of their lung status is necessary. Sometimes the amount of oxygen in the blood is measured during therapy to see if any abnormalities are present. In some rehabilitation sites, it may be possible to include a lung rehabilitation program within the person's disease-specific rehabilitation program. Usually, pulmonary rehabilitation programs emphasize instruction in breathing techniques, pacing of physical activities, and exercises and relaxation techniques to assist in activities of daily living.

The goal of rehabilitation is to improve function, which is usually attained through the efforts of the multidisciplinary team of health professionals working together to identify and address potential barriers to effective function. Factors that have an important bearing on the outcome of rehabilitation are the nature and extent of the limitation, the person's motivation, and the presence of adequate daily supervision.

CHAPTER 9

TAKING MEDICATIONS

In the United States, 25 percent of prescription drug use is accounted for by people who are older than 65—that is, 12.6 percent of the population. This fact, along with a greater understanding of how older people are more likely to experience adverse drug reactions, has prompted increased interest in how aging affects the ways our bodies handle drugs. Government recommendations now require that older people be included in the testing of medications before they are released to the public. Despite these recommendations, there is still a surprising lack of information concerning the principles and practices of drug treatment in older people.

In this chapter we will review how aging affects the ways our bodies respond to, process, and eliminate drugs. We will learn about the adverse effects of drugs and how to reduce our chances of experiencing an adverse drug reaction.

Pharmaco-kinetics

The word *pharmacokinetics* (from the Greek, meaning "drug" and "movement") refers to the ways a drug travels to its destination. This includes the processes of drug absorption, distribution throughout the body, and elimination from the body. Information

Table 4. Factors That Alter Drug Disposition in Old Age

PHARMACOKINETIC FACTORS	PHYSIOLOGIC CHANGES	SIGNIFICANCE
Absorption	Reduced stomach acid; reduced small bowel surface area	Little change in absorption with age
Distribution	Reduced total body water; reduced lean body mass; increased body fat	Higher concentration of drugs that distribute in body fluids; increased distribution and often prolonged elimination of fat-soluble drugs
Liver metabolism	Decreased enzyme activity; reduced liver mass; reduced liver blood flow	Decreased metabolism of some drugs
Kidney elimination	Reduced blood flow and filtration	Decreased kidney elimination of drugs; marked variation in individual cases

Source: Adapted from Vestal RE. Aging and pharmacokinetics: impact of altered physiology in the elderly. *Physiology and Cell Biology of Aging*, vol. 8. New York: Raven Press; 1979:198. Reprinted with permission.

about the age-related changes in the body affecting pharmacokinetics is helpful for determining the appropriate dosage of medications. (See Table 4 for factors that alter pharmacokinetics with aging.) The absorption of medications generally changes very little as we age. However, some drugs that we take by mouth are rapidly filtered out of circulation by the liver, which metabolizes drugs toward elimination from the body. The liver performs a number of important functions including altering chemicals and nutrients absorbed into the blood, regulating blood sugar, and manufacturing and storing proteins and vitamins. Any reduction in the liver's ability to extract a drug can result in an increased amount of the drug remaining for longer times in the general circulation. Medications that have been shown to circulate for longer times include labetalol, propranolol, and lidocaine. However, there is no uniform effect of age on the initial extraction of drugs from the circulation by the liver. In other words, no general guidelines are available for assessing age-related liver function.

The distribution of drugs is also affected by changes in our bodies including the relative increase in body fat and decrease in body water and lean muscle mass. Drugs are either fat or water soluble; drugs that dissolve in fat are distributed more widely than those that dissolve in water. However, increased distribution of fat-soluble drugs can delay their elimination from our body, and this may prolong the effect of a single dose. This is particularly important for drugs that are given in single doses on an intermittent basis such as some pain relievers and sleeping medications. For example, it may take up to 90 hours for an older person's body to eliminate the drug diazepam whereas it may only take 24 hours for younger people.

While distribution may increase for fat-soluble drugs, it may decrease for water-soluble drugs. For example, the volume of distribution of digoxin, a water-soluble digitalis compound, is decreased with age. When the body contains less water, as is the case with older persons, the dosage required to obtain a specific concentration of a drug in the blood is less than it would be in a younger person's body, where water volume is higher. Thus, the initial amount of digoxin needed to produce a given blood level in people with heart disease is 30 percent lower in older people than in younger people. For similar reasons, older people may be at an increased risk of intoxication from alcohol because there is less water in the body to dilute the alcohol.

Changes in the Binding of Drugs with Body Proteins

Some drugs bind very strongly to proteins in the blood, limiting their full effectiveness of circulation throughout the body. Thus the amount of the drug that is free (unbound) is more relevant than the total amount in the body. Aging can affect the quantity of binding proteins and thereby change the amount of the drug that circulates unbound. Examples of drugs showing this effect include phenytoin, warfarin, and many nonsteroidal anti-inflammatory drugs (NSAID).

Liver Metabolism of Drugs

Most drugs are absorbed, metabolized, and prepared for elimination from the body by the liver. For some drugs, the rate of blood flowing to the liver is what determines this absorption and elimination. For other medications, however, this depends upon the rate of the liver's ability to chemically metabolize them. Some drugs fall in between so that their absorption and elimination depend upon both the rate of the liver's metabolism and the rate of blood flow to the liver. Because of this, age-associated reductions in liver metabolizing ability and liver blood flow can change drug processing.

As we age, the kidney's ability to eliminate drugs is reduced. The filtering rate and the function of the kidney tubules generally decline. The effect of age on drug metabolism varies widely as aging is only one of many factors that affect our metabolism of drugs. For example, cigarette smoking, alcohol intake, dietary modification, other medications, viral infections, the amount of caffeine taken in, and other unknown factors also seem to affect the rate of drug metabolism. In addition, there is remarkable variation (up to sixfold) among individuals in the rate of drug metabolism that is thought to be genetic in origin. Therefore, unless an effect of age is very large and consistent, it may be hidden by these other factors.

In addition to the factors that determine the drug concentration at the site of action, the effects of a given drug also depend upon the sensitivity of the target organ. This target organ sensitivity is called pharmacodynamics (from the Greek, meaning "drug," "power"). The influence of aging on the biochemical and physiologic effects of drugs and how they work is largely unknown. In part, this is because it is very difficult to determine drug effects accurately using the non-invasive techniques usually required in clinical studies.

Changes in Pharmaco- dynamics with Aging

In general, drugs function by binding with a receptor and by modulating the activities of individual cells. Age-related changes on this cellular level can occur at many different steps, including binding to the receptor and translating either the receptor's response into some biochemical reaction or the cellular response to a biochemical event. In some tissues, the receptors will respond, but the desired chain of results may not be fully realized. Therefore, as we age, defects in receptor responsiveness may occur at more than one location in the cell.

Most drug effects in older people are either similar to or greater than those in younger people. In other words, we become more sensitive to drugs. Moreover, these effects may be magnified if we have a disease that alters the drug's elimination from the body or the body response to the drug.

Adverse Drug Effects

We are at increased risk for adverse drug reactions from certain classes of drugs as we grow older. Following is a review of some of these adverse reactions to illustrate a few of the mechanisms of increased drug toxicity with aging. (See also Medication Problems in Chapter 26.)

Adverse Reactions of Cardiovascular Drugs

Cardiovascular drugs are a common group of medications that sometimes cause adverse reactions. Decreased dosages of digitalis compounds are generally needed for older people who have heart disease. This is because of the age-related reductions in our body's water and muscle mass and reductions in the clearance rate of the drug, as discussed above. Excessive dosing probably accounts for much of the adverse effects caused by digitalis including nausea, loss of appetite, and changes in mood. Fortunately, digitalis can be safely withdrawn in those of us who have had it prescribed for either mild heart failure or swelling of the legs that has no clear origin. Therefore, if you are taking digitalis, you should review the condition for which it was originally prescribed, and discuss with your physician whether it could be stopped.

Diuretics rank high among the classes of drugs that can cause side effects. These "fluid pills" can cause dehydration and low potassium, sodium, and magnesium in the blood, making one feel weak, tired, and run down. Such adverse effects are poorly tolerated because of the changes in our body's organs and regulating systems that occur with advancing age. You can help to compensate for this by drinking plenty of fluids (at least eight to ten eight-ounce glasses a day) and asking your doctor about having your blood checked at regular intervals.

The drugs that are sometimes prescribed to prevent irregular heartbeats can also cause problems. Because these antiarrhythmics have a very narrow range between their useful and toxic effects, careful dosing and judicious monitoring of blood levels are required. The side effects that these medications can produce in people of any age—drowsiness, slurred speech, confusion, and numbness and tingling in the arms and legs—are increased as we age. Not all of the antiarrhythmic drugs cause these problems, but the likelihood of side effects is high enough that you should always check with your doctor if you feel there is a complication.

Medication for depression and anxiety is particularly likely to cause adverse effects as we age. The initial doses of these medicines should be very small, as they increase your risk of a drop in blood pressure as well as your level of sedation; therefore, low doses of high-potency drugs such as haloperidol are often favored. However, drug-induced Parkinsonism occurs more commonly with the use of high-potency compounds. You should also be aware that the incidence of abnormal body motions called tardive dyskinesias is due to antipsychotic medication. The frequency of other movement side effects also increases with age.

We also become more vulnerable to adverse effects of antidepressants as we age, such as a fall in blood pressure, the inability to void, disturbances of the heart rhythm, confusion, and sedation.

Benzodiazepines are sometimes prescribed for anxiety; certain drugs in this class take longer to be removed from your body (examples include chlordiazepoxide, diazepam, flurazepam, and alprazolam). However, lorazepam, oxazepam, and temazepam are metabolized more readily. Any of these drugs, however, can greatly increase sedation and your risk of falls. Some experts suggest that they should not be used at all in elderly people because of their tendency to cause memory problems and falls.

Adverse Effects of Drugs Used for Depression and Anxiety

Older people use pain-relieving agents more frequently than any other age group. Although the liver's ability to metabolize acetaminophen for elimination from the body may decline slightly, dosage adjustments are not usually necessary.

Our ability to metabolize some nonsteroidal anti-inflammatory drugs (NSAIDs) is decreased, but it is not clear that these differences alone increase the risk of toxicity. Bleeding in the gastrointestinal tract is related to the use of NSAIDs for all age groups and increases in significance as we get older. Recent or current users of these medications are more likely than nonusers to suffer significant gastrointestinal bleeding.

Adverse Effects of Pain Relievers

The drug metabolism of the anticoagulant warfarin does not appear to change as we age. The clinical benefit of this drug remains the same for a number of conditions. Therefore, unless you have a significant risk for bleeding, such as from falls, unsteady gait, poor

Adverse Effects of Blood Thinners (Anticoagulants)

compliance with medicines, or a tendency to bleed, you should not avoid using this medicine just because of your age. Another blood thinner called heparin must be injected and is generally used for hospitalized people with certain conditions that predispose them to blood clotting. The anticoagulant effect of this drug remains unchanged with age.

Aging Changes That Modify Drug Effects

Drugs can place stress on a number of the body's systems that may have changed with aging, thereby producing adverse effects, and interfering with the way the body regulates itself. For example, a common side effect of some medications is a fall in blood pressure when a person stands up. Drugs can also affect heart function or the regulation of body fluids to further accentuate this fall of blood pressure with change in position.

As we age we are also susceptible to medications such as barbiturates and benzodiazepines that can increase the risk of a very low body temperature (hypothermia). Medications given to people with psychiatric illness can also produce these effects. (Alcohol use can also cause a drop in your body temperature.) People who are known to have a low body temperature or who have had a previous episode of very low body temperature may be at risk for significant drug-induced hypothermia. (See page 440 for more on hypothermia.)

A low level of sodium in the blood (hyponatremia) is a common complication of diuretics, usually within the first week of therapy. The symptoms you might experience depend upon how low your sodium is and how fast it declined, but mild reductions may not produce symptoms. Common symptoms are fatigue, lethargy, muscle cramps, loss of appetite, confusion, and nausea. Symptoms of severe declines in sodium are coma and seizures. For thiazide diuretics a low sodium occurs in part because of age-related impairments in kidney function. A low sodium in the blood is a complication of other drugs such as chlorpropamide, nonsteroidal anti-inflammatory drugs, and high-dose narcotics. A low potassium in the blood caused by diuretic therapy occurs with increased frequency as we age. An elevated potassium in the blood also occurs as a side effect of drugs or because of such conditions as diabetes mellitus, kidney failure, and other kidney diseases.

Nonsteroidal anti-inflammatory drugs need to be used with caution as we get older, because of the risk of gastrointestinal bleeding and kidney impairment. Aging puts us at risk for kidney problems due to the changes in kidney blood flow caused by these drugs. This adverse effect is most likely to occur if we have congestive heart failure, liver disease, or certain types of kidney disease.

A cardinal principle of treatment is to avoid drugs that might adversely affect preexisting medical conditions. Table 5 lists some of the disorders that are associated with the risk of an adverse drug effect. Because the conditions that are listed in this table commonly occur as we age, a cautious approach to drug treatment is warranted. If you are taking medication, you should ask and be informed about the potential adverse side effects and promptly seek medical advice if any of these effects appear.

Drug and Disease Interactions

An episode of sudden confusion, called delirium, is often due to medications. (Delirium is discussed in detail in Chapter 13.) The drugs that are known to cause delirium are divided into two groups, depending upon whether they affect specific receptors within the brain, called muscarinic receptors (named for the substance muscarine, which was first isolated from the poisonous mushroom *Amanita muscaria*).

Drug-Induced Confusion

Antimuscarinic toxicity caused by drugs can be difficult to recognize. Many of the essential features—warm, dry skin; dilated pupils; or a fast heart rate—may be less evident in older people than they are in younger people. Medications such as narcotics, antidepressants, antipsychotic agents, drugs used to relieve spasms in the bowel, and many other nonprescription medications, such as antihistamines, have appreciable antimuscarinic effects. These drugs frequently cause confusion, and individuals with Alzheimer's dementia are especially susceptible.

These drugs may also cause more subtle changes than obvious episodes of delirium. For example, and paradoxically, antimuscarinic drugs may relieve agitation and paranoia in people who have Alzheimer's disease. But they may also reduce a person's self-care activities, presumably because of further declines in the cognitive function caused by the drug. Therefore, if you notice any decline in function, such drug side effects should be considered as a possible cause.

Table 5. Some Important Drug/Disease Interactions in Older Persons

DISEASE	DRUG	ADVERSE EFFECT
Dementia	Psychotropic drugs, levodopa, antiepileptic agents	Increased confusion, delirium
Glaucoma	Anticholinergic drugs	Acute glaucoma
Congestive heart failure	Beta-blockers, verapamil	Acute cardiac collapse
Heart rhythm disorders	Tricyclic antidepressants	Slowed heartbeat
Hypertension	NSAIDs	Increase in blood pressure
Peripheral vascular disease	Beta-blockers	Intermittent leg pain with activity
Chronic obstructive pulmonary disease	Beta-blockers; opiate agents	Wheezing; respiratory depression
Chronic renal impairment	NSAIDs, contrast agents, some antibiotics	Acute kidney failure
Diabetes mellitus	Diuretics, corticosteroids	Elevated blood sugar
Prostatic hypertrophy	Antimuscarinic agents	Urinary retention
Depression	Beta-blockers, some antihypertensives, alcohol, benzodiazepines, steroids; Digoxin	Precipitation or exacerbation of depression; Cardiac arrhythmias
Peptic ulcer disease	NSAIDs, anticoagulants	Gastrointestinal bleeding

NSAIDs, nonsteroidal anti-inflammatory drugs.

Source: Cusack BJ. Polypharmacy and clinical pharmacology. In: Beck JC, ed. *Geriatrics Review Syllabus: A Core Curriculum in Geriatric Medicine*, 1st ed. New York: American Geriatrics Society; 1989:134. Reprinted with permission.

Drugs without significant antimuscarinic effects can also cause confusion and delirium. Drugs used in the management of Parkinson's disease are common offenders and can cause confusion when used together or alone. Others include corticosteroids, cardiovascular drugs, NSAIDs, and some antibiotics. These medications are given just as examples; any drug should be suspected when an episode of acute confusion occurs.

In summary, medications can have beneficial and adverse

effects. Aging tends to increase our vulnerability to side effects. As we age we lose body water and muscle and increase our proportion of body fat. This change in body composition means that a given dose of a water-soluble drug gives a higher concentration since it is dissolved in a smaller amount of water. Drugs that are fat soluble have more prolonged effects. Changes in the liver and kidneys tend to reduce the metabolism and elimination of drugs. Any sudden change in our function should raise our suspicion of an adverse drug reaction, although side effects can also appear gradually and undramatically. We should always consider an adverse drug reaction for any new or unexplained symptom. (For more information, see pages 447 to 453.)

CHAPTER 10

LONG-TERM CARE

The most difficult issues we face as we age deal with loss or partial loss of independence. For most of us, the fear of becoming a burden on family members is stronger than the fear of death. Long-term care is the range of services that addresses the health, personal care, and social needs of individuals who need assistance in caring for themselves. The specific site and nature of this long-term care vary according to individual circumstances. While nursing home care comprises the most easily recognized form of long-term care, home care and community services accommodate a much larger percentage of the population.

No matter where the services are provided, the goals of long-term care remain the same and involve the restoration and maintenance of health and function. This includes preventive services as well as the management of sudden illnesses. The scope of services an individual requires depends upon the extent of disability and underlying illnesses, the availability of support, and the person's potential for recovery.

About one-third of people who receive long-term care live in an institutional setting, while the remaining two-thirds remain in the community. This means that for every older person living in a nursing home there are two similar people living in the community who may require equal levels of assistance. Of the elderly people who live in institutions, over 90 percent live in nursing homes, while the remainder live in mental institutions or chronic disease hospitals. Most older adults live in the community in a family setting, although the proportion decreases with age. Thirty percent of community-living older people live alone, the great majority of them women. In fact, 40 percent of older women compared with only 15 percent of older men live alone. About 80 percent of older people have living children and, of these, two-thirds live within 30 minutes of a child and share weekly or more frequent visits with their children. About three-quarters have weekly or more frequent telephone conversations with children.

The use of long-term care services increases steadily with increasing age. In 1990, approximately seven million people used some form of long-term care, which includes institutional services such as nursing homes, and community-based services such as home care services, chore services, Meals on Wheels, and adult daycare, as well as informal care by family and friends. By some projections, by the year 2040 the number of people who will require long-term care services will increase to about 18 million.

The best long-term care system for you must not only respond to your physical needs for assistance but must also consider a wide variety of possible changes in your mental function and behavior. For example, as you might expect, nursing home residents have more cognitive and psychological impairments than the rest of the elderly population. Although mental health needs are obviously great, the number and diversity of long-term services to handle behavioral problems are limited.

In addition to your physical, psychological, and emotional situations, the extent of your social supports has a significant impact on your long-term care situation. As we grow older, we are more likely to live alone or with a relative other than a spouse. As our need for personal care assistance increases, so does our dependence on others. This creates tensions in the complex web of interpersonal relationships that shapes our lives and gives them meaning.

An effective match between your needs and available services is

Institutional and Home Care

often the critical factor in determining the site of long-term care. Transportation, legal and psychological counseling, special housing, and in-home specialized medical care are a few of the unmet needs that are frequently identified by older people who need long-term care. Accessibility may be related to personal and public financing (or a lack thereof); this may also be affected by a lack of knowledge among ourselves or our families and even among professionals and discharge planners about the scope of health care services that are available.

Comprehensive Geriatric Assessment

Comprehensive geriatric assessment by an interdisciplinary health care team is increasingly being recognized as a way to coordinate care more effectively and to overcome some of the problems of availability and accessibility of long-term care. The team includes doctors, nurses, social workers, and other professionals such as dentists, physical and occupational therapists, psychiatrists, pharmacists, and nutritionists. Most medical schools support comprehensive geriatric assessment, and some community hospitals are making these services available.

Importance of Caregivers

Of all the factors that determine if and when a person will require institutionalization, the availability of a caregiver is among the most critical. Contrary to commonly held perceptions, care given by family members or friends accounts for most of the care provided in the community. Formal sources of care such as paid home health care, homemaker or chore services, and adult daycare account for only 15 percent of community care for the disabled elderly age group. Generally, caregivers are women (about 75 percent)—usually wives, daughters, or daughters-in-law who often forgo employment (about a third are employed) and other familial obligations to provide primary care to a relative. About a third of these caring women live in poverty. The average age of informal caregivers is 57 years. Three-quarters of the caregivers share households with the care recipient (whose average age is 78 years), and have been providing assistance for several years, usually seven days a week. Caregivers help with household tasks such as shopping and transportation and assist with personal hygiene. The importance of these figures is that the responsibility of care weighs heavily on many families and women in particular. Without relief or counseling, many families are stressed to the point of disintegration. Assistance from an interdisciplinary team can be crucial in helping to deal with these stresses.

Despite the availability of home care services, the benefits of home-based care compared with institutional care are not obvious. In fact, the use of home care has not yet been shown to improve mortality, physical or mental function, or to increase life satisfaction. In addition, the assumption that home care significantly shortens nursing home stays or postpones institutionalization altogether has not been borne out. It appears that people who are most likely to be institutionalized are those who are extremely difficult to sustain in the community.

Although the nursing home is but one option for long-term care, it deserves special mention because of its unique place in society. The diversified highly regulated nursing home of today is a far cry from the nursing home of 30 years ago or the unsupervised, limited service, privately financed home for the poor that was common at the turn of the century. Much of the structural and functional changes in nursing homes are due to the Social Security Act of 1935 and the Medicare and Medicaid programs that were enacted in the mid-1960s. Additional changes include the growth of the older age group and the age-dependent increases in disability. The overall percentage of older adults who live in nursing homes is approximately 5 percent, but this number increases dramatically with age, ranging from about 1 percent for people 65 to 74, 6 percent for persons 75 to 84, and 22 percent for people over the age of 85.

Nursing Home Care

The nursing home has traditionally been removed from the medical mainstream. There is almost no instruction in nursing home care during medical school and residency training, so that the physician has little practical experience in which to discern fact from fiction. Less than one-half of all practicing physicians ever visit nursing homes, and a much smaller percentage are in attendance on a regular basis. Fortunately, interest in long-term care, and in nursing homes specifically, has blossomed recently due to powerful economic and social forces that have created a need to accommodate large numbers of ill, functionally disabled elderly persons outside the hospital.

The nursing home must fulfill two seemingly conflicting roles, those of a health care facility and those of a home. Not only does each role carry with it different goals and expectations, but each also raises a variety of different social, administrative, legal, and environmental issues.

Although most nursing homes model themselves after hospitals, their staffing patterns are very different. Nursing homes typically have significantly fewer nurses than hospitals. Half of the work force is made up by nurses' aides who provide most of the care, and who are not required to have any special professional credentials. However, nursing home care does involve highly trained professionals and includes physicians, social workers, dietitians, pharmacists, rehabilitation specialists, and administrators. In nursing homes, a team approach to care is critical, and the nurse oversees the coordination and implementation of clinical services.

Choosing a Nursing Home. If a nursing home care becomes necessary, you or your family will face the difficult issue of choosing the appropriate facility. No nursing homes are perfect, and even the better ones will be very different from your current living situation.

Your doctor may recommend a few nursing homes; other professionals such as home health nurses and social workers can provide additional referrals. In general you should be concerned with quality, the range of service, convenience, and costs. Checklists have been developed to help with this process (see Table 6).

Try to visit as many places as you can to get a sense of the environmental characteristic, overall atmosphere, and quality of care. Your visit may last an hour or two to provide time for discussions with the admissions officer, nursing home administrator, head nurse, and social worker.

Your family's involvement is important to your health and well-being. Nursing homes may often be scary and depressing, and moving into one can fill us with a sense of betrayal and failure. Contrary to the stereotype, families do not abandon their loved ones following institutionalization. In fact, only a minority of nursing home residents are truly without a family. You should encour-

Table 6. Nursing Home Checklist

1. Is the facility clean and free of odor?

2. Is it well maintained?

3. Do residents look well cared for?

4. Are the rooms adequate?

5. What recreational and private space is available?

6. Are there appropriate safety features, such as railings and grab bars?

7. Is the home licensed by the state and certified in Medicaid?

8. What is the staffing ratio of nurses to residents?

9. Do the administrators and professionals have special training in geriatrics or long-term care?

10. Are key professionals full-time or part-time?

11. How long have administrators and professionals been with the nursing home?

12. What type of medical coverage is provided?

13. How close is the facility to family members? How close is it to the nearest hospital?

14. What is the food like?

15. How much do basic services cost? What services are covered?

16. What additional services are available and what is their cost?

17. What happens if a person runs out of money and needs medical assistance?

age your family to visit you regularly. Through such visits, your family becomes an important participant in your total care. Your family may offer companionship and assistance with the basic activities of daily living, and may be an advocating voice for your rights.

Medical Care Issues in the Nursing Home. Many of the problems that residents of a nursing home suffer from require specific diagnosis and treatment. These problems commonly include infections, urinary incontinence, falls, fainting, depression, confusion, malnutrition, and pressure ulcers. The approach to these problems often differs from that found in the hospital or the clinical office setting. The goals of medical intervention may vary enormously from one person to another, ranging from pure comfort measures to aggressive diagnostic and treatment efforts.

In the nursing home, infection is the most common sudden medical problem leading to hospitalization. Ironically, the rate of infection in nursing homes is equal to that found in most hospitals. Unfortunately, many hospital admissions of nursing home residents occur as a consequence of clinical and social factors that are not directly linked to the underlying illness. Such factors include a lack of adequately trained staff, an inability of the nursing staff to administer intravenous therapy, a lack of diagnostic services such as X rays, physician convenience, and pressure from both staff and family to transfer older persons with "difficult" complications. In the best of worlds it should be possible to have these services available in the nursing home, which would make it possible for the nursing home resident to stay in the facility while receiving treatment.

The transfer of older people back to the nursing home is also frequently a problem, due to the often delayed or incomplete transfer of information from the hospital, a situation that jeopardizes continuity of care. This is an especially important issue in nursing homes where the attending physician is different from the physician who is providing the care in the hospital. The failure of hospital physicians to fully appreciate the limits and benefits of nursing home care has resulted in the often hasty discharge of patients to nursing homes, only to result in readmission to the hospital within a short time. Physician involvement in nursing homes, and in all of long-term care, will almost certainly increase in response to the needs of one rapidly aging population.

Home Care, Assisted Living, and Continuing Care Retirement Communities

Although most of us would prefer to stay in our own homes, a practical concern is that home care services have not yet evolved in all communities as a viable option to nursing homes. Fortunately, home care is one of the fastest-growing segments of the health care system.

Home care services predominantly involve help with household tasks and providing home health services. Household chores include meal preparation, house cleaning, and laundry; help with personal care such as feeding, toileting, or bathing is sometimes included. Home health services are provided by nurses, physical therapists, or speech therapists. To be eligible under Medicare for these services you must be home-bound, need this intense level of care, and be expected to benefit from it over a reasonable period of time. In other words, these are generally time-limited services. Your doctor can help you arrange for home services or can direct you to the appropriate professionals in your community.

Assisted living means living in a facility offering a combination of home care and nursing home facilities. It gives you a greater sense of control, independence, and privacy by providing more choice within an institutional setting. Many people live in the facility, but each person's bedroom and bathroom can be locked by the resident. Dining and recreational facilities are usually shared. This approach to long-term care is especially appealing for people with good mental function.

A relatively new living arrangement for healthy, moderately affluent elderly people is the continuing care retirement community. The appeal of these communities is that future health care needs are covered in a setting that is an attractive residential campus where numerous cultural and recreational activities are available. Entrance fees can be substantial (over $250,000 at the upper end) and monthly maintenance fees average around $1,000. While these communities appeal to individuals who do not want to burden their children with their care, for some people it signals the beginning of an empty future. Memorial services are a regular occurrence and social networks may not be as emotionally supportive as they appear. Nonetheless, some individuals feel a sense of added security and peace of mind.

Long-term care is an area that most of us would rather not address because of its myths and stereotypes and the accompanying range of complex emotions it may evoke in us. Nursing homes are generally neither as bad as we fear nor as good as we would like. The care issues center around maximizing autonomy and minimizing complications and dependency. Other care options such as home care and assisted living are rapidly growing and provide an increasing array of alternatives.

PART III

LEGAL, ETHICAL, AND FINANCIAL CONSIDERATIONS

CHAPTER 11
ETHICAL ISSUES AND CONCERNS

Your care may involve ethical concerns that cannot be resolved solely by scientific expertise and clinical experience, but rather require choosing among conflicting responsibilities, values, and principles. As an example, for a person with dementing illness the desirable goals of safety and independence may be incompatible. Moving into an institution would increase safety but reduce independence; staying in the home maintains independence but at an increased risk of injury. A number of guidelines have been written that address such dilemmas and have clarified the terminology, analyzed the justifications for different positions, and suggested various approaches. Despite these guidelines, it is often a difficult task to reach decisions in individual circumstances.

Medical decisions should be made by capable, informed patients in concert with their physicians, based on the ethical principle of respect for their autonomy. Except for extraordinary circumstances, you have the legal right to make decisions about your body and about your medical care. The doctrine of informed consent follows from our societal respect for autonomy and self-determination.

Respecting Your Choices

Informed Consent

The legal doctrine of informed consent states that you have the power to choose among medically feasible plans for your care. Informed consent requires effective communication between you and your doctor. However, in order for you to make informed choices, you need to discuss with your doctor your diagnosis and the outlook, the nature of the recommended test or treatments, the various alternatives, the risks and benefits of each alternative, and the likely outcomes. Both of you should share your questions and concerns, and repeat these discussions as often as needed.

Informed consent does not mean that you can dictate your care. If a person requests tests or treatments that the medical profession considers useless or harmful, physicians have no obligation to comply. They do have a duty to use their technical expertise to benefit you, or at least not to harm you. When disagreements of this kind occur, further discussion is needed to clarify the concerns and to reach a mutually acceptable decision.

Decision-Making Capacity

The process of informed consent is only meaningful if you have the capacity to make informed decisions. Strictly speaking, all adults are presumed to be competent to make decisions at a specific age (usually 18 years), and this presumption continues until the court determines that an individual is incompetent. Practically speaking, however, physicians are sometimes asked to evaluate a person's decision-making capacity. If a physician believes that a person lacks the ability to make informed decisions about medical care, that person is deemed "incapable." This determination is significant because decisions will then be made by someone other than the patient. The term *incompetence* refers to a judgment by a court of law.

A process called a "sliding scale" has been recommended for assessing a person's capacity to make medical decisions. A sliding scale affords patients of questionable capacity more protection when the potential harm resulting from the decisions is greater. Therefore, except in the case of an unconscious or a severely demented person, it makes more sense to speak in terms of capacity for specific tasks, "decision-specific" capacity, than capacity in a general sense. You may be capable of making decisions about medical care, but not about finances, or vice versa.

Your ability to make medical decisions may fluctuate. For example, a person with delirium may be mentally clear in the morning but confused in the evening. Imagine having a high fever that clouds your thinking and disorients you. Choices that are made when you are capable of making informed decisions should be recorded and respected. If possible, decisions should be deferred until you have regained your decision-making capacity.

Your capacity to make decisions about medical care requires that you realize that there are choices, the nature of the recommended care, the alternatives, the risks and benefits of each, and the likely consequences.

One frequent error physicians make regarding decision-making capacity is their overemphasis on mental status testing. Often, when the capacity of a person is questionable, a mental status examination is administered. Even if you perform poorly on a mental status test or have impaired memory, you may still have the capacity to make informed decisions. It is essential to assess very directly your understanding of the risks, benefits, and consequences of the alternative plans of care. Another mistake is to equate decision-making capacity with rational decisions. Requiring rationality would disqualify people who make highly personal or unconventional decisions. As one court declared in a case that involved the refusal of treatment, beliefs that are "unwise, foolish, or ridiculous" do not render a person incompetent.

If you are unable to participate in the decision-making process, someone will have to make decisions on your behalf. The decision-making hierarchy for surrogate decisions places your expressed wishes as paramount. These wishes can take the form of advanced directives, living wills, and durable powers of attorney for health care. Expressed wishes take precedence over substituted judgments or acting in your best interest.

Surrogate Decision Making

Whenever possible, your physician should respect the informed choices that you have expressed while you were still capable of making decisions. Following advance directives demonstrates respect for your individuality and self-determination and is preferable to following the choices of others, such as family members or other caregivers unless that is your wish.

Advance Directives

Your conversations with relatives, friends, or health care workers—the most common form of advance directives—are valuable but should be documented carefully so that the information is available later. Since a few state courts have ruled that oral statements may be legally challenged if they are not sufficiently explicit, and since written statements clearly reflect your intention to direct future health care, you should give written advance directives whenever possible.

Living Wills. Laws that authorize living wills (also called natural death, death with dignity, or right-to-die laws) have been enacted in almost all states. Some states that do not have living will statutes grant individuals comparable rights under court opinions. Generally, these laws allow you to direct doctors to withhold or withdraw life-sustaining treatment if you become terminally ill or have another condition that is specified in the statute and are no longer capable of making decisions. In a few states, an individual may also appoint proxy decision makers. Legal immunity is given to caregivers who comply with the living will made in accordance with the statute.

Living wills, however, only apply to terminal illness and may not extend to severe dementia, severe stroke, or what is called a persistent vegetative state, where the person is in a form of coma. These are not considered terminal illnesses. Another important drawback of the living will is that an individual in some states is permitted to decline only treatments that "merely prolong the process of dying," a category that is difficult to define. Furthermore, many living will statutes do not allow the refusal of artificial feedings and hydration, although this restriction has been overturned in some state courts. Obviously, you need to be familiar with the laws in your state, because the specific provisions and procedural requirements vary.

Durable Power of Attorney for Health Care. Because it is more flexible and comprehensive than the living will, the durable power of attorney for health care is the preferred advance directive. It allows you to designate a surrogate, presumably a friend or relative, to make the medical decisions if you lose decision-making capacity. (While you are still capable, you give your own informed consent or refusal.) It is advisable for you to guide the surrogate, by indicating what types of treatment you would or would not want in a specific situation. Unlike most living wills, the durable power of attorney for health care can apply to all situations—not just terminal illness—in which the person is incapable of making decisions.

Problems with Advance Directives. Advance directives have limitations because you may not fully understand treatment options or appreciate the consequences of your choices. Advance directives may also be too vague to guide clinical decisions. For example, general statements rejecting "heroic treatments" do not indicate whether you want a particular treatment for a specific situation, such as antibiotics for pneumonia following a severe stroke. On the other hand very specific directives for future care may not be applicable to unanticipated circumstances. Furthermore, after expressing advance directives, people may change their minds without informing anyone, or medical circumstances may change as new or experimental therapies become available. You and your doctor can do a great deal to resolve these problems by discussing advance directives with each other.

Because most older people want to express their preferences regarding life-sustaining treatment, but few have done so, you and your physician should routinely share information on advance directives. A straightforward question to your doctor may open the topic: "Can we talk about how decisions will be made for my medical care in case I am too sick to talk to you directly?"

To improve communication, which can resolve many problems posed by advance directives, you should ask your physician about situations that commonly develop in your particular illness or condition. Ask clarifying questions about the various treatments and treatment options. In addition, check to make sure that the directives are taken seriously, including the designation of a surrogate decision maker as well as an indication of how much discretion that surrogate should be allowed and how you will make known any changes of mind. It is also important for you to have ongoing discussions about these issues with family members and friends.

Words such as *heroic* and *extraordinary* care are frequently, although not wisely, used in discussions about life-sustaining treatment. Highly technical, invasive, or expensive treatments like dialysis or mechanical ventilation are sometimes regarded as heroic or extraordinary, as opposed to "ordinary" care like antibiotics and intravenous fluids. These distinctions, however, are ambiguous, confusing, and best avoided, since every treatment has benefits and drawbacks that need to be evaluated for each individual. Decisions should not be based on the nature of the treatment but rather on whether the benefits to you outweigh any disadvantages.

Choosing a Surrogate Decision Maker. Traditionally, family members act as surrogates for incapacitated individuals, because presumably they best know the person's preferences and will act as an advocate. Family members are normally consulted by the physician; however, the physician may sometimes decide that decisions by family members are questionable because of conflicting personalities, values, or interests. In addition, relatives may be estranged or unwilling to make decisions or may disagree among themselves. In other cases, elderly people have no surviving relatives.

When there are no relatives or friends to represent the person, it may be that your physician is the next best choice as surrogate decision maker. The physician will understand the medical procedures and your condition. Your lawyer is another possibility. But consider that the courts are cumbersome, expensive, and slow, and the adversarial legal system and media publicity may polarize families and doctors, or lead to medically unrealistic decisions.

Acting in Your Best Interests

When incapacitated individuals have not given advance directives or appointed a surrogate, ethicists have recommended basing decisions on the best interest of the person by weighing the benefits and burdens of treatment. This is, however, a complicated and often controversial process that requires addressing such factors as the person's pain and suffering, safety, and loss of independence, privacy, and dignity. Well-meaning third parties may disagree on how to weigh these factors, which are often summarized in the ambiguous phrase "quality of life." Because individuals commonly assess their own quality of life in making medical decisions, judgments that follow the person's values are appropriate. Quality-of-life judgments that follow the assessments of other people are prone to cause problems, since they may be biased or discriminatory, particularly if social worth or economic productivity is considered. For example, life situations that would be intolerable to young, healthy people may be acceptable to older, debilitated individuals, and vice versa.

Courts have relied on the doctrine or the legal dictum of substituted judgment to link their decisions to the preferences of the individual. Searching for the person's preferences is always an appropriate first step, but in many cases the person's wishes are unknown or unclear. Thus, in reality many decisions in clinical practice and legal rulings are based on an assessment of the person's best interest.

Preventing Harm

Doctors have a duty to use their expertise for the benefit of the people in their care, although this duty may conflict with the duty to respect refusals of care by informed capable individuals. You retain the right to refuse treatments that your doctor considers to be in your best interest. Frank discussions can improve your mutual understanding of risks, benefits, and underlying beliefs.

Placement Issues

Preventing harm to an individual is frequently an issue in decisions regarding nursing home placement. Believing that living independently is too unsafe for a person, family members or caregivers may seek to override one's desire to remain at home. It is appropriate to try and arrange in-home supportive services first, but the crucial ethical issue is whether an older person is capable of making an informed decision about where to live; if so, his or her decision should be respected, even if others believe that it is unwise or foolish and even if it puts that person at greater risk.

Abuse of Elderly People

In cases of possible abuse, the duty to protect older people justifies some interventions, since they may be unable to protect themselves, not know how to get help, fear retaliation, or be ashamed to admit the abuse. A doctor who suspects abuse has the ethical duty to intervene to determine if the victim has the capacity to make decisions, is informed, and is not coerced. Some states require caregivers to report suspected abuse to a protective service agency. If the person is severely incapacitated, support interventions may be appropriate, such as installing home care services, counseling the abusive caregiver, or moving the older person to another residence. Family members can sometimes feel overwhelmed by their responsibilities, lack caregiving skills, have no respite, and become abusive. Supportive services should be offered, although capable individuals may refuse the assistance. If a person is not capable and the abuse seems clear, the physician must consider a report to adult protective service agencies or a petition to the court for a new guardian.

Guardianship

Some older people cannot manage their finances or provide themselves with food and shelter. Sometimes relatives or friends make informal arrangements to help these individuals. In other cases, the person, when he or she was capable, had executed a durable power of attorney that appointed another person to handle his or her affairs. In still other cases, it is necessary to ask the courts to appoint a guardian, as when property must be managed or sold to pay for long-term care.

All states allow the courts to establish limited guardianships (sometimes called conservatorships) and unlimited guardianships (called committeeships). A limited guardianship empowers the guardian to act in a specific area that corresponds to the areas of the person's life in which he can no longer function as determined by the court. An unlimited guardianship strips the older person of all legal authority and permits the guardian to make all the decisions about the older person's life in matters that affect property, residence, medical care, and personal relationships. Since an unlimited guardianship requires that the court find that the person is incompetent (this legal judgment requires that the person receive the protection generally afforded to a child), most states have a statutory preference for limited guardianships.

In guardianship hearings, petitioners—usually the relatives, but possibly social service agencies or even a health care provider—must demonstrate that the person is no longer able to manage her affairs and provide for her needs safely. If the person is found incompetent, the court appoints a guardian.

Decisions for People in Nursing Homes

Nursing home residents may need additional safeguards when decisions about life-sustaining treatments are made. They may not have close relatives to act as their advocates, the physician-patient relationship may be superficial, and there are fewer caregivers involved in the decision making in this setting than there are in hospitals. In addition, substandard care is sometimes a problem. Whether to transfer nursing home residents to a hospital when their condition worsens is a common dilemma, since for many of the residents the goal of treatment may be to relieve discomfort rather than to prolong life. If individuals or their surrogates decline the transfer to a hospital, their wishes should be respected. It should be a routine part of nursing home care to discuss these decisions well in advance.

Advances in medical technology have created medical dilemmas, because not all of the goals of care can be achieved. For example, in a seriously ill person a sudden worsening or complication of the person's condition may be reversible, but restoring function and improving the underlying disease may be impossible. In such a context, life-sustaining treatment may be appropriately withheld in several situations.

Life-Sustaining Treatments

The physician has no obligation to provide treatment if there is no specific medical rationale for it, if it has proven ineffective for the person, if the person is unconscious and will likely die in a matter of hours or days even if the treatment is given, or if the expected survival is virtually zero. The doctor's discretion in these matters may vary widely given the range of jurisdiction across the nation.

An informed person who is capable of making medical decisions may refuse life-sustaining treatment, such as cardiopulmonary resuscitation, intensive care, transfusions, antibiotics, and artificial feedings. An informed refusal should be respected, even if the person's life may be shortened as a consequence and even if the person is not terminally ill or in a coma. As for people who are not capable of making decisions, two questions need to be considered: What standard should be used? And who should make the decisions?

Cardiopulmonary resuscitation (CPR) may be an effective treatment for unexpected sudden death, but it is not effective for people whose death is expected. The outcomes after CPR are generally poor for older people, because of serious illnesses and decreased functional status. Less than 10 percent of people over 70 are discharged from the hospital alive after CPR. Few data exist on

Do-Not-Resuscitate Orders

outcomes after CPR in nursing homes. In addition, many long-term care facilities do not have the technical capability to perform CPR effectively.

When CPR is medically futile and thus ethically inappropriate, a patient should not be offered the choice between CPR or no CPR, but instead the physician should explain why CPR is not indicated, and a do-not-resuscitate order is generally written. In some settings, however, a statute may require that physicians offer the option of CPR even when it would be futile.

When CPR might be of benefit, the doctor must make sure that all concerned appreciate the fact that the likelihood of survival is low even if CPR is administered. Many people with chronic illnesses do not want CPR, and their informed refusal should be respected. The attending physician should also indicate the reasons for the order and plans for further care in the medical record.

Strictly speaking, a do-not-resuscitate order means that only CPR will not be performed; other treatments may still be given. Discussions with your doctor about do-not-resuscitate orders are excellent opportunities to review the total plan of care, including supportive care and appropriate treatments that would be continued after the do-not-resuscitate order takes effect.

Withdrawing Treatment

Strange emotional feelings are a natural part of decisions to withdraw or withhold care. We are torn between our impending sense of loss of our loved ones and our desire that their suffering be relieved and their dignity maintained. When a treatment has proven ineffective, there is little point in continuing it. Often, a distinction is made between stopping treatment and not starting it in the first place (for example, some people are willing to withhold mechanical ventilation, but are reluctant to discontinue it once started), although logically, ethically, and legally, there is no difference. If you feel that there is an important emotional difference between stopping a treatment and not starting one, you should explicitly discuss this with your physician.

Tube Feedings

In severely demented or debilitated individuals who cannot or will not eat, artificial nutrition and hydration are ethically and legally controversial. The feeding of helpless people is laden with symbolic and emotional significance, and it is possible that these individuals may suffer hunger or thirst if tube feedings are withheld. Tube feedings clearly benefit people if they provide the time to treat underlying conditions or to clarify the situation, and if the person wants the feedings.

The benefits are less clear in severely demented individuals who consistently refuse feedings offered by hand or who are unlikely to suffer hunger or thirst. Tube feedings may also have adverse consequences, such as pneumonia if the feedings are aspirated into the lungs. Moreover, because individuals often pull out the feeding tubes, demented individuals on tube feedings are often restrained, thereby compromising what little dignity and independence they retain. This causes a special problem because patients cannot comprehend how the treatment benefits them. Restraints are also difficult to reconcile with the goal of humane care. Sedation or "chemical restraints" might seem more acceptable on the surface, but they are also undignified and often associated with unacceptable side effects. Therefore, when a person pulls out a feeding tube, everyone involved should reconsider whether the feeding tube is appropriate. If so, other less obtrusive or more permanent measures, such as tubes placed in the stomach or intestine, should be considered. However, if the goal is to provide comfort, giving the person more direct attention and affection may be preferable to trying to increase the intake of nutrients.

Active Euthanasia

Active euthanasia (mercy killing) is illegal. Requests for it generally arise because individuals suffer uncontrolled pain, demand more control over their care, or fear abandonment. Many terminally ill people who have requested euthanasia change their minds after symptoms of pain have been relieved. It is relevant to note that experiments with self-administered pain medications indicate that the feeling of control is central to a person's comfort.

There is great potential for abuse with active euthanasia, especially in a society that has a less than perfect history when it comes to protecting the vulnerable, disadvantaged, or disabled. Because of this, opponents assert that allowing voluntary euthanasia might all too easily lead to involuntary euthanasia of helpless people. Others feel that the administration of active euthanasia is incompatible with the role of physicians and may undermine other people's trust in their doctors. However, in exceptional cases in which severe symptoms can be relieved only by causing unconsciousness, some people believe that it may be more compassionate to carry out a person's request for active euthanasia than to have the person continue an existence that is degrading. Active euthanasia should be distinguished from the withholding or withdrawal of treatment (which is sometimes termed "allowing to die" or "passive euthanasia"). Thus, the concern that active euthanasia is unethical should not lead doctors to continue futile treatments or to reject requests by informed individuals to withhold treatment.

Assisted Suicide

Statistically, elderly white men are at a greatly increased risk for suicide. Most suicides are impulsive acts that are not well thought out, so the person who seriously considers this act usually suffers from depression. Because individuals who are incapacitated by depression cannot make informed decisions, family and friends are quite likely to intervene and seek medical advice. Physicians have traditionally felt it their duty to intervene in order to prevent suicide.

For some people, however, suicide might be considered a rational choice, as, for example, in the case of those with widespread cancer who might have debilitating symptoms despite having received optimal treatment. Believing that a progressive illness of this type would be degrading and wishing to have control over their death, they might ask the physician how to end their life or request the medications with which to do so. These are matters of individual conscience. Many physicians believe that assisted rational suicide is unethical, for the same reasons that they oppose active euthanasia—they feel that there is a great danger of abuse, it is incompatible with the role of the physician, and it undermines a person's trust in doctors. In any case, in most states the law prohibits it.

CHAPTER 12

FINANCING HEALTH CARE

Health care financing is one of the most complicated and rapidly changing aspects of the entire delivery of care. This chapter will give you some of the basics to help you make an informed choice about health insurance. We will review the Medicare and Medicaid programs and explore other methods of paying for health care.

A unique aspect of financing health care for older people is the high proportion of funding that comes from public sources (65 percent versus 30 percent for those who are younger than 65). The rationale for establishing public funding such as Medicare (for people over 65) and Medicaid (for people below poverty line) was the large number of older people who are below the poverty line and the need to improve access to care. Between 1965 and the present, the proportion of people over age 65 who live below the poverty line has dropped dramatically from 25 to 12 percent. However, because of the increase in the cost of medical care for older people, the proportion of income that older people pay out-of-pocket for health care actually increased from 15 percent to 18 percent. Most people are not able to finance their own health care.

Medicare
The federal government program Medicare was enacted in 1966 as a provision (Title XVIII) of the Social Security Act, and it is today the nation's largest insurance program for older people. Health care under the Medicare program is not free. You must pay a percentage of the charges. Even if you are eligible for Medicare, you must apply for the benefits; enrollment is not automatic. Fortunately almost anyone over age 65 can enroll in Medicare; few are refused. But, if you have not paid enough social security, you may have to pay a little over $200 per month to buy into the program. A free book called *The Medicare Handbook* can help answer your questions on eligibility and benefits. You can obtain one by calling (800) 234-5772 or by visiting your local social security office.

The Health Care Financing Administration (HCFA) is the executive branch agency in the federal government that oversees and administers the Medicare and Medicaid programs. HCFA contracts with private firms, mainly insurance companies, to process the claims and to make payments to providers. These contractors are either "intermediaries" (part A of Medicare) or "carriers" (part B). The coverage for hospital services (part A of the Medicare program shown in Table 7) originated in the movement toward national health insurance in the late 1940s. By contrast, coverage for physician services (part B of Medicare shown in Table 8) was actually offered by some members of Congress as an alternative to part A. Table 9 lists some additional services that are usually covered by Medicare; some of the services that are not covered by the program are listed in Table 10. As a result of these separate origins, the financing, administration, participation, reimbursement, and data collection for the two parts of the program are separate.

In part A, the hospital insurance pays for all hospitalization costs after you pay a deductible ($716 in 1995). In a few special circumstances part A will also pay for 150 days of skilled nursing home care, home care, and hospice care. The expenditures for part A are paid out of the hospital insurance trust fund and are financed through the social security tax. Part B provides medical insurance and pays for 80 percent of the approved doctor's fee. Part B covers outpatient hospital services, diagnostic tests, ambulance transportation, and medical equipment such as wheelchairs. Expenditures for part B are paid out of a different fund, which is financed by

**Table 7. Coverage for Services
Under the Medicare Program, Part A**

Coverage	Services Included	Conditions That Must Be Met	Deductible (D) Copayment (C)	Reimbursement
Inpatient hospital care	Semiprivate room, special units, laboratory, x-ray, medication, supplies, blood (except for first 3 units), meals, nursing (not private duty)	Care ordered by physician; care can only be provided in hospital for stay approved by peer-review organization	d: $716 for each benefit period* c: $179 per day for days 61–90; $358 per day for days 91–150; no coverage beyond day 150	Prospective payment modified per case by DRG
Nursing facility	Semiprivate room, rehabilitation services, meals, nursing, medications, use of appliances	Must follow within 30 days of a 3-day or longer hospital stay, for a condition related to reason for NF admission; care ordered by physician	d: none for 1–20 days c: $90 for days 21–100; no coverage beyond day 100	Reasonable cost up to a limit
Home health care	Part-time skilled nursing, PT, ST, OT; part-time home health aide and medical equipment also covered if skilled nursing, PT, ST needed	Skilled nursing, rehabilitation, PT, ST ordered by physician	d: none c: 20% only for durable medical equipment	Reasonable cost up to a limit
Hospice	Inpatient and outpatient nursing, physician, drugs, PT, ST, OT, homemaker, counseling, inpatient respite (5 days), medical and social services	Patient certified by a physician as "terminally" ill; patient chooses hospice over standard Medicare benefits for terminal illness	d: none c: $5 for drugs and 5% of inpatient respite care; total coverage limited to 210 days	Daily fixed rate per case for up to 210 days

DRG, diagnostic-related group; NF, nursing facility; PT, physical therapy; ST, speech therapy; OT, occupational therapy.
*Benefit period begins with day of admission and ends 60 consecutive days after patient has been out of the hospital or nursing facility.

Table 8. Coverage for Services Under the Medicare Program, Part B

COVERAGE*	SERVICES INCLUDED	CONDITIONS THAT MUST BE MET	DEDUCTIBLE (D) COPAYMENT (C)	REIMBURSEMENT
Physician services	Medical and surgical services, diagnostic procedures, radiology, pathology, drugs and biologicals that cannot be self-administered	Care medically necessary for diagnosis and management of acute or chronic illness	d: $100 deductible covers all part B services c: 20%	Approved standard fee or actual charges, whichever is lower
Mental health services	Outpatient therapy for mental illness conducted by a physician, a psychologist, or in a comprehensive rehabilitation outpatient setting	As above	d: SAPS c: 50%	As above
Hospital outpatient services	Ambulatory surgery services incident to the services of a physician, diagnostic tests (laboratory/X ray), ER, and hospital-based medical supplies	Care ordered by physician	d: SAPS c: SAPS	Varies by type of service
Independent laboratory services	Clinical diagnostic laboratory	Tests ordered by physician	d: none c: none	Approved standard fee
Durable medical equipment	Wheelchairs, oxygen equipment (but not oxygen)	For use in home; to serve a medical purpose for people who are either sick or injured	d: SAPS c: SAPS	Approved standard fee

MEI, Medicare Economic Index; ER, emergency room; SAPS, same as physician services.

*Beneficiaries must pay a monthly premium for coverage.

general tax revenues and premiums paid by beneficiaries. Tax revenues make up 75 percent while premiums make up 25 percent. The premiums paid by older persons finance less than 10 percent

**Table 9. Additional Services Usually Covered by
Medicare—Parts A and B**

Ambulance transport

Ambulatory surgical services

Blood (patient must pay for first 3 units)

Hepatitis B vaccine

Immunosuppressive drugs

Kidney dialysis and transplants

Liver transplants

Outpatient physical and occupational therapy

Pneumococcal vaccine

Prosthetic devices (not dental)

Radiation therapy

Rural health clinic services

of the entire Medicare program. To participate in part A of the program, beneficiaries need only to be eligible for social security, whereas participation in part B is voluntary and requires that the beneficiary pay an additional payment of a monthly premium ($46.10 in 1995).

Despite the costs, 95 percent of the people who are eligible to participate do so in part B (you should too!). Other differences between the two parts of the program relate to their reimbursements, which are shown in Tables 7 and 8. You may be able to save money if your doctor has agreed to accept Medicare's approved amount as full payment. Doing this is called accepting Medicare assignment; about half of the doctors in the United States accept assignment. This approach saves you money because the charge is less and your doctor submits the insurance form. A list of participating doctors is available free from your Medicare carrier. Check *The Medicare Handbook* for the name of your carrier. If Medicare refuses to pay for a particular service (called denying the claim),

Table 10. Services Not Covered by Medicare

Chronic (ongoing) home care services

Chronic nursing home services

Cosmetic surgery

Eyeglasses, hearing aids

Immunizations (except pneumococcal or hepatitis vaccine or if required by injury)

Prescription medications (except those administered in hospital or in some circumstances in nursing facility or physician's office)

Preventive foot care

Routine (preventive) history and physical examination

you can appeal. It is very important to note the time limit for appealing decisions printed on each denial notice. These time limits are strictly enforced and you could lose an important opportunity to appeal. The appeal process is complicated and legal assistance is helpful.

A major problem with the future financing of part A of the Medicare program is that it depends totally on revenues from the social security payroll tax. Even with very optimistic projections, it seems likely that Medicare expenditures will be depleted shortly after the turn of the century.

Medicaid   Medicaid, which was created in 1966 as part of the Social Security Act (Title XIX), is a joint federal and state program financed almost totally from state and federal taxes. The Medicaid program is complicated because it is administered by the state. States have discretion in deciding which services will be reimbursed so that no two programs are the same. The federal government pays from 55 to 80 percent (the average is 60 percent) of the cost, the percent of federal payment depending upon the state's per capita income relative to the national per capita income. Eligibility for this program depends upon your income or assets being below a specified level, and access to this fund is limited to people with low income who qualify for certain "categorical" programs. Fewer than 40 percent of people whose incomes are below the federal poverty level are currently covered by Medicaid.

Unlike members of other age groups, if you are 65 and older, you are eligible for Medicaid under provisions made for those who are "blind, disabled, or aged." Thus all people who are 65 and older can receive Medicaid if their income including social security benefits falls below a certain federally set level.

This broad eligibility enables most people age 65 or older with moderate or low incomes and limited assets who need nursing home care to qualify for Medicaid. Because of this, services to people 65 and older comprise nearly 40 percent of the program's expenditures in 1989 (the vast majority of payments went to chronic nursing home care).

One of the critical considerations in approaching the financing of long-term care is the issue of Medicaid "spend-down," which is when people admitted to nursing homes have to spend down their personal assets to Medicaid income levels in order to be poor enough to qualify for Medicaid during their nursing home stay. One recent innovation is the program introduced in Connecticut and pending in several states to allow people who purchase private long-term care insurance to exclude from the assets considered in determining eligibility for Medicaid coverage an amount equal to the benefit paid by the private insurance company.

Private Insurance Policies

Obviously Medicare was not designed to cover all of your health care costs. As we have seen, it covers sudden catastrophes requiring hospitalization. But you have other health expenses, and for all your health care bills Medicare will only pay about half. To cover those expenses not paid by Medicare, private companies sell insurance, sometimes called Medigap. You may not need Medigap insurance if you are covered by Medicaid because Medicaid pays almost all health care expenses. In addition, you may have group health insurance if you remain employed and may be able to connect it to a supplemental Medicare policy.

If you decide to buy supplemental Medigap insurance, your first step is to understand exactly what Medicare does and does not cover so that your supplemental policy fills the coverage gap. As a general rule you will need only one supplemental policy—having more than one is a waste of money. Ideally, supplemental policies should cover all out-of-pocket expenses you might be required to pay before Medicare pays (the deductible expense) and the amount of the bill not covered by Medicare. Unfortunately, ideal policies do not exist. Most supplemental policies do not cover services such as private duty nursing care, rest home care, or routine health care that Medicare does not cover. You should be very cautious in purchasing a policy to take the place of one you already have. Your new policy may not cover any diseases you already have. You should always pay for the policy by a check made payable to the insurance company. Never pay cash and never make out the check to the insurance agent. Also, it makes no sense to buy a disease-specific policy that pays for treatment of only one disease such as cancer.

Because of the high cost of long-term care and the low likelihood that the government will expand Medicare coverage to include nursing home costs, there has been a growing interest in private long-term care insurance. Although the impact of private insurance on nursing home financing is still very small (about 1 percent), the number of long-term care insurance policies has increased from fewer than 100,000 in 1986 to more than 2 million policies in 1990, with about 5 percent of those over age 65 now having some type of long-term care insurance.

Over 40 percent of all people will need some stay in a nursing home during their lifetimes. Those who enter a nursing home stay an average of 2.8 years at an average annual cost, as of 1993, of $27,600. Although averages are useful for overall planning purposes, they hide the significant variation of risk by sex and length of stay. For example, women face an average lifetime cost of $37,500 compared with $15,900 for men. The 9 percent of people who stay more than five years account for 65 percent of the total cost at a rate of over $115,000 per person.

The biggest factor in trying to decide whether to buy a long-term care policy is the cost of the coverage. Your policy must be able to adjust the amount paid to correspond to rising costs (this is sometimes called an inflation adjustment). If your financial status is secure and substantial, a long-term care policy may provide good protection of your estate. Those with more moderate means should consider transferring assets to family members at least 30 months before nursing home care is needed. Transferred assets do not count in determining Medicaid eligibility provided the transfer takes place 30 months before entering the nursing home. When resources have been thus depleted, Medicaid will cover the cost of nursing home care.

PART IV

CONDITIONS THAT AFFECT OLDER PEOPLE

CHAPTER 13

MEMORY AND THINKING: DEMENTIA, DELIRIUM, AND AMNESIA

Overview

Classifying Dementias

Dementia Management

Delirium (Sudden Confusion)

Amnesia

Memory problems, or dementia, represent an acquired loss of intellectual ability that occurs over a long period of time and affects many areas of cognitive functioning. Problems in thinking and memory may be caused by a variety of diseases, including Alzheimer's disease, Pick's disease, and vascular causes. Although memory loss is one feature of dementing illness, it is usually accompanied by an impairment in at least one of the following areas: language; recognizing spatial relationships; other areas of thinking (such as calculating numbers or abstract thinking); executive functions such as making lists or planning; or a change in personality. The degree of intellectual loss is generally severe enough to interfere with social and occupational functioning. Dementia is differentiated from sudden memory problems by its long time course. While sudden states of confusion (called delirium) progress in hours to days, dementia progresses over months to years. In addition, dementia does not usually affect the person's level of consciousness, but sudden confusion generally does. Other features that distinguish dementing illness from acute confusional states are listed in Table 11.

Dementia affects less than 10 percent of people who are older than 65, but increases to approximately 15 to 20 percent for people at the

Overview

Epidemiology

Table 11. Clinical Characteristics of Dementia Compared with Delirium

CHARACTERISTIC	DEMENTIA	DELIRIUM
History		
Onset	Insidious	Sudden
Duration	Months to years	Hours to days
Motor Signs	None (until late)	Muscle shakes or tremors
Speech	Normal	Slurred
Mental Status		
Attention	Normal	Fluctuating, inattention, easily distracted
Memory	Impaired recent memory	Impaired by poor attention
Language	Difficulty finding the right word	Normal; misnaming may be prominent; writing difficulty often prominent
Perception	Abnormalities not prominent	Visual, auditory, and/or tactile hallucinations may be clear
Mood/effect	Apathetic and/or loss of impulse control	Fear and suspiciousness may often be prominent
Other systems	No involvement of other organ systems	Systemic illness (fever, chills, weight loss, poor appetite) or toxic exposure may be present

Source: Cummings JL, Benson DF. *Dementia: A Clinical Approach.* Boston: Butterworth; 1983:13. Reprinted with permission.

age of 85. A much higher prevalence of Alzheimer's disease may occur in older age groups.

Evaluation If you are having problems with memory or other cognitive abilities, you should have an interview and complete physical examination by a physician trained in geriatric medicine. Memory assessments can also be performed by neurologists, psychiatrists, or primary care physicians with appropriate training. By paying close attention to memory, language, visual and spatial function, and additional skills, the physician can usually tell if you have a dementing illness and define the type of dementia and whether any other neurologic abnormalities are present.

Formal, detailed neuropsychological testing that involves such activities as interpreting stories, drawing objects, remembering words, and so on may be helpful in some circumstances. Such testing is especially useful for those people who, despite a history of functional decline, have very mild dementing illnesses or who have such a high intelligence that the extent of their dementing illness remains unclear on examination. Further testing can also be helpful in establishing a reference point for people with uncertain diagnoses and in determining if depression is a contributing factor to any cognitive or functional decline.

The diagnostic use of neuroimaging studies that show the brain structures such as computed tomography (CT) scans or magnetic resonance imaging (MRI) remains controversial. The vast majority of these examinations do not identify potentially treatable lesions; however, they may detect characteristic patterns of atrophy, in some of the less common dementias. For example, both Huntington's and Pick's diseases can be identified by the location of atrophy in the brain. (These conditions are discussed later in this chapter.) Imaging studies may also detect structural abnormalities such as tumors, strokes, hydrocephalus, subdural hematomas (bleeding beneath the membrane tissue covering the skull), and other conditions. Imaging studies are not necessarily needed for people who begin to show signs of dementia. When dementia results from one of these structural abnormalities, it may be partially reversible. Other potentially reversible causes of dementia are sometimes detectable through a complete blood count and a routine set of blood tests. These include tests of kidney and liver function, thyroid function, vitamin B_{12} and folic acid levels, and a test for syphilis. Sometimes an electroencephalogram (EEG) can be helpful. Its use is restricted to situations where there is a high suspicion of a condition that produces EEG abnormalities, such as Pick's disease or Creutzfeldt-Jakob disease. In general, the usefulness of examining the spinal fluid in the evaluation of dementia is limited and a spinal tap is only recommended in certain circumstances: when dementia begins in a relatively young person; when

Table 12. Causes of Dementing Illness

CAUSE	EXAMPLES
Degenerative	Alzheimer's disease Pick's disease
Depression	Depression
Infectious	AIDS Neurosyphilis
Metabolic	Thyroid disease Vitamin B_{12} deficiency
Toxins	Alcohol Heavy metal exposure Drugs
Vascular	Multiple strokes
Others	Trauma (head injuries) Cancer Subdural hematoma

the disease progresses very rapidly; in people who have a positive blood test for syphilis; for very unusual symptoms; for signs and symptoms of meningitis; or other underlying diseases that may involve the nervous system.

Classifying Dementias

Dementing illnesses are usually categorized according to their suspected cause as degenerative, vascular, infectious, toxic, or metabolic. There are also a variety of miscellaneous conditions (see Table 12). Autopsy series suggest that about 50 percent of all cases of dementia are due to Alzheimer's disease, the predominant degenerative dementia. Between 10 and 15 percent are due to vascular causes such as small strokes, and an additional 10 to 20 percent to a combination of Alzheimer's disease and multiple small strokes. A smaller percentage of dementias is due to alcoholism, trauma, brain tumors, and miscellaneous causes. There is now an increased awareness and recognition of the AIDS-dementia complex.

Over two million Americans have Alzheimer's disease, a type of dementing illness named after the German physician who first described its pathologic features.

With Alzheimer's disease, nerve loss is usually seen in a number of important brain regions. In particular, there appears to be a marked reduction in those structures that use acetylcholine as their primary neurotransmitter (neurotransmitters enable nerve cells to communicate with each other).

Causes of Alzheimer's Disease. Increasing age and a history of the illness in other family members are risk factors for the development of Alzheimer's disease. Women are more prone to develop the disease, and proposed risk factors that have not been proven include prior head trauma, age of mother at time of delivery, and the aluminum and other trace metal content in drinking water. Various subtypes of Alzheimer's disease have been proposed based on age of onset, family history, the presence of shaking or movement disorders, and particular neuropsychological profiles.

One of the two characteristics of Alzheimer's disease on microscopic examination of the brain at autopsy is the presence of dying nerves called neuritic plaques. At the core of these nerves are amyloid deposits. Amyloid is a poorly soluble material (resembling silk) that is sometimes deposited in blood vessels. A specific type of protein appears to be the primary building block of amyloid, and deposits of this protein have recently been found in people with Alzheimer's disease and Down syndrome. These deposits may be seen in parts of the brain that are not associated with the neuritic plaques and are thought to represent an earlier change in brain structure in people who have Alzheimer's disease. The other characteristic feature of Alzheimer's disease seen under the microscope are neurofibrillary tangles, which are thought to contain abnormal microtubular proteins. Normally these microtubules are used as scaffolding within the cells, providing structure. Despite these hallmarks, however, both neuritic plaques and neurofibrillary tangles are found in the brains of many elderly people who had no evidence of Alzheimer's disease.

Considerable interest has been focused recently on the genetics of Alzheimer's disease. It seems that there is a variety of

Alzheimer's disease that is primarily familial (genetic). At present, the prevalence of the disease and the lack of complete family medical histories make it difficult to distinguish between genetic and nongenetic cases. Extensive research is under way to determine the causes of the entity we call Alzheimer's disease and whether it is actually one or several diseases.

Symptoms of Alzheimer's Disease. People with Alzheimer's disease usually show a subtle and progressive worsening of their memory; in contrast to people with other forms of dementia or age-associated memory impairment, they respond very poorly to cues (or "reminders"). Language difficulties are also a consistent feature of Alzheimer's disease. Early in the course of Alzheimer's disease, affected individuals may have difficulty finding the right word. This can later progress to more severe difficulties in understanding language and in speaking. The content of language in Alzheimer's disease is sometimes characterized as empty or impoverished; it carries very little meaning. While the ability to repeat words is relatively well preserved, naming and comprehension abilities are impaired as the disease progresses.

People with Alzheimer's disease may have difficulty in recognizing objects, drawing simple designs, and locating objects. A common complaint of caregivers is that the demented person gets lost, even in the immediate neighborhood. Executive functions such as the ability to organize and plan and to think abstractly are frequently impaired. These disabilities usually interfere with the capacity to make appropriate social and occupational judgments.

Behavioral and psychiatric symptoms are also common features of Alzheimer's disease. These include wandering, aggressive behaviors, visual hallucinations, and delusions. These delusions may often involve concern that others are stealing objects from them or being unreasonably suspicious of other people's intentions. Misidentification of familiar people or locations may also occur, and irritability and anxiety may develop as well as features of depression. Despite these significant deteriorations in cognitive function, the ability to perform physical activity is remarkably preserved until late in the course of the disease. Very late in the illness some people develop stiffness in their arms and legs.

Table 13. Criteria for Clinical Diagnosis of Alzheimer's Disease

1. The criteria for the clinical diagnosis of *probable* Alzheimer's disease include:

   dementia established by clinical examination and documented by the Mini-Mental State Examination, Blessed Dementia Scale, or some similar examination, and confirmed by neuropsychologic tests;

   deficits in two or more areas of cognition;

   progressive worsening of memory and other cognitive functions;

   no disturbance of consciousness;

   onset between ages 40 and 90, most often after age 65; and

   absence of systemic disorders or other brain diseases that in and of themselves could account for the progressive deficits in memory and cognition.

2. The diagnosis of *probable* Alzheimer's disease is supported by:

   progressive deterioration of specific cognitive functions such as language (aphasia), motor skills (apraxia), and perception (agnosia);

   impaired activities of daily living and altered patterns of behavior;

   family history of similar disorders, particularly if confirmed neuropathologically; and

   laboratory results of normal lumbar puncture as evaluated by standard techniques, normal pattern or nonspecific changes in EEG such as increased slow-wave activity, and evidence of cerebral atrophy on CT with progression documented by serial observation.

3. Other clinical features consistent with the diagnosis of *probable* Alzheimer's disease, after exclusion of causes of dementia other than Alzheimer's disease, include:

   plateaus in the course of progression of the illness;

   associated symptoms of depression, insomnia, incontinence, delusions, illusions, hallucinations, catastrophic verbal, emotional, or physical outbursts, sexual disorders, and weight loss;

   other neurologic abnormalities in some patients, especially with more advanced disease and including motor signs such as increased muscle tone, myoclonus, or gait disorder;

   seizures in advanced disease; and

   CT normal for age.

4. Features that make the diagnosis of *probable* Alzheimer's disease uncertain or unlikely include:

   sudden, apoplectic onset;

   focal neurologic findings such as hemiparesis, sensory loss, visual field deficits, and incoordination early in the course of the illness; and

   seizures or gait disturbances at the onset or very early in the course of the illness.

5. Clinical diagnosis of *possible* Alzheimer's disease:

   may be made on the basis of the dementia syndrome, in the absence of other neurologic, psychiatric, or systemic disorders sufficient to cause dementia, and in the presence of variations in the onset, in the presentation, or in the clinical course;

   may be made in the presence of a second systemic or brain disorder sufficient to produce dementia, which is not considered to be *the* cause of the dementia; and

   should be used in research studies when a single, gradually progressive, severe cognitive deficit is identified in the absence of other identifiable cause.

6. Criteria for diagnosis of *definite* Alzheimer's disease are:

   the clinical criteria for probable Alzheimer's disease and histopathologic evidence obtained from a biopsy or autopsy.

7. Classification of Alzheimer's disease for research purposes should specify features that may differentiate subtypes of the disorder, such as:

   familial occurrence;

   onset before age of 65;

   presence of trisomy 21; and

   coexistence of other relevant conditions such as Parkinson's disease.

EEG, electroencephalogram; CT, computed tomography.

Source: Stadlan EM. Clinical diagnosis of Alzheimer's disease. In: McKhann G, Drachman D, Folstein M, et al, eds. Report of the NINCDS-ADRDA Work Group under the auspices of Department of Health and Human Services Task Force on Alzheimer's disease. *Neurology.* 1984;34:940. Reprinted with permission.

Generally, people with Alzheimer's disease have little insight into their own disabilities and as the disease progresses, they may require increasing help with very basic daily activities. Even with the marked individual variation in the rate of disease progression, most people experience severe disability within 8 to 12 years of onset. The severity of the dementia is strongly related to survival. Wandering, falling, urinary incontinence, and behavioral problems such as suspiciousness or paranoia, agitation, and hallucinations are also associated with a poor outlook.

Evaluation of Alzheimer's Disease. The diagnosis of Alzheimer's disease is based on a complete evaluation by a very skilled interviewer and diagnostician. The clinical criteria for Alzheimer's disease are shown in Table 13. If established by these criteria, the diagnosis of probable Alzheimer's disease has an 85 to 95 percent correlation with autopsy studies (which are the only way to make a diagnosis with certainty). Nonetheless, the differentiation of Alzheimer's disease from other dementing illnesses is usually difficult.

Treatment of Alzheimer's Disease. There is presently no cure for Alzheimer's disease. Useful management approaches are given later in this section.

Pick's Disease

Pick's disease, named after the 19th-century neurologist Arnold Pick, is a rare disease that usually afflicts people who are between the ages of 40 and 60, although it can occur in a person as old as 80 or as young as 21.

Cause of Pick's Disease. The cause of Pick's disease is unknown, although about 20 percent of affected individuals have a family history of it. Pick's disease and Alzheimer's disease may initially appear to be similar, but the brain degeneration is different in these two dementing illnesses. Localized atrophy of particular sections of the brain, especially the frontal and temporal lobes, is characteristic. In addition, when brain tissue is examined under the microscope at autopsy, there are two abnormalities that are unique to Pick's disease: "balloon cells," which are swollen nerve cells, and "inclusion bodies." Other degenerative changes in the brain include loss of nerve networks and atrophy of the areas involved with language, memory storage, and thought processing.

Symptoms of Pick's Disease. The first symptoms of Pick's disease are personality changes, emotional disturbances, impaired judgment and insight, and socially inappropriate behavior. Speech disturbances are common. People sometimes have a cluster of three symptoms called the Kluver-Bucy syndrome: blunted emotional responses including lack of fear, inappropriate sexual behavior, and unusual oral behavior, such as putting objects into their mouths. Curiously, people tend to retain their memory function and the ability to calculate numbers until the disease is advanced.

Pick's disease often progresses rapidly and as the disease progresses, loss of memory and speech difficulties increase; ultimately, the person eventually becomes mute. Death usually occurs from between 2 and 15 years after symptoms begin.

Treatment for Pick's Disease. There is no known cure for Pick's disease, although some of the behavior abnormalities do respond to selectively appropriate treatment as outlined in the management section.

Dementias Caused by Vascular Disease

The precise definition of dementia caused by blood vessel diseases is not well established even though vascular disease is the second most common cause of dementia after Alzheimer's disease. Cognitive ability is damaged, it appears, by multiple small strokes that decrease blood supply to various parts of the brain. In vascular dementia there is sometimes a sudden onset of difficulty followed by abrupt deterioration of function. The location of the vascular damage is an important factor in whether or not stroke patients develop dementia; dementing illness is most likely when a blood vessel at the back of the brain is damaged.

Cortical multi-infarct dementia refers to a syndrome of multiple small strokes caused by vascular disease or the migration of blood clots arising in the *large* feeding arteries to the brain. A person with this condition may have several neurological difficulties that, depending on their location, may include loss of the use of one-half of the body, sensory loss, speaking difficulties, difficulty organizing things, difficulty naming objects, and other specific difficulties.

Multi-infarct dementias of deeper brain structures are caused by lack of blood flow in *medium to small* vessels. These blood vessel problems form little holes in the brain, called lacunae (from the Latin, meaning "pit" or "gap"), that are most often found deep in the brain. People with this situation have difficulty swallowing, difficulty speaking, fluctuating emotions, slow movements, urinary incontinence, and a small-step gait.

Dementias Caused by Infections

While much less common than Alzheimer's or vascular disease, infections can also be the cause of dementing illness. One infectious disease called Creutzfeldt-Jakob disease (named for two German psychiatrists) is a rare disorder occurring in about one in one million demented individuals. The infection is thought to be due to a very slow growing virus, which, unlike other viruses, does not provoke an inflammatory response from the body. This virus is resistant to conventional treatments. As a result of these differences from true viruses, physicians hypothesize that the cause is really an infectious protein particle called a prion.

The onset of Creutzfeldt-Jakob disease usually occurs in people aged 50 to 70 and is marked initially by subtle changes in behavior such as fatigue, difficulty concentrating, and depression. Eventually, multiple cognitive difficulties develop. Muscle jerks are common, and the person may develop difficulty with coordination. This illness proceeds rapidly to a state where the person cannot move. The final stages are characterized by seizures.

In a significant percentage of the patients with AIDS, the human immunodeficiency virus (HIV) may infect the brain directly and cause a slowly progressive dementia. Most people affected in this way are forgetful and demonstrate inattention and slowing of their thought processes. They may appear to be withdrawn, apathetic, or depressed, and psychiatric symptoms may be present. Within the brain, the white matter below the brain surface and basal ganglia are the structures most severely affected. Cognitive dysfunction in people with the HIV virus can also be due to additional infections with a number of other organisms.

Reversible Dementias

Of all people with dementing illness, about 5 to 10 percent may have partially reversible dementia and 3 percent have totally reversible dementia. Drug toxicity heads the list of partially and completely reversible causes of dementia. (Adverse drug reactions are discussed in Chapter 9.)

Alcohol-Associated Dementias. A chronic dementia can also be associated with alcoholism. People with alcohol problems experience acute confusion and memory disorders. This dementia usually occurs after more than ten years of alcohol abuse. Difficulty with the memory alone and not in other areas suggests this disorder. Cognitive problems may vary but nonverbal skills are usually more affected than verbal skills.

Depression. Sometimes called pseudodementia, depression that is associated with intellectual decline is a potentially reversible cause of dementing illness in older people. Forgetfulness, slowness to respond, poor attention, and disorientation are common characteristics, as are a depressed mood and feelings of worthlessness or guilt. A clinical evaluation characteristically reveals no language difficulties, word-finding difficulties, or poor coordination. Usually there is an overall slowing down of movement, although some people may have restlessness and agitation. Clues to depression usually include sleep disturbances, problems with appetite, and a lowered sexual drive.

It is important to recognize that depression and dementia may exist together and that some people who initially respond to antidepressant medication may subsequently develop the symptoms of an irreversible dementia. (Depression is covered more extensively in Chapter 15.)

Thyroid Disease. Both overactive and underactive thyroid glands can cause dementia. The neurologic signs of an overactive thyroid gland include tremors, muscle weakness, seizures, and eye problems. A dementia caused by thyroid disease is usually characterized by anxiety, restlessness, irritability, and poor attention and memory; there may also be depression, apathy, and other psychiatric symptoms. Hypothyroidism, or an underactive thyroid, may result in muscle weakness, clumsiness, and seizures. Mental difficulties include lack of attention, lethargy, and impaired ability to think abstractly. With appropriate treatment to restore the thyroid hormone level to normal, the changes in mental function caused by both overactive and underactive thyroid conditions may improve, sometimes dramatically.

Vitamin B₁₂ Deficiency. The neurologic signs of vitamin B_{12} deficiency include dementia, atrophy of the nerves in the eye, and changes in the nerves in the arms and legs. The dementia is characterized by slowness, apathy, irritability, and confusion. The mental status changes may fluctuate, and agitation and depression may also be present. Within the brain, there is degeneration and a swelling of the lining around the nerves. Treatment with intramuscular vitamin B_{12}, if started early, can reverse the changes in the nervous system and can stop the progression of dementia in long-standing cases.

Normal-Pressure Hydrocephalus. Normal-pressure hydrocepalus is the condition caused by an increased fluid pressure inside the brain causing a gait disturbance, dementia, and urinary incontinence. The problem seems to be due to difficulty in reabsorbing spinal fluid generated by past trauma or inflammations at the base of the brain. Stiffness of the legs and difficulty in starting to walk contribute to the gait disturbance. The gait problem has been described as a "magnetic gait." The person seems to have feet that are stuck to the floor as if wearing magnetic shoes on a metal floor. There is also difficulty in standing straight, and falls are frequent. The degree of mental change ranges from minor inattention, decreased spontaneity, and generalized slowing, to more significant memory disturbances, apathy, withdrawal, and poor judgment. Brain imaging shows very large fluid spaces in the brain without shrinkage of the tissue. Treatment consists of placement of a neurosurgical shunt, a catheter or tube that goes from the brain to the abdomen to help divert the accumulation of spinal fluid. Drainage of spinal fluid through this tube sometimes improves the cognitive problems.

Neurosyphilis. Neurosyphilis occurs about 15 years after the primary infection with syphilis. Prior to the introduction of penicillin, this accounted for 15 to 30 percent of admissions to mental institutions. Psychiatric features of neurosyphilis are common and include grandiose delusions, a hyperactive state, depression, and hallucinations. In addition, there are many cognitive defects including disorders of memory, attention, language, and organizing and sequencing tasks. There is brain shrinkage, especially in the frontal and temporal areas. At autopsy, the lining of the brain looks thick and dulled. Although it is a rare disorder today, cases of neurosyphilis are increasing particularly in people who also have the AIDS virus.

Dementias Caused by Poisons. In addition to alcohol, a number of other toxic substances may cause cognitive dysfunction especially with exposure over long periods of time. Examples include arsenic and heavy metals such as lead, thallium, manganese, and mercury. A number of industrial solvents and insecticides have also been found to cause dementia.

When a dementing illness has a potentially reversible cause, treatment of the underlying disease is undertaken to attempt to halt progression of the illness and possibly reverse the decline of mental function. It is also important to review carefully any medications that may contribute to mental dysfunctions. If possible, visual and hearing difficulties should be corrected since sensory difficulties can contribute to cognitive problems. Early in the illness, memory-helping techniques such as note taking can be useful. Speech and physical therapy can help.

Dementia Management

Caregivers concerned with management of people suffering dementia should keep in mind that people do better with ongoing sensory and social stimulation tailored to their skills and that regularity of daily routines provides security for most people with dementia. Stimulants in the evening such as coffee are not recommended since they can produce or aggravate sleep disturbances. Additional helpful strategies include simplifying the environment, removing clutter, and providing better lighting. Sessions where people can reminisce about any life events they still remember can emphasize cognitive abilities and help maintain self-esteem.

Because people with Alzheimer's disease have complex mental dysfunction and because they have a high rate of motor vehicle accidents, they should not be allowed to drive under any circumstances.

The general principle is to preserve a person's autonomy as much as possible without compromising anyone's safety.

There is currently no treatment that consistently improves memory in people with Alzheimer's disease. While a number of compounds have been studied, there is no evidence that any of them has a lasting effect. The drug tacrine, which increases the concentration of one of the brain's neurotransmitters, may set back the clock of cognitive decline by six months in some people with Alzheimer's disease, but decline is at the same rate. The drug is very expensive and causes substantial liver toxicity, requiring frequent blood tests.

In Alzheimer's disease and other dementing illnesses, caregivers need to consider the best methods for managing the patient's mood and behavior. Characteristically, Alzheimer's victims suffer from depression, anxiety, hallucinations, or aggressive behavior. They can wander and get lost and become very agitated at night. The first challenge for caregivers is to identify which, if any, of these problems is significant enough to warrant intervention. Then it is important to develop a treatment plan for each specific problem while realizing that other difficulties may not improve. One helpful way to think about these problems is to determine how aware the person is of his surroundings and the consequences of his actions; the capacity for controlling impulses; the amount of arousal exhibited; and the outlets for self-expression. Categorizing the difficulties in this way can lead to creative solutions.

Another principle of treatment is for caregivers to learn about behavior patterns that can be anticipated and environmental modifications that might be beneficial. For example, it may become important to take the knobs off of the stove to prevent cooking accidents or to lock doors to prevent wandering and getting lost. In addition, caregivers should look out for and, if possible, reduce any factors that might aggravate or produce a behavior problem, such as stress in the household or medical problems in addition to Alzheimer's disease. In some cases, drug treatment may be necessary to modify discomforting or difficult behavior. Because individuals suffering from dementia may not be able to verbalize the side effects they are experiencing, caregivers should obtain information about possible adverse drug effects (pharmacists are an excellent source) and should be on the alert for their manifestations.

Wandering, a common complication that affects up to one-half of people with severe dementia, can have one or more causes. A demented person may get lost, especially if she has recently moved to an unfamiliar location. Agitation, depression, hallucinations, boredom, the need for more frequent toileting, or pain can also cause the demented individual to wander, and sometimes no specific cause for wandering is evident. Regular exercise is often helpful. Provide the person with an armband or a nonremovable identification bracelet so she can be promptly identified and returned if she becomes lost. Drug treatments and physical restraints do not cure wandering and usually increase agitation and irritability, but in very rare circumstances they may be necessary to maintain a person's safety.

The psychiatric complications of dementia, such as paranoid or accusatory beliefs, delusions, and hallucinations, need not be treated if they are mild. If, however, these conditions are disruptive to the person or cause very agitated, aggressive, or hostile behavior, medication may be necessary. Aggressive behavior can take many forms and range from cursing and spitting to direct physical attack. Maintaining composure, using distraction, and modifying the environment all can be helpful. For example, soothing music can sometimes help to relieve stress. In addition, spending more time completing a potentially disruptive task, such as bathing, may help reduce this sort of behavior.

Confusion or agitation that occurs in the early evening or night is referred to as "sundowning." Dementia clearly predisposes a person to sundowning but the extent of this problem is unknown. The primary management involves establishing soothing environmental conditions such as a quiet room with reduced (but not absent) sensory input—lighting, music, television. Special cues such as talking quietly to the agitated person can be helpful. Although it is occasionally necessary to administer sedative medications, it is important to appreciate that such medications also have the potential to increase a person's confusion.

In caring for a person with a dementing illness, a caregiver undergoes a tremendous amount of stress and is vulnerable to depression, drug and alcohol abuse, and stress-related problems. These consequences appear to be more closely related to the characteristics of the caregivers, such as their level of morale, health, and coping mechanisms, than they are to the cognitive or functional status of the older people for whom they are caring. It is important for caregivers to know about the patient's illness and its likely course, the type of therapy that may be required, and any difficulties in function and behavior that may be encountered because it helps caregivers not to place unrealistic demands upon the demented person. Education and informed and effective assistance improve the quality of care and help reduce caregiver stress and burnout. The Alzheimer's Association, with chapters throughout the United States, is a useful source of information and support groups.

Finally, in caring for people with dementia it is important for families and other caregivers to know of all of the available community services that might provide assistance, including caregivers' relief opportunities. Obviously, all decisions regarding management can become very difficult, especially those regarding possible placement in nursing homes. It is also important to discuss the issues of power of attorney, guardianship, and end-of-life issues, such as advanced directives for treatment options and life-sustaining measures (see Chapter 11 for a more detailed discussion) and, if feasible, information about arrangements for an autopsy. An examination of the brain after death may be important to help understand the cause of the dementing illness and to provide useful information for family members.

Delirium (Sudden Confusion)

A sudden change in mental function, or acute confusion, is the most common complication of hospitalization in older people. In the past, this condition was known by a variety of names including sundowning, toxic psychosis, and metabolic encephalopathy. The preferred medical term is delirium. Table 14 lists the medical criteria for the diagnosis of delirium.

What Causes Delirium?

Delirium is often caused by changes in the chemical transmitter between nerves—acetylcholine. Relatively small reductions of oxygen or glucose in the brain can significantly reduce the amount of acetylcholine made in the brain. Medications that block acetylcho-

Table 14. Clinical Criteria for Delirium

A.	Reduced ability to maintain attention to external stimuli and to appropriately shift attention to new external stimuli
B.	Disorganized thinking, as indicated by rambling, irrelevant, or incoherent speech
C.	At least two of the following: 1. Reduced level of consciousness 2. Perceptual disturbances: misinterpretations, illusions, or hallucinations 3. Disturbance of sleep-wake cycle, with insomnia or daytime sleepiness 4. Increased or decreased psychomotor activity 5. Disorientation of time, place, or person 6. Memory impairment
D.	Development of clinical features over a short period of time; tendency for them to fluctuate over the course of a day
E.	Either (1) or (2): 1. Evidence from the history, physical examination, or laboratory tests of a specific organic factor (or factors) judged to cause the disturbance 2. In the absence of such evidence, a causative factor can be presumed if the disturbance cannot be accounted for by any other mental disorder

Source: American Psychiatric Association. *Diagnostic and Statistical Manual of Mental Disorders.* 3d ed (rev). Washington, D.C.: American Psychiatric Association, 1987. Reprinted with permission.

line can produce delirium. People who have Alzheimer's disease can experience delirium in addition to dementias and appear to lose the cells in the brain that make acetylcholine.

While an interruption of these nerve signals via acetylcholine cannot explain all episodes of delirium, it is important to remember this chemical transmitter because a number of medications can affect its functioning. For example, medications given to nearly 60 percent of nursing home residents and about 25 percent of people living in the community are potentially capable of blocking at least some acetylcholine transmission.

Other substances, such as cortisol, endorphins, and small proteins have also been considered as potential causes of delirium. Information concerning these substances and their relation to delirium is very limited.

Conditions That Produce Delirium

Virtually any medical condition is a potential cause of delirium. For example, delirium may be the initial presentation of a serious life-threatening illness such as a heart attack. Often there is more than one potential cause identified in a given person with delirium. The most common causes in people who are in the hospital include problems in body chemistry, drug toxicities, infections, low blood pressure, and reduced oxygen in the blood (hypoxemia). In only a small number of people is delirium due to a sudden change in the nervous system such as a stroke, brain tumor, or an infection in the nervous system.

Delirium can also result from sensory deprivation. In one study, delirium after an operation occurred twice as often in intensive care units without windows as compared with those with windows. In addition, a form of delirium that occurs at night (sundowning) may, in part, be due to sensory deprivation. Problems with vision and hearing may make it more likely for the person to misperceive stimuli and increase their susceptibility to delusions or hallucinations.

Drugs are a leading cause of delirium in the hospital. Common drugs causing this condition include narcotics (and other pain relievers), sedatives, corticosteroids, and drugs that affect acetylcholine in the brain.

Alcohol abuse is frequently overlooked as a cause of delirium in older people. Delirium can be produced by either intoxication or an abrupt withdrawal from alcohol. Alcohol-withdrawal delirium appears to be as common in elderly people with alcoholism as in their younger counterparts. Alcohol withdrawal has an increased mortality rate in elderly people, about 25 percent in one study. Another underappreciated cause of delirium is withdrawal from sedatives.

Delirium After Surgery

Delirium after an operation is one of the most frequent conditions seen in the surgical setting, and it can be mistaken for depression. This postoperative delirium in older people leads to longer hospital stays, a higher death rate, and a greater need for nursing home care after discharge. The type of operation determines the risk for delirium. Five to 15 percent of people have delirium after cataract surgery, and over 50 percent of older people who undergo hip surgery will have delirium. Trends in surgical practice also affect one's chances of having delirium. For example, a decrease in the rates of delirium after heart surgery has been attributed to shorter time spent on the heart bypass machine and improved monitoring during surgery.

If a person has dementing illness or depression before surgery, they are at higher risk for postoperative onset of delirium. Delirium may be the initial observable manifestation of a number of medical complications that can arise after surgery, such as infection, heart difficulties, or drug toxicities.

A diagnosis of delirium is based on careful observation, awareness of changes in the person's usual mental state, and knowledge of the current physical problems. An attempt at conversation with the person reveals wandering attention, poor ability to follow directions, and easy distraction. The content of the person's speech itself may reflect disorganized thoughts and problems with perception. The person may appear restless and move a lot, and the level of consciousness may change frequently. Various disturbances may occur at night. Sometimes the muscles jerk and twitch and there can be a flapping movement of the hands, called asterixis, which is known to occur only in delirium. While asterixis is characteristic of delirium, it is a relatively uncommon occurrence.

Symptoms of Delirium

The person's difficulty in thinking may not be obvious to a casual observer, and sometimes physicians ask a series of simple standardized questions to try to evaluate mental function. The use of standardized questions makes it possible to monitor subsequent progress, to a certain extent. However, these verbal tests do not identify the key symptoms of the delirium, which usually include a lack of attention, a rapid onset, and a fluctuating course. Sometimes more sophisticated testing is recommended in order to determine and monitor these features.

The electroencephalogram (EEG) observes brain waves through electrodes placed on the scalp. It is a useful test if delirium is suspected because test results are always abnormal in this disorder.

The reason for the delirium cannot always be determined from the EEG, but if the EEG is normal, then the person does not have delirium.

Differentiating Delirium from Look-alike Conditions

Delirium can be mistaken for dementing illness or for psychiatric diseases such as schizophrenia. While much less common than delirium, certain forms of epilepsy can also closely resemble delirium.

Generally, psychiatric conditions occur in early adult life before the age of 40. *Any sudden and acute change in a person's behavior after that age should initially be considered as delirium until examination or testing proves otherwise.*

Other features that may help separate psychiatric diseases from delirium are the character of any hallucinations the person may have. Psychotic patients typically hallucinate that they are hearing voices or sounds. People with delirium usually experience visual hallucinations. In addition, the physical characteristics that are typical of delirium, such as the hand flapping, asterixis, EEG changes, and the evidence of an acute medical illness, are generally absent in psychiatric disorders.

Like delirium, dementing illness may produce memory and thinking problems. One key difference is that dementia has a much longer onset and generally fluctuates over a period of weeks to months. In addition, demented individuals generally remain aware of their environment until very late in the illness.

The two conditions can occur together, however, and delirium occurs more frequently in demented than in nondemented individuals. Up to half of demented people manifest evidence of delirium during a hospitalization for medical illness. Whenever there is a sudden deterioration in behavior or thinking in a demented person, particularly when the person is hospitalized, the cause is likely to be delirium. Sudden confusion may be due to epilepsy rather than delirium. Most of the time, when this is the case, the person is known to have a seizure disorder but in the case of some older people, sudden and acute confusion may be the initial manifestation of epilepsy.

Treatment of Delirium

Delirium is a true medical emergency and immediate medical evaluation and treatment should be obtained. The cornerstones of medical management include prompt recognition of the condition, identifying the specific cause, managing any agitation or disruptive behavior, and providing general supportive care. Because delirium can be caused by so many different things, no simple strategy for this evaluation can be given here.

Generally, the physician looks for any underlying conditions. Unless they are absolutely necessary, all drugs are generally stopped and specific laboratory tests are ordered to check for any underlying conditions.

People with delirium may have brain abnormalities that will show up on brain-imaging studies such as computed tomography or magnetic resonance imaging. However, the imaging frequently uncovers a preexisting condition that may have predisposed the person to delirium. A comprehensive medical evaluation is still needed to identify any precipitating illness, which is usually apart from the nervous system.

At times, people with delirium can be so agitated or disruptive that their behaviors must be controlled promptly to prevent them from harming themselves or others. Regretfully, there is no ideal solution to this problem.

Because sedatives do not reverse the underlying abnormalities that cause delirium, they are never to be used in people who are drowsy or not easily aroused. Furthermore, these drugs can bring on delirium. Because of this, they are usually only given for short periods of time, and their use is limited only to those people whose agitation seriously interferes with their care.

Supportive care for people with delirium includes careful attention to medical, environmental, and social situations. Medical complications include disorders of body chemistry, aspiration, malnutrition, pressure ulcers, joint stiffness, and any other conditions that might result from immobility and a reduced state of consciousness. Management of the environment involves continually helping the person feel oriented, avoiding unnecessary moves from one room or space to another, and leaving on dim lights at night to decrease delusions or hallucinations. Eyeglasses or hearing aids can help to diminish sensory isolation. Family members, close friends, or even paid assistants can participate as sitters to reduce the fear and anxiety that accompanies delirium. Professionals in social work and nursing are often quite skillful in helping the person with delirium. Decisions about nursing home care should be made cautiously because the person's hospital behavior may not accurately reflect the capacity to function in a stable, familiar environment. In addition, the delirium may be slow in resolving.

There is no evidence that using physical restraints on people with delirium is effective in reducing falls or other accidents. Furthermore, restraints increase immobility and thus the risk of contracting pneumonia, developing pressure ulcers, and even accidental strangling. Unfortunately, the harsh realities of personnel shortages in the hospital or in nursing homes (especially at night) and concerns about institutional liability in the event that residents injure themselves often make the use of physical restraints seem appealing.

Finally, treatment may be complicated by medical and legal issues. The use of restraints and strong medications constitutes a common form of involuntary treatment of an agitated person. Furthermore, civil commitment procedures are generally followed in the involuntary treatment of behaviorally disturbed people; they are not considered necessary or appropriate in treating people with delirium.

The Outlook for People with Delirium

Approximately 25 percent of people aged 70 or more who are admitted to a general medical hospital have delirium. For most of these people delirium was one of the symptoms of their medical illness. The risk of delirium is influenced by a number of factors and increases in people who are demented, dehydrated, taking drugs known to affect the nervous system, or who are judged to be severely ill by their doctor. In these older people, the delirium is not typically characterized by disruptive features (the person may be quiet and withdrawn) and may be missed by doctors or else mistaken for dementing illness.

Delirium is an underappreciated source of disability and death. Death rates are significantly higher; the relative risks for death are from 2 to 20 times greater for people with delirium than for those without it. The short-term death rate appears to be higher because of the presence of significant underlying medical problems; the longer-term death rate probably reflects the underlying frailty that predisposes a person to delirium.

Amnesia is a relatively rare memory disorder in older people that is characterized by the inability to learn or recall any new information, even though there is normal attention, memory for past events, and generally good intellectual function.

All conditions that produce amnesia share a common underlying change in the brain: a disorder located in deep brain structures. In most cases, the abnormalities must be on both sides of the brain to produce a permanent amnesia. The most common causes of amnesia include the Wernicke-Korsakoff syndrome (named for the 19th-century German professor Carl Wernicke and for Sergiei Korsakoff, a Russian neurologist), rare forms of stroke, head trauma, brain infections with the herpes virus, a period of very low blood sugar, brain tumors, and prolonged cardiac arrest that impairs blood supply to the brain. The Wernicke-Korsakoff syndrome results from thiamine depletion and is most commonly observed in patients with alcoholism. It can occur in other settings, especially with other causes of chronic nutritional depletion.

Causes of Amnesia

People with amnesia fail to learn dates and locations and are sometimes disoriented as to time and space. They cannot learn word lists for later recall. The amnesia may extend back from a few minutes to at most a few years from the onset of the memory disturbance. It is interesting that people generally do not lose their identity or forget their names. A complete loss of personal identity, such as the complete amnesiac portrayed in the movies, almost never occurs and usually indicates the presence of a severe psychiatric condition. People with amnesia do not benefit from cues to help them remember such as multiple-choice lists. Making up farfetched stories is common in the sudden onset periods of amnesic disorders. People with this condition can supply sensible and often seemingly autobiographical but totally inaccurate information in response to questions that they cannot answer accurately.

Symptoms of Amnesia

Although there is no specific therapy for amnesia, most amnesic individuals experience some degree of spontaneous recovery. Those who recover completely are never able to remember that period during which no learning occurred. Those who make a

Treatment of Amnesia

partial recovery may experience some ongoing degree of difficulty in learning. The severity of brain damage is reflected in the length of the amnesic interval of which the person remembers nothing. This may serve as a useful guide to the likelihood of recovery of function.

CHAPTER 14

NEUROLOGIC DISORDERS

Overview

Neurologic conditions are extremely common in elderly people and are a major source of disability. When cells of the nervous system disappear after severe injury, they are lost forever because they cannot reproduce; however, remaining nerve cells tend to compensate for lost neurons by growing new connections. This process resembles the growth of trees in a forest: If a tree is lost, the remaining trees sprout new branches to restore the canopy. Additional compensatory mechanisms are also available.

Neurologic problems seen in older people can be grouped into three categories: cerebrovascular disorders (those caused by problems in the blood supply to the brain), degenerative disorders (when a part of the brain atrophies), and other conditions such as brain tumors or seizures. Numerous medical conditions and a huge number of medications can affect neurologic function.

Changes in neurologic function result from diseases and cannot be ascribed to normal aging. Because of this, any new change in function must be carefully evaluated.

SYMPTOMS
Dizziness

Dizziness is used to describe a variety of unpleasant sensations that often interfere with balance and walking. It is one of the most common complaints mentioned by people over age 65. People sometimes use "dizziness" to describe unpleasant faintness, light-headedness, or poor balance. Blurred vision, double vision, and changes in blood pressure may also be interpreted as dizziness. Age-related deterioration of the balance mechanisms makes any disorder of the inner ear particularly distressing to older people. Because of this variety of symptoms, a key aspect of the evaluation involves determining exactly what a person means by "dizzy." Disequilibrium, light-headedness, and vertigo (a spinning sensation) may all be reported as dizziness, but the approaches needed for evaluation and treatment usually differ. A simple classification is dizziness without spinning sensation and dizziness with spinning sensation.

Dizziness Without Spinning Sensation

Several disorders, such as disequilibrium (unsteadiness) and light-headedness, may interfere with walking, but do not cause a spinning sensation. A person may complain of poor balance or dizziness.

Causes of Dizziness Without Spinning Sensation. Disequilibrium in elderly people may be caused by deficiencies in sensory perception. Poor vision, arthritis, and foot problems may contribute to this condition of altered sensation. A previous stroke can produce sensory problems that are experienced as a balance problem or dizziness. Some people who complain of dizziness actually mean light-headedness. In this condition, the problem is rarely in the nervous system and it is almost never caused by small strokes. A few people with epilepsy may have this complaint, but the most likely causes of light-headedness are changes in blood pressure with standing (orthostatic hypotension), irregular heartbeat, near fainting, anxiety, depression, and severe narrowing of a heart valve.

Management of Dizziness Without Spinning Sensation. The management of such disequilibrium begins with avoiding medications that could be contributing to the problem. A cane can help stabilize the person's walking by adding an extra sense of the ground. Proper glasses and a hearing aid may be helpful for people with vision and hearing problems. Keeping the lights on at night helps to prevent falls by increasing sensory input. Management of heart and blood pressure problems is tailored to the specific condition.

Vertigo is defined as a spinning sensation, a distortion of orientation, or the erroneous perception of motion. It may be present all the time or brought on by certain positions.

Dizziness with Vertigo, a Spinning Sensation

Causes of Dizziness with Vertigo. Stroke and transient ischemic attacks (TIAs) involving the circulation in the base of the brain can cause sudden vertigo. A stroke or bleeding in the cerebellum can cause sudden vertigo, but this is usually associated with sudden arm or leg clumsiness or a staggering gait. This condition occurs abruptly and often the person cannot walk. Vomiting is a frequent sign of this disorder, but headache is not common.

Disorders of the inner ear (the labyrinth) are usually the cause when vertigo is the only neurologic symptom. A prominent feature of this is a rhythmic oscillation of the eyes called nystagmus. A person with inner ear problems may have experienced similar vertiginous attacks in the past. While not life-threatening, inner ear problems can be disabling. People complain of spinning (usually away from the side of the affected ear), difficulty walking, nausea, and vomiting.

Inflammation of the inner ear, known as neurolabyrinthitis, is characterized by the sudden onset of very severe vertigo continuing for up to 24 hours. There are no changes in hearing and no other neurologic findings. It is a benign condition that can occur as a single episode or can recur. It is thought to be caused by a viral infection of the nerves in the ear.

Benign positional vertigo is severe vertigo that occurs with a particular head position or on turning. It can be brought on if a person tilts the head back and sometimes occurs again when sitting up. If this maneuver is repeated many times in succession, the intensity of the vertigo may decrease. While this condition generally gets better on its own, it can recur. The person can generally avoid further attacks by learning to change positions slowly. The condition is caused by abnormalities in the middle ear.

People with problems in the cerebellum or brain stem may also have vertigo when they change positions. In such cases, vertigo begins immediately with the change of position and lasts longer than 30 to 40 seconds. It does not get better after repeated movements.

Recurrent vertigo with progressive hearing loss is called Ménière's disease (after the 19th-century French scientist, Prosper Ménière, who first described vertigo related to the inner ear). It is characterized by episodes of severe vertigo, nausea, and vomiting that may last for a week or more and may be disabling. Between episodes are often mild dizziness and ringing in the ears. The disorder worsens, eventually leaving the older person deaf and in some cases with impaired balance and gait. An interesting phenomenon early in the course of the illness is that people traveling in an airplane often describe improvement in their symptoms, possibly due to the decrease in atmospheric pressure.

Management of Vertigo. Older people with sudden vertigo may require hospitalization to prevent dehydration due to vomiting. Treatment generally consists of rest and mild sedation. People usually tolerate positional vertigo without medicines once they have learned to adapt their movements.

Fainting (Syncope)

The medical term for loss of consciousness, or fainting, is syncope (pronounced SIN-co-pee, from the Greek meaning "to cut off"). Syncope involves a transient loss of consciousness accompanied by unresponsiveness and loss of muscle tone followed by a spontaneous recovery. It occurs in response to a sudden loss of blood flow to the brain; it is not considered a disease in itself, but rather a symptom of one or more possibly serious conditions.

Syncope occurs in about 2 percent of people between the ages of 65 and 69. It increases to about 12 percent in those over age 85.

About 6 percent of people in institutions have syncope and about one-third of these people have multiple attacks. The death rate for people who have syncope is about 1½ times that for people who do not have syncope. This is probably due to the underlying disease itself rather than the loss of consciousness.

People over the age of 65 who have experienced loss of consciousness due to heart disease have a 33 percent risk of death after one year. This death rate is compared to the 6 to 12 percent rate for those who experience loss of consciousness due to other causes. For those people with no clear cause of syncope, the death rate is about 6 percent. Syncope does not produce a significant increase in death rate for older people in nursing homes, but it is an important risk factor for accidents, such as falls.

Causes of Syncope

Loss of consciousness may be due to normal cardiovascular aging (as described below) or to underlying diseases or medications that can interfere with normal blood pressure control. Generally, when we stand up, between one and two pints of blood become temporarily pooled in our legs. In younger people this reduction in circulating blood volume is detected by receptors in the lungs and large blood vessels in the neck. These receptors alert the nervous system, which, in response, signals the blood vessels in the legs to contract, and the heart to beat faster. This protects the person from having any large drop in blood pressure. With aging, there is a progressive decrease in the heart's ability to beat faster after a change of position, a period of exercise, a loss of blood volume, or in response to other stimuli. Consequently, the heart does not always respond promptly or adequately to signals from the nervous system telling it to beat faster in response to reduced blood volume and, ultimately, our blood pressure drops. This age-related decline in maximum heart rate leaves us vulnerable to a drop in blood pressure and possible syncope.

The kidney's decreasing ability to retain sodium coupled with a blunted thirst response to dehydration predispose us to dehydration and a drop in blood pressure as we age. An additional factor is that the aging heart does not relax quite as effectively between beats. Because of this, our heart must have as much blood returned to it as possible to maintain a normal blood pressure. Therefore, we become increasingly vulnerable to a drop in blood pressure if our blood volume is reduced or if medications cause our blood vessels to dilate.

Blood flow to the brain is also reduced with aging and if relatively common diseases like congestive heart failure or blood vessel disease to the brain (carotid artery disease) are superimposed, this can cause a further reduction in blood flow. These conditions can bring the blood flow to the brain close to the critical threshold required to maintain consciousness. Because of this increased vulnerability, relatively mild disturbances such as rapid breathing or mild dehydration can lead to a drop in the blood flow to the brain and produce syncope. Furthermore, since high blood pressure may have conditioned the blood vessels in the brain to adjust to a higher level of blood pressure, older people with high blood pressure may require this increase in pressure to maintain adequate levels of blood flow to the brain.

The causes of syncope, as shown in Table 15, can be classified as orthostatic hypotension (low blood pressure syndromes), abnormalities in the composition of the blood, heart disease, and primary brain disorders.

Orthostatic Hypotension. A drop in the blood pressure with changing position from lying to standing is called orthostatic hypotension.

Table 15. Causes of Fainting (Syncope)

ABNORMAL BLOOD COMPOSITION	
BRAIN DISORDERS	
Blood vessel disease	Seizures
HEART AND CIRCULATORY DISEASES	
Heart attack	Pulmonary embolism
Heart rhythm problems	Heart valve problems
ORTHOSTATIC HYPOTENSION (LOW BLOOD PRESSURE)	
Blood vessel dilation	Volume depletion
Drugs	

This is a common cause of syncope. Estimates of how common orthostatic hypotension is vary widely, but probably around 5 percent of older people with normal blood pressure have significant orthostatic hypotension. For people with high blood pressure, this prevalence may increase to 20 to 30 percent. The strictest definition of orthostatic hypotension is a drop in the blood pressure of 20 millimeters of mercury or more, with standing, and is associated with symptoms such as light-headedness, dizziness, or unsteadiness. Orthostatic hypotension suggests an underlying inability to maintain blood pressure that predisposes the person to a further blood pressure reduction as a result of dehydration, blood loss, or medications.

There are several causes of orthostatic hypotension. The adverse effects of medications are the most common cause of orthostatic hypotension in older people. Drugs used to treat depression or high blood pressure are common offenders. Sometimes the blood pressure will drop immediately after eating and this may be further worsened by taking blood pressure medications just before meals. Prolonged bed rest can also result in a drop in blood pressure when a person rises from bed to a standing position. This is probably caused by deconditioning of the cardiovascular system.

Orthostatic hypotension can also result from disease states of the nervous system. The symptoms that suggest such diseases include dizziness on standing, visual problems, urinary incontinence, an inability to sweat, difficulty tolerating the heat, constipation, chronic fatigue, and impotence. Parkinson's disease, multiple strokes, and other vascular problems are common central nervous system disorders that are associated with orthostatic hypotension and problems maintaining the blood pressure. (See Table 16 for approaches to managing orthostatic hypotension.)

Other Causes of Syncope. In some cases syncope can be explained by increased sensitivity of pressure sensors in the neck, which can be further aggravated by tight collars, neck turning, and various drugs.

In people who have other risk factors, urinating, passing a bowel movement, and coughing can produce loss of consciousness. This syncope occurs as a result of the combined effects of impaired return of blood flow to the heart, nervous system reflexes, and of

**Table 16. Management of
Orthostatic Hypotension**

NONPHARMACOLOGIC INTERVENTIONS

Substitution or discontinuation of offending medications

While recumbent, exercising the legs and feet prior to standing

Wearing full-length elastic stockings

Maintaining a high-salt diet (in absence of fluid overload or heart failure)

Elevating the head of the bed 5 to 20 degrees

age-related changes in the ability of the heart to speed up and to constrict the blood vessels in the legs. Syncope after a meal may represent a drop in blood pressure due to blood pooling in the abdomen.

Severe narrowing of one of the heart valves, called aortic stenosis, is the most common change in the structure in the heart. In this condition, fainting during physical activity depends on how tight the narrowing is. In older people, loss of consciousness is sometimes the sole symptom of a heart attack, representing injury-related reductions in the ability of the heart to pump blood. Irregular heart rhythms can also produce loss of consciousness by reducing blood flow to the brain. It is rare for syncope to occur as the result of a primary problem in the brain such as a stroke or epilepsy; but when it does, there are usually other severe neurologic changes. Seizures, however, may accompany syncope regardless of its cause.

How Syncope Is Evaluated

Even after an extensive evaluation, the cause of syncope is not always clear. About one-third of people evaluated have a specific disease-related cause such as heart disease; another third have low blood pressure caused by orthostatic hypotension, eating, or medications; and in the last third no clear cause is ever discovered. The evaluation includes documentation of factors that led up to the loss of consciousness, the time it began, how long it lasted, and how the person recovered. Knowing about additional symptoms can also be helpful. Any prescriptions or over-the-counter medications must be evaluated.

A physical examination includes measuring blood pressure while the person is in different positions, including lying, sitting, and standing. The intensity, rhythm, and quality of the pulse measured in the neck, arms, and legs are evaluated. The person is further examined for signs of heart disease, gastrointestinal bleeding, decreased blood volume, and diseases of the nervous system. People aged 70 or older often have syncope in association with an irregular heartbeat. A common procedure is to check for this condition with an electrocardiogram monitor that can record heartbeats for 24 hours while the person carries on normal activities, and in particular the activities performed at the time of loss of consciousness. On the other hand, since so many people aged 75 and older have irregularities in their heartbeat rhythm, arrhythmia by itself, when there is no loss of consciousness, is not necessarily a dangerous symptom.

Management of Syncope

It may be possible to treat older people for a specific cause of syncope, but, more often, multiple potential causes may need to be treated. An important decision is whether to discontinue or change the doses of medications potentially causing low blood pressure. A person using medication for high blood pressure may need to adjust the dosing schedule, particularly at mealtimes, because some older people develop low blood pressure after eating.

Seizures

A seizure may occur as a single event that is produced by a specific problem and that recurs over time with varying frequency. This recurring type of single seizures is called epilepsy. Seizures can also be continuous, consisting of sequences of fits separated by minutes or seconds—a condition called status epilepticus. In about 90 percent of elderly people with the new onset of seizures, there is an identifiable brain problem.

Types of Seizures

The various types of seizures are classified and defined according to their characteristics as noted by a physician and the results of an electroencephalogram (EEG) test (sometimes called a brain wave test). Generalized seizures cause the person to lose consciousness while convulsive movement occurs on both sides of the body.

Generalized major seizures, called grand mal seizures, are the ones most commonly seen in elderly people. Petit mal seizures are also encountered in adults. These cause a momentary loss of awareness without any major movement. The person stares off into space for a few seconds and then returns to consciousness (sometimes completing the sentence started just prior to the onset of the seizure). Focal or partial seizures are ones that emanate from a particular part of the brain and are manifested by a sudden change in movement, sensation, or behavior. The person usually remains conscious during this sort of seizure. In one variation, called complex partial seizures, there can be an alteration in consciousness. Complex partial seizures arise from an abnormality in the temporal lobe of the brain, the part of the brain just above the ear. The temporal lobe seizure syndrome varies but it often involves psychiatric phenomena such as hallucinations, illusions, panic states, and bizarre activity of the arms and legs. Partial seizures can also develop into generalized seizures.

Causes of Seizures

About half of the seizures that older people experience for the first time are caused by strokes that occurred earlier in the person's life. These strokes are usually small and may have been forgotten or never clinically identified. In another 12 percent of people, seizures occur at the onset of an acute (sudden) stroke caused by a blood clot that has traveled into the brain, called an embolus. Seizures can also occur during the rehabilitation phase in about 15 percent of individuals suffering from an acute stroke. About 10 percent of people who have had a stroke suffer a recurring seizure disorder that requires treatment with medications. Bleeding within the brain and hemorrhages in the brain lining frequently cause seizures during the acute phase of the event.

Seizures that are caused by any structural problem within the brain may be provoked by an underlying infectious illness or a change in body chemistry. Focal seizures in elderly people can be caused by brain tumors, brain abscesses, and previous head trauma. People who have meningitis or encephalitis can also have generalized seizures. About 25 percent of people in the late stages of Alzheimer's disease can have generalized seizures. Multiple strokes that cause dementia may also produce seizures.

The temporary neurologic dysfunction that occurs after a focal seizure can sometimes be confused with that of a transient ischemic attack (TIA). (TIAs are discussed later in this chapter.) They represent a transient disability that completely resolves in a few minutes to hours. Focal sensory seizures can cause temporary numbness or other subjective feelings of abnormality, for example, vision shifts, funny smells, or strange sounds. A person may also move differently, whether or not he or she experiences the sensory phenomena. Intermittent rhythmic moving of a hand or foot, facial twitching, or other jerky movements are all possible indications of an underlying seizure. When the focal movement problem spreads, the person loses consciousness and develops a generalized seizure. If the focus of the seizure is in the part of the brain that controls movement, the person may, at the cessation of the seizure, develop mild paralysis (called Todd's paralysis, for the American neurologist Eli Todd) that usually disappears within a few hours. Sometimes the Todd's paralysis can last a day or so and create the misleading impression that the person has had a stroke. Fortunately, in most instances the paralysis disappears with no aftereffects.

The Evaluation of Seizures

Because seizures can be associated with so many different disorders, the physician's evaluation is comprehensive. A complete medical and neurologic examination can sometimes show sudden illnesses that precipitated the seizure. A spinal tap may be necessary if the physician suspects meningitis because of the presence of fever, changes in mental function, or a severe or persistent headache. Brain imaging, such as a CT scan or an MRI scan, is usually suggested to identify abnormalities in the brain such as tumors, abscesses, or blood clots. The MRI is usually better than a CT in identifying these abnormalities.

The electroencephalogram (EEG) can sometimes be helpful in identifying the focal point of the seizure activity. An EEG is not needed to detect that a person is having or has had a grand mal seizure—these seizures speak for themselves. However, in more subtle seizures the EEG can help to identify the abnormal brain waves that explain the person's behavior while the seizure is taking place. Elderly people with recurrent seizures can have abnormal EEG tracings that reflect an abnormality in the brain structure. However, people who have had a single seizure due to effects of medication or a change in body chemistry may have a normal EEG after the seizure. The amount of abnormality on the EEG does not tell much about the severity of the underlying cause.

Treatment for Seizures

The first step in the management of a person with recurrent seizures is to correct any underlying process that might be provoking the seizures. A brain abnormality that might be the cause of seizure might also be impossible to remove, but it still may be possible to improve the person's state of health. Common problems of body chemistry that can induce or aggravate seizures include having a low level of sodium in the blood, a low calcium level, low blood sugar, and alcohol toxicity.

Drug treatment is usually the next step in management. The choice of a particular drug is less important than its correct use. It may take a while for a medication to stop the seizures, and dosages should be changed only after appropriate blood levels of the medication have been maintained at a steady state and have failed to stop the seizures. In older people, side effects can occur at much lower doses than they do in younger people. For example, some medications used to control seizures may diminish cognitive function in older people and in some individuals doses can impair memory and cause changes in behavior. Because of this, the medication initially chosen should be given in an adequate dose for a period long enough for the drug to reach its steady state in the blood before it is replaced by another medication or another medication added to the regimen. If possible, the medication should be taken in once-a-day dosages in order to simplify the routine. Such once-a-day dosing should be adhered to if it is at all possible.

Recurring seizures that are caused by problems in the brain, such as strokes or brain tumors, are more difficult to control than those seizures that occur in the late stage of Alzheimer's disease. The person with Alzheimer's disease may have a single seizure as the result of some other illness; there is no need to treat such a seizure unless it recurs. People with Alzheimer's disease have an increased chance of developing a hemorrhage and subsequent blood clot in the space between the brain and the skull, a condition called a subdural hematoma. This condition may cause and thus reveal itself through a seizure.

A tremor is medically defined as the involuntary vibrating movement across a joint caused by muscle contractions. Tremors are generally described in terms of how rapid they are, how much shaking appears, and whether the tremor occurs without movement at rest or whether it occurs with action. All tremors get worse with emotional stimulation, and they all disappear with sleeping.

Tremors

Tremors are classified as either resting tremors or action tremors. In "resting" tremors, the shaking worsens when the body rests and actually goes away with movement. In contrast, with the "action" tremor, no tremor is evident at rest, but it appears when the body part is moved and often gets much worse as the body part moves away from the body. Resting tremors are caused by Parkinson's disease, which produces dysfunction of deep structures in the brain called basal ganglia. Action tremors are often seen in diseases of the cerebellum, the back portion of the brain that helps coordinate movement.

Types of Tremors

Normal, healthy people have a very rapid fine-action tremor—called physiologic tremor—that can easily be observed by placing a piece of typing paper on one's outstretched fingers. The edge of the paper exhibits a very fine movement indicative of this normal vibration. This normal tremor may become more evident in states of anxiety, exercise, sleep deprivation, or by stimulant drugs so that it can be seen clinically. This is the tremor of nervousness or stage fright.

An action tremor that originates in the central nervous system, called essential tremor, is a tremor that is somewhat slower and more pronounced than the physiologic tremor and is more evident on action. Usually this tremor affects the arms more than the legs, and it sometimes produces head bobbing. There is often a family history of a similar tremor.

Mild sedation may help the person with an essential tremor. Initially, alcohol diminishes the tremor, but once alcohol has been metabolized, the tremor may become worse. The prescription drug

Treatment of Tremors

propranolol is sometimes used to reduce the amount of vibration produced by the essential tremor.

Speaking Difficulty (Aphasia)

The difficulty in speaking, called aphasia, involves a diminished language capacity produced by a specific problem in the brain. Aphasia is different from mutism, which is a state where no sounds are produced. It is also to be distinguished from dysarthria, which is a disturbance that reflects the loss of control over the voice box and other parts of the speech production apparatus. Dysarthria is characterized by slurring words, imprecise articulation, and a distortion of sounds.

Types of Aphasia

Aphasias are generally classified according to the person's fluency of speech, comprehension of spoken language, and ability to repeat words and phrases. This classification also helps the examiner to deduce the site within the brain of the problem causing the abnormality. Since most aphasias include naming problems, difficulty with this task is a useful way of identifying an aphasic disturbance from other speech problems. On the other hand, it is not helpful in telling the type of aphasia since it is common to all types. Writing abnormalities almost always mirror the characteristics of the person's spoken voice, but reading aloud and reading comprehension are affected differently in various types of aphasia and are usually evaluated separately.

The characteristics of spontaneous, verbal output help determine whether the aphasia is fluent or nonfluent. Nonfluent aphasias are characterized by a relative lack of speech, effortful speech production, problems with pronunciation, decreased phrase length, and problems with grammar, but what the person says conveys useful information. In addition, there are few paraphasic errors. Paraphasic errors may be literal, where sounds or homonyms are substituted, or they may be verbal, where one word is substituted for another, or they may be nonsense words. The fluent aphasias are characterized by normal-sounding speech or even an increased amount of speech. The speech production seems to require little effort and the phrase lengths sound normal. Other characteristics include normal speech melody and inflection, but the content is empty with very little information, and there are a number of paraphasic errors. Fluent aphasias may also be associated with difficulties doing calculations, telling right from left, identifying fingers, and problems in establishing the order of various tasks.

Aphasia may occur with any disorder that involves the left side of the brain (in the area near the left ear) in people who are right-handed and for most people who are left-handed. Aphasia is observed in people who have had strokes, brain tumors, trauma, and in dementing disorders such as Alzheimer's disease and Pick's disease. The nonfluent aphasias usually result from carotid or middle cerebral artery disease, while fluent aphasia usually results from emboli, blood clots that travel to the brain and obstruct an artery.

Causes of Aphasias

An evaluation of a person with aphasia generally involves testing spontaneous speech, comprehension, repetition, naming, reading, and writing. Comprehension is often assessed by asking people to follow simple instructions such as to point to objects in a room and to answer yes or no questions. Attention is tested by asking the person to repeat words, phrases, and increasingly long sentences. The ability to name objects is evaluated by pointing to various objects in a room, body parts, or items of clothing. Reading is usually assessed by having the person read aloud and follow written commands. Writing is evaluated by having the person write words, phrases, and sentences.

Evaluation of Aphasias

Management first involves identifying the cause and then specifying the treatment. Partial recovery from aphasia is the rule. Speech and language therapy produce improvement in function. Aphasias involving the least loss of speech functioning are generally associated with the best long-term improvement.

Treatment of Aphasias

Huntington's disease (named after the American doctor, George Huntington, who described it) is an inherited dementing illness. This disease affects the nervous system and is characterized by abnormal movements and psychiatric symptoms. Virtually all of the cases of this disease in the U.S.A. have been traced back to six individuals who emigrated from England in 1632. The illness usually begins when the person is between 30 and 40, but it may occur before the

CONDITIONS
Huntington's Disease

173

age of 15. About a quarter of cases occur after 50. It affects between 3 and 7 people per 100,000 people in the population at large.

Cause of Huntington's Disease

Atrophy in two deep brain structures called the caudate and putamen are characteristic of the disease. The genetic defect for Huntington's disease is on the short arm of chromosome 4.

Symptoms of Huntington's Disease

Mental difficulties may precede or follow the movement disorder in Huntington's disease. The movement disorder is characterized by writhing, jerky movements; it usually begins in the hands and face and eventually involves the limbs, neck, and trunk; abnormal movements of the eyes are frequently seen. Individuals may become depressed or irritable, aggressive, and impulsive; occasionally, a major psychiatric illness may develop. As the disease progresses, thought processes slow, impairment of insight and judgment occurs, and people display an inability to maintain a set of activities or to organize their thoughts. There may be impaired memory, especially for skilled activities.

Treatment of Huntington's Disease

Currently Huntington's disease has no satisfactory treatment. However, genetic research holds considerable promise for a cure at some point in the future.

Parkinson's Disease

Parkinson's disease (named for the English physician who first described it in 1817, James Parkinson) is the second most common degenerative disease of the nervous system—the most common is Alzheimer's disease. Parkinson's disease is a slowly progressive disease of the nervous system that is associated with an average survival of about 14 years, although people can live considerably longer. It is fairly common in people between 60 and 65 years of age and is most common among those aged 75 and older.

Causes of Parkinson's Disease

In Parkinson's disease, there is a loss of the nerve cells in the brain that contain a dark pigment. These pigmented cells normally produce a substance called dopamine, which acts as a chemical messenger between nerve cells. Dopamine production is markedly reduced in the parts of the brain that contain these pigmented neurons. No one knows why these neurons are lost in Parkinson's disease.

Long-term exposure to the metal manganese can cause a syndrome that resembles Parkinson's disease, but in most cases it has not been possible to relate the disease to a specific environmental toxin. Research on possible environmental factors continues.

The principal feature of Parkinson's disease is slowing of movement (bradykinesia). This slowing occurs not only in the initiation of movement but also in a reduction in speed during the course of movement. This slowness starts on one side of the body and usually ends up involving both sides. The slowness progresses from the hands toward the body. Very early in the condition, the arm fails to swing normally when the person is walking. Late in the disease there is almost no movement in the body at all. The slowness of a single arm or leg in early Parkinson's disease can be confused with paralysis, but a person with Parkinson's disease has normal power of movement if given enough time. In addition to this slowed movement, people with Parkinson's disease have stiffness in the muscles so that if the arm or leg is moved passively by another person, there is a fluid resistance to movement. To the examiner, the arm feels like it is being moved through a sea of cold molasses.

Symptoms of Parkinson's Disease

Most people with Parkinson's disease have a distinctive coarse tremor at rest. The tremor begins at the fingers with a pill-rolling movement and over time begins to involve the hands and then the arms. The combination of the resting tremor, the muscle stiffness, and the lack of movement represents the hallmark of Parkinson's disease. The lack of movement interferes with walking, producing the characteristic bent-over shuffling gait. Generally, people are not prone to falling early in the course of the disease, but as it progresses they develop an increasingly unstable gait. Another feature is softening of the voice so that late in the course of the illness, the person speaks in a whisper. Fine movements of the hands, such as buttoning shirts or tying shoelaces, may be impaired. Some people notice that their handwriting gets smaller and smaller as the disease progresses.

Depression and dementing illness are other important components of Parkinson's disease. As many as 40 percent of Parkinson's victims have some type of depression, which may be due to changes in the chemical breakdown of certain brain substances and not simply due to despair over the loss of function.

Constipation is another common symptom of Parkinson's disease. Contributing factors include decreased physical activity, disease-related changes in bowel function, and the effect of drugs. Treatment for this usually involves forcing fluids, modifying the diet, and using laxatives. Another common feature is drooling, caused by the person's infrequent swallowing and posture, which is usually bent forward. People can lose weight during their illness, and this weight loss is not always due to a decrease in appetite. Excessive oily dandruff on the scalp and eyebrows and dry eyes and dry skin are other complaints.

Treatment of Parkinson's Disease

The management of Parkinson's disease requires careful cooperation with the primary physician. The mainstay of treatment is levodopa (L-dopa), which the body converts to the missing substance, dopamine. L-dopa is usually combined with another medicine called carbidopa, which keeps this conversion from happening outside of the brain, allowing more of the L-dopa to be delivered to the brain. Elderly people are often started on 25 milligrams of carbidopa and 100 milligrams of L-dopa administered twice a day. The dose is gradually increased until symptoms decrease or side effects appear. Usually a total daily dose of 75 to 100 milligrams of carbidopa is necessary to reduce the side effects of L-dopa: nausea, diarrhea, low blood pressure, and irregular heartbeat.

However, the most significant adverse reactions to these medications in elderly people are the precipitation of sudden psychosis and hallucinations. People who are taking L-dopa can also develop other movement problems such as writhing of the arms or neck, which they seem to tolerate better than the slowness or cessation of movement. Another medication, called selegiline, helps to increase the effects of L-dopa and lengthen its action. This medication is a weak antidepressant; the antidepressant effects may contribute to its effectiveness. In addition, several studies suggest that selegiline may actually help prevent loss of nerve cells.

Amantadine, a drug used for influenza, has been helpful in some people. It is not clear exactly how it works, but it seems to influence the release of dopamine. Amantadine is usually given with L-dopa, but it is common for the beneficial effects to wear out after a few months. Sometimes hallucinations and delirium occur as side effects to amantadine.

Occasionally, bromocriptine, a dopamine stimulant, is added to the L-dopa and carbidopa regimen. Bromocriptine is particularly apt to cause psychosis in elderly people, so the initial dosage is usually extremely low. Pergolide is another dopamine stimulant that is associated with the same adverse effects as bromocriptine.

When used alone, drugs that block acetylcholine, a different chemical messenger, or neurotransmitter, may reduce the symptoms of Parkinson's disease. These drugs can also be added to a regimen if L-dopa and carbidopa fail to relieve the person's symptoms adequately. The side effects associated with these drugs include dry mouth, constipation, difficulty voiding, lethargy, and psychosis or delirium.

Disorders Similar to Parkinson's Disease

While a number of disorders produce a condition that resembles Parkinson's disease, telltale differences can help distinguish them. Progressive supranuclear palsy is a degenerative disorder that causes slow movements and sometimes a tremor; however, this disease usually progresses much more rapidly than Parkinson's. A person with progressive supranuclear palsy falls early in the course of the disease and experiences difficulty with the tongue, mouth, and other muscles around the face. Difficulty speaking and swallowing are early findings. In addition, stiffness usually occurs in the body and then spreads to the arms and legs, rather than starting in the arms and legs and spreading to the body as in Parkinson's disease. However, the most distinctive feature of progressive supranuclear palsy is the onset of difficulty in moving the eyes up and down and later from side to side. While people with Parkinson's disease may have some mild limitations of eye movements, they experience this to a much lesser degree.

An illness called Shy-Drager syndrome causes a combination of slow movements, significant nervous system dysfunction, clumsiness, and additional findings that are not seen in Parkinson's disease. Another way to differentiate these conditions is that neither Shy-Drager syndrome nor progressive supranuclear palsy responds to L-dopa.

Although people who have many small strokes appear to be slow moving, a physician can usually tell that they are only slow to begin movement but not slow to execute the movement. They generally do not have tremors and show signs of increased muscle tone (spasticity) rather than stiffness (rigidity).

Movement Problems Caused by Drugs

The drugs used to treat psychiatric diseases (antipsychotic drugs) often interfere with dopamine release and are among the major causes of movement disorders in elderly people. The factors that determine the severity of the movement problem are the dosage of the drug, the length of time the person has been on it, being older, and being female.

Parkinsonism (conditions that look like but are not Parkinson's disease) is an expected effect of the long-term use of antipsychotic drugs. Some people with drug-induced parkinsonism do not have the muscle stiffness that is seen with Parkinson's disease. The manifestations of drug-induced parkinsonism usually disappear when the drugs are stopped, but years of high-dose therapy may produce parkinsonism that does not disappear.

Tardive dyskinesias are movement disorders that develop after months or years of taking antipsychotic drugs. These movements consist of rapid irregular muscle contractions that cause the person's lips, tongue, face, and neck to move constantly and purposelessly. Tongue movement can be especially evident and can protrude from the mouth in a "fly-catching" motion. The lips can smack and form many odd facial expressions.

Sometimes long-term antipsychotic drug treatment causes extreme restlessness and an inability to remain still. Antipsychotic drugs can also cause sudden muscle reactions in any part of the body. The person usually complains of cramps and other pains as well as severe stiffness.

Usually, these reactions are transient in nature, but they can be relieved immediately with specific medications. Movement disorders—tardive dyskinesia—that are a much-delayed reaction to long-term antipsychotic drug therapy become initially worse when the antipsychotic drug is stopped. However, they diminish within a month or so. The abnormal movements also decrease when the dose of these drugs is increased but they usually reappear shortly.

People with this condition seldom complain of the mouth and tongue movements, although they are quite disfiguring. In managing tardive dyskinesia, the older person and the physician together have to weigh the benefits and risks of the antipsychotic medicine. Clearly, using the lowest effective dose for the shortest period of time reduces the chance of precipitating a tardive movement disorder.

Stroke

A stroke is an injury to brain tissue that occurs when the blood supply to the brain is inadequate due to disease or obstruction of arteries in the head and neck. The part of the brain involved is unable to transmit signals to other parts of the nervous system, thus affecting any number of body functions (see Figure 12).

Over the past 40 years, the incidence of stroke has declined in people who are younger than 70. The reasons for the decline are not completely understood, but more aggressive treatment of high blood pressure may be a factor. However, the risk of stroke remains 12 times greater for people in their late seventies compared with the risk for those in their late fifties.

Causes of Strokes

Three mechanisms can produce a stroke: (1) a clot can form within a large or small artery supplying blood to the brain, a condition called thrombosis; (2) a clot can travel from the heart or neck up into the brain where it obstructs an artery—this is an embolus; (3) an artery can burst and hemorrhage inside the brain. Determining which of these three causes has produced a stroke is often difficult and can elude even the most sophisticated clinical examination. Generally speaking, about 35 percent of strokes are hemorrhages, 15 percent are due to emboli, and the rest are thought to be due to thrombosis.

Large-Artery Strokes

A stroke due to an obstruction or narrowing of a large artery is often preceded by a period of reduced blood supply to the brain.

Cause of Large-Artery Strokes. Hardening of the arteries, called atherosclerosis, is the most common cause of carotid artery narrowing, but a tear in an arterial wall, a constricting tumor, or other diseases involving the arteries must be considered.

Symptoms of Large-Artery Strokes. Reduced blood flow in a large artery is manifested by changes in function and sensation in the hands and face and usually lasts less than 15 minutes. If the left side of the brain is affected, then sudden difficulty in speaking can occur. This transition disability that completely resolves in minutes to hours is called a transient ischemic attack (TIA). About 50 to 75 percent of the time, a stroke due to obstruction of the main artery supplying blood to the brain (the carotid artery, which runs up the neck) is preceded by one or more transient ischemic attacks. However, among all stroke types, a preceding TIA occurs only about 10 percent of the time. The TIA may be followed by a sudden deficit in a person's ability to function normally or fluctuating deficits that develop over a period of 12 to 48 hours. About 20 percent of the time, a stroke occurs suddenly without any warning or fluctuation. The carotid artery is the site of the clot in about 5 to 6 percent of all strokes caused by decreased blood flow to the brain. After the initial stroke, there is an 8 percent chance that a second stroke will occur within the first month.

If the blood clot affects blood circulation in the back of the head (in the region of the basilar artery), the progression of symptoms goes from dizziness to headache and finally to coma. Depending on the severity of the stroke, people may have difficulty speaking, numbness on one half of the body, double vision, weakness of the face, and weakness on both sides of the body. These manifestations may be temporary, or they may fluctuate. If they become worse, the person may not survive.

The number or severity of TIAs does not reliably predict the severity of a potential stroke. Nonetheless, a TIA must be taken as a signal for a possible stroke, and the person who has had a TIA should be thoroughly evaluated to determine the source of the problem.

Evaluation of Strokes

Physicians have many tests available to look for narrowings or plaques in the carotid artery, and the choice of the appropriate procedures must be individualized. A conventional angiogram—injecting radiographic dye into a blood vessel and then taking X rays—remains the definitive method for evaluating vascular changes and for examining the rest of the circulation within the brain. This is often a necessary procedure for people who are considering surgical options. The risk associated with angiography is directly related to the person's overall condition and to the experience of the radiologist performing the procedure. Frequent evaluations are necessary for people whose neurological findings keep changing in order to determine the direction of change. For people who have thrombotic strokes (due to blood clots without TIAs), a functional problem that gets better and then worse usually signifies that the functional problem will become permanent and irreversible. However, the fact that the stroke has a gradual progression sometimes allows for treatment before a person has permanently lost the capacity to function.

Treatment of Strokes

Surgery to remove a plaque or to open a narrowed artery is an option for healthy people who have many symptoms related to the tight arterial narrowing of at least 70 percent or more. The use of blood thinners, called anticoagulants (heparin and coumadin), is another option to prevent strokes in people with recurrent TIAs or symptomatic carotid artery narrowing. These drugs are generally used for several months. Treatment does not appear to be necessary for people known to have carotid artery disease but who have no symptoms.

Aspirin and other drugs that affect blood platelets also seem to help prevent TIAs and subsequent strokes. Aspirin reduces the risk of stroke due to carotid artery disease from approximately 19 to 12 percent over a three-year period. Though the recommended dose of aspirin varies, one regular aspirin (300 mg) a day seems sufficient.

In a stroke, the aim of the initial therapy is to prevent or reduce the extent of injury to brain tissues. If it is clear that bleeding is not present (usually determined by a brain imaging study such as a computed tomography or CT scan) anticoagulation with heparin is sometimes started. Large strokes sometimes cause fluid retention, and consequent swelling in the brain can occur during the first 36 hours. Lethargy, coma, and sometimes death follow this rise in increased pressure caused by the swelling within the head. With such large strokes, it is likely that the person will not be able to function independently.

Figure 12. Brain Areas Affected by Strokes

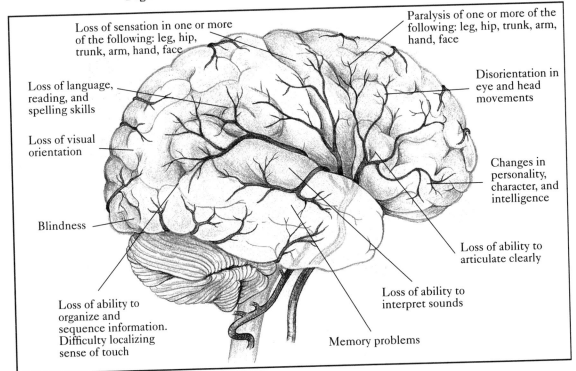

Loss of sensation in one or more of the following: leg, hip, trunk, arm, hand, face

Paralysis of one or more of the following: leg, hip, trunk, arm, hand, face

Loss of language, reading, and spelling skills

Disorientation in eye and head movements

Loss of visual orientation

Changes in personality, character, and intelligence

Blindness

Loss of ability to articulate clearly

Loss of ability to organize and sequence information. Difficulty localizing sense of touch

Loss of ability to interpret sounds

Memory problems

After a stroke has occurred, careful physical and neurologic examination supplemented by special X ray procedures, such as a CT scan or MRI, can identify the location of the stroke and the arteries involved.

Small Blood Vessel Strokes

The tiny end-branches of the large blood arteries penetrate deep within the brain to serve the basal ganglia, the thalamus, the white matter below the cortex, and the brain stem. Blood clots in these small vessels (thrombosis) can cause small areas of damaged brain tissue called lacunae. In most cases, long-standing high blood pressure is responsible for this condition. Lacunar strokes, which become worse in a matter of hours, often have a fluctuating course. About 25 percent of the time, people have a history of TIAs. The TIAs of these small blood vessels cannot be reliably distinguished from those from large blood vessels without special studies. However, strokes caused by these small vessels usually have a distinctive pattern. About 60 percent of persons suffering lacunar strokes will have weakness or paralysis on one side of the body without any changes in body sensation. Other characteristic symptoms include changes only in sensation, hand function, speaking, coordination, or weakness. About 2 percent of those who have had a lacunar stroke will have a recurring stroke within a month. Over time, many of these small strokes can result in a decline in thinking ability, a condition called multi-infarct dementia (*infarct* means damaged tissue). Controlling high blood pressure can prevent these strokes.

Embolism of a blood clot to the brain accounts for about 25 to 30 percent of strokes. The extent of the neurologic damage depends upon the size of the clot. If the clot is small, the damage is localized to the end-branch areas of the vascular territory. Clots can break off from a larger clot in the heart, a clot on the valves of the heart, or from large arteries such as the carotid artery. In some people, emboli are documented without a clear source of the clot. An irregular heartbeat, called atrial fibrillation, is associated with a 14 percent risk of embolism when the rhythm first starts. The risk remains about 5 percent per year afterwards. About 2 percent of people older than 60 have this condition.

Strokes Caused by Embolism

Symptoms of Strokes Caused by Embolism. The onset of strokes caused by embolism is very sudden in 90 percent of cases, resulting in maximal functional difficulties in only a few minutes. A fluctuating course of functional capacity or intermittent changes in function are rarely seen in this type of stroke. A person's medical history and examination will help a physician identify the source of the original clot.

Treatment of Strokes Caused by Embolism. The high rate of early recurrence after an embolus (over 10 percent the first two weeks) forces most physicians to prescribe anticoagulants (blood thinners) unless there is a very strong reason not to or unless the stroke is very large. Mild anticoagulation seems to be effective in preventing strokes in people who have atrial fibrillation. Use of anticoagulant medications requires individual therapy to balance the benefits and risks.

Strokes Due to Bleeding in the Brain

Brain hemorrhages occur less often than other types of strokes and are often seen with high blood pressure.

Cause of Strokes Due to Bleeding in the Brain. A change in the walls of the blood vessels is a predisposing factor in brain hemorrhage in some older people. A silklike substance called amyloid makes the vessel wall more fragile.

Symptoms of Strokes Due to Bleeding in the Brain. The symptoms of people with brain hemorrhage are so similar to those of persons who have had strokes due to blood clots that the distinction between the two kinds of strokes cannot be made without special brain imaging (with CT scan or MRI) to identify the hemorrhage.

Decreased alertness and vomiting are signs that a brain hemorrhage is occurring. Hemorrhage in the brain stem can cause coma. Bleeding into the cerebellum is a neurologic emergency, because the resulting blood can cause brain stem compression and death. Symptoms of this hemorrhage include severe headache, dizziness, clumsiness, difficulty moving the eyes, and paralysis of parts of the face. Removal of the blood clot can result in recovery if it is done before the brain stem is compressed.

Treatment of Strokes Due to Bleeding in the Brain. Except when the cerebellum is involved, treatment of brain hemorrhage is aimed at preventing the aspiration of stomach contents into the lungs, keeping the person from becoming dehydrated, and managing the underlying medical problems.

In strokes due to hemorrhage, the outlook is determined by the size and location of the bleeding. Generally when hemorrhaging produces a blood clot larger than 5 centimeters—about the size of an egg—the outlook is very poor.

Stroke Rehabilitation

The death rate within 30 days after a stroke is between 20 and 30 percent. In any type of stroke, the outlook depends upon the size and location. Stupor, coma, severe weakness, and difficulty moving the eyes indicate large strokes and therefore predict an unfavorable outcome. The person's functioning before the stroke is also a critical factor in determining her ultimate independence. Age by itself does not limit the potential for a good outcome, but it is a factor that contributes to a higher probability of coexisting illness and shorter survival.

People who have had strokes involving the brain stem or those who have had many strokes often have difficulty swallowing, detected through observation. Sometimes signs of the difficulty are subtle, and special X ray studies can be helpful in uncovering the problem. The person should not be fed until it is clear that regular feeding does not present an unacceptable risk of aspiration of food into the lungs.

Depression that is caused by the stroke is a complication in up to 60 percent of people. If not treated, the depression may persist for many years following the stroke. It can interfere with appetite, sleep patterns, energy level, and extent of cooperation with rehabilitation. Treatment with antidepressant medications can improve performance and rehabilitation, increasing functional capacities. Specialized stroke rehabilitation units may not improve the final neurological problem in stroke victims, but they do appear to improve the person's ability to function. Functional independence is limited in people who have complete paralysis of one half of the body, problems with vision or perceptions, and severe brain stem involvement. Rehabilitation is discussed more completely in Chapter 8.

Meningitis

Meningitis is a bacterial or viral infection of the covering, or meninges (from the Greek and Latin, meaning "membrane"), around the brain and spinal cord.

Causes of Meningitis

In older people, meningitis is most often caused by bacteria and occasionally by viruses. Because of this, any older person who has signs of meningitis should be assumed to have bacterial meningitis until it is proven otherwise. Generally the organisms that cause meningitis in older people are the same as those in younger people. Other organisms can also cause older people to contract meningitis, and a thorough and careful assessment by the physician is always important.

Symptoms of Meningitis

Most older people show the typical features of meningitis: high fever, significant changes in mental function, headache, and a stiff neck. However, some people may not show these changes and may show only an unexplained low-grade fever, changes in mental function, or seizures. This is a serious medical problem and any older person suspected of having meningitis should see a physician right away.

Evaluation of Meningitis

The physician makes the diagnosis of meningitis after performing a spinal tap and examining the spinal fluid. The changes in the spinal fluid that are characteristic of meningitis do not differ in older people compared with younger people.

Treatment of Meningitis

The treatment of bacterial meningitis depends upon the specific laboratory findings, but intravenous antibiotics are always necessary. People usually recover from meningitis if appropriate treatment is given promptly.

CHAPTER 15

PSYCHOLOGIC CONCERNS

Overview

Anxiety

Depression

Alcohol Abuse

Drug Dependency

Your mental health will significantly influence your level of function and social activities, and even the course of medical illness. Over 25 percent of older people have significant mental illness and more than 90 percent of institutionalized elderly people have some psychologic problems.

Psychiatric illnesses can occur on their own or as coexisting with other medical problems. Because elderly people often have a number of illnesses, it is important to monitor the interactions between physical and psychologic conditions and their treatments. If you are experiencing emotional suffering, you should seek help; most psychologic problems are treatable and can be relieved with appropriate therapy.

Overview

Anxiety is a common experience in later life. While anxiety can be specifically associated with panic attacks, phobias, and other psychiatric conditions, most anxiety is called generalized anxiety disorder (GAD). Anxiety can be a signal of problems that a person has difficulty managing with his usual coping strategies. It may signal that a person has inner psychological conflicts of which she may not be aware. It may also indicate concerns about life's circumstances.

Anxiety

Many older people may become anxious because of several simultaneous problems such as physical illness, personal loss, psychological distress, and environmental stress.

Symptoms of Anxiety

The essential feature of a generalized anxiety disorder is unrealistic or excessive anxiety and worry about multiple problems in one's life. This may include worrying about misfortune to children and grandchildren, finances, or physical health. Obviously, if there is only one area of worry, or when the worry may be realistic, this is not a generalized anxiety disorder but a normal reaction to an unpredictable situation.

Anxiety influences our physical and psychological states; the signs fall into three categories. The first is tense muscles, which lead to shaking and trembling, muscle restlessness, and easy tiring. The second category is increased nervous system activity indicated by such things as shortness of breath, rapid heart rate, sweating, dry mouth, dizziness, nausea and diarrhea, flushes or chills, frequent urination, or difficulty swallowing. The third category involves being excessively vigilant, feeling keyed up or on edge, having exaggerated responses to startling phenomena, having difficulty concentrating, trouble falling asleep or staying asleep, or feeling irritable.

In a community survey of people 55 years or older, over 15 percent of men and 20 percent of women suffered such significant anxiety symptoms to be candidates for some form of treatment. Anxiety is generally inversely related to physical health: As health status deteriorates, anxiety increases.

Causes of Anxiety

In older people, symptoms of anxiety are not as clearly defined as they are in younger people—this makes it more difficult to determine if a person requires clinical attention. Clinically significant anxiety is more likely to occur concurrently with states of depression, in dementia, or as a consequence of physical illness or drug treatment. However, in some cases it may be impossible to distinguish between anxiety and normally appropriate worry and concern about the present or future.

Anxiety can be one symptom of several medical disorders in later life including heart disease, lung disease, thyroid and other

**Table 17. Differential Features of
Anxiety and Depression**

DEPRESSION	ANXIETY
Persistent mood problems	Episodic mood problems
Severe in the morning	Progressive worsening during the day
Slow movement hurts	Normal movement hurts
Excessive guilt	Panic attacks
Suicidal thoughts	Phobic symptoms
Family history	No family history

Source: Adapted from Avant RF. Anxiety and depression: determining the predominant disorders. *Family Practice Recertification.* 1984;6(3 suppl):24. Reprinted with permission.

endocrine problems, neurologic illnesses, psychologic illnesses, dietary problems (such as excess caffeine intake or vitamin B_{12} deficiency), and drug-related disorders, including medication side effects and symptoms of withdrawal from alcohol or drugs.

In older adults, symptoms of anxiety and depression tend to accompany each other; this may make it difficult to determine which disorder is dominant. Both of these conditions may cause older people to complain, seek help, or talk about their physical symptoms or lack of memory. Table 17 shows useful features to help determine whether anxiety or depression is the major disorder.

Generalized anxiety can be confused with panic disorders. People with panic disorders—a sudden state of extreme and uncontrollable hyperarousal—are usually convinced that they will die or lose control. Older people who have a history of panic attacks are most likely to experience these, as it is very uncommon for panic attacks to occur for the first time in late life. Some people develop a form of anticipatory anxiety, which is a constant fear of recurrent panic attacks. One coping mechanism to avoid panic attacks is to remain home, which leads to extreme avoidance behavior called agoraphobia (from the Greek, *agora,* "meaning gregarious").

Anxiety may accompany an obsessive-compulsive disorder, which does not commonly develop in the elderly but often persists into old age from an onset earlier in life. Obsessions are persistent ideas, thoughts, impulses, or images that one may experience, at least initially, as being intrusive or senseless. Compulsions are repetitive, purposeful, and intentional behaviors that are sometimes performed in response to an obsession or in a stereotypical fashion. The goal of this compulsive behavior is to avoid discomfort and anxiety. An example is repetitive hand washing.

Anxiety is a regular feature of delirium and may also be present in dementing illnesses. It needs to be distinguished from agitation in these conditions, since elderly people with either delirium or dementia often appear apprehensive, fearful, and may have indications of anxiety. Anxiety can exist simultaneously with agitation, but agitation is distinguished by the presence of physical motor restlessness. This excessive purposeless movement characterizes agitation in contrast with the inner subjective apprehension that defines anxiety.

Treatment of Anxiety Disorders

Approaches that do not rely on medications may be ideal for anxiety in the older adult. These approaches include reducing the stimulus that produces the anxiety and counseling and relaxation techniques. These techniques are usually quite effective and older people benefit from them in the same ways that younger people do.

Doctors sometimes prescribe antianxiety drugs when a person's symptoms interfere with the ability to function or if they aggravate another illness. This is often encountered in older people who are facing a crisis such as the stress of hospitalization, grief, or a change in living circumstances. Sometimes antianxiety medications are useful for people who have a long-standing psychiatric illness that has responded to these medications in the past. The group of drugs most commonly used are called benzodiazepines. They are classified according to their chemical properties, but there is no evidence to suggest that one benzodiazepine is better than any other. The ones that do not linger long or accumulate quickly in the body are usually preferred. These short-acting compounds provide flexible dosing, but it is important to remember that rebound anxiety can result from their use.

Rebound anxiety occurs after the effects of the medication have worn off, and it can be more intense than the original anxiety. This rebound anxiety may occur because the medication replaces and increases the amount of certain anxiety-restraining substances ordinarily produced in the body, which signals the body's production to slow down. Consequently, when the medication wears off, there is a complete deficit of the anxiety-restraining substances and anxiety rebounds with a vengeance. Regardless of the choice of antianxiety drugs, their use in older people must be very carefully monitored.

Because our central nervous system becomes more sensitive to the effects of anxiety-reducing drugs with age, older people are more likely to exhibit side effects at doses that are generally nontoxic in younger adults. Any coexisting physical or emotional illness can further predispose the elderly person to increased drug toxicity. For example, any central nervous system disorder, such as stroke, Parkinson's disease, or dementia, may increase one's sensitivity to these drugs.

Another potential source of increased toxicity of anxiety-reducing drugs in older people is the interaction with other medications that the person may be taking. Medications with sedating properties may especially increase the central nervous system toxicity of anxiety-reducing drugs.

Generally, four side effects of anxiety-reducing drugs—sedation, clumsiness and staggering, mood difficulties, and impaired thinking—may occur in older people at much lower doses than those given to younger adults. These effects are increased by alcohol use or concurrent use of other medications affecting the central nervous system, and are often worse at night. Specific symptoms of toxicity include a staggering gait, difficulty speaking, uncoordination and unsteadiness, slowed reactions, and diminished accuracy of various motor tasks. The thinking impairment caused by anxiety-reducing drugs is characterized by difficulty remembering, increased forgetfulness, and decreased attention. This cognitive impairment may resemble the early stages of a dementing illness, and some older people who take these drugs for a long time seem to be losing their memories because of this commonly overlooked side effect. Generally, the cognitive impairment is reversible, however, and discontinuing the drug usually results in improved memory, attention, and concentration.

Depression

Depression refers to a variety of disorders that are grouped together by symptoms, genetic predisposition, environmental triggers, and responses to treatment. Mild depressive symptoms, however, should be distinguished from a more severe depression because the causes, outlook, and treatment are very different.

Older people frequently experience temporary changes in their moods, usually as a result of some identifiable stress or loss. These changes respond to support when they are mild and, given time, generally get better on their own without any further intervention. However, when compared with the same symptoms in younger people, depression in older people is more likely to result from a medical condition or some dementing illness. Medical problems can aggravate the normal fluctuations in mood, leading to significant disruption of a person's ability to function socially as well as in other productive activity. Mood changes in older people can also be the first symptom of an illness, such as Alzheimer's disease or thyroid disease.

In contrast to the temporary and common fluctuations in mood, severe depression (called major depression) is relatively uncommon in people who are over 60. In a community survey, over 25 percent of older adults reported symptoms of depression although only 1 percent had major depression. Major depression is more often seen in the hospital and in long-term care settings where it may be seen in 10 to 15 percent of older people. However, just because severe depressive episodes in elderly people are less common than in younger people, this does not diminish their importance. Suicide rates in older white men are higher than those of any age, sex, or racial group in the United States. These severe depressive disorders usually occur spontaneously and are not caused by or related to medical or social problems.

Frequently, major depression is seen in dementing disorders such as Alzheimer's disease, dementia caused by multiple strokes, and Parkinson's disease. Among older people who have dementing illness, between 20 and 40 percent also have a major depression. Depression may be commonly seen in the early stages of a dementing illness, although transient and even severe mood swings are seen in the later stages as well.

Table 18. Diagnostic Criteria and Characteristics of Depressive Disorders

	DURATION	SYMPTOMS	HEREDITARY PREDISPOSITION	RESPONSE TO SOMATIC INTERVENTIONS
Major depression	2 weeks or more	Significant symptoms Subtypes: Melancholia Seasonal pattern Psychosis Recurrent depression	Yes (particularly melancholia)	Yes (particularly melancholia, psychosis, and seasonal pattern)
Dysthymia	2 years or more	Less prominent depressive symptoms May be secondary to a physical disorder (e.g., diabetes)	Probable	Probable
Adjustment disorder	Onset within 3 months of stressor and duration no longer than 6 months	Maladaptive response or overreaction to stress that does not persist	None	None

Source: Compiled from American Psychiatric Association. *Diagnostic and Statistical Manual of Mental Disorders*, 3d ed (rev). Washington, DC: American Psychiatric Association; 1987:213; 329. Reprinted with permission.

The categories of mood disorders are shown in Table 18.

Major Depression. Among these disorders, major depression has several distinct characteristics. At least five of the following symptoms must be present on a day-to-day basis for at least two weeks to warrant the diagnosis, and at least one of the symptoms must be depressed mood or loss of interest or pleasure.

- Depressed mood
- Loss of interest or pleasure
- Significant weight change or change in appetite
- Sleeping difficulty

Types of Depression in Later Life

- Severe restlessness or agitation or significant slowing of movement
- Decreased energy, fatigue easily
- Feelings of worthlessness or excessive guilt
- Decreased ability to think or concentrate
- Recurrent thoughts of death or suicide

Melancholia: If a person has symptoms that meet the criteria for major depression, it is useful to consider if the person suffers from melancholia. The term *melancholia* as used clinically refers to the type of depression that is most responsive to medication. At least five of the following nine symptoms must be present on a day-to-day basis.

- Loss of interest or pleasure in most activities
- Lack of reaction to pleasurable stimuli
- Variation during the day with the depression being worse in the morning
- Early-morning wakening
- Slow movements or severe agitation
- Significant weight loss
- No change in the personality before the onset of the depression
- A previous history of a major depression with good recovery
- A previous good response to treatment for the depressive episode

Psychotic Depression: Another type of major depression is that which is characterized by the presence of *psychotic symptoms.* These psychotic symptoms usually occur late in the course of the disease, following a significant period of depression. The psychotic symptoms may be delusions or hallucinations that have a depressive (nihilistic) quality or tone. Psychotic depression occurs relatively more frequently in the later stages of life.

Seasonal Depression: People with a seasonal pattern of depression often report a relationship of their depression to a distinct two-month period of the year (usually the winter), with the occurrence of at least three episodes of the illness in three separate years. Although seasonal variation in mood is common in late life, it occurs relatively less frequently in older people than in younger ones.

Dysthymia. Another depressive condition is called dysthymia. It is seen in about 2 percent of older people and is distinguished from major depressions by less severe symptoms than those associated with major depression and by having symptoms that last at least two years. Two or more of the following criteria need to be met.

- Poor appetite or overeating
- Change in sleep pattern
- Low energy or fatigue
- Low self-esteem
- Poor ability to concentrate or difficulty in making decisions
- Feelings of hopelessness

Dysthymia may occur either by itself or with another psychiatric or medical disorder. When it starts in late life, dysthymia may derive from a loss of self-esteem. The degree to which a person experiences this loss depends upon a number of complex factors, including social expectations, individual personality characteristics, and specific life events. When the personality characteristics make up lifelong patterns that interfere with an individual's ability to function, they are called personality disorders. Sometimes dysthymia can occur because of personality disorders or other situations such as substance abuse or severe anxiety. However, a more common cause of dysthymia is having another serious medical illness with accompanying loss of function and independence.

Adjustment Disorders. Adjustment disorders with depressed mood may follow the onset of a sudden medical illness. In such a reaction, initially there is doubt, surprise, and wonder. Statements of denial or disbelief are common at this stage. Then there is an intense flooding of anxiety, which leads to feelings of confusion and the inability to solve the problem. The person may not be able to function very well, but over time the person begins to adjust, and if the underlying illness is corrected the dysthymia tends to resolve.

Usually a depressive reaction to some stress is classified as an adjustment disorder when it is maladaptive, when there is an impairment in the level of functioning, when symptoms go far beyond what people would normally expect, or when the reaction occurs within three months of the onset of the stress. Clearly, there is room for subjective interpretation as to what is an adjustment disorder and what is a normal reaction to a specific stress. In elderly people, the four most common stresses are physical illness, reactions to the death of loved ones, retirement, and moving into an institutional setting. When the reaction to the death of a loved one is judged to be "normal," involving appropriate grief, psychiatrists call this "uncomplicated bereavement" rather than a psychiatric disorder.

Depression and Loss of Vitality. One type of depression that is not easy to describe with the existing classification system is the chronic depression that sometimes coexists with the loss of vitality and extreme weight loss. The symptoms of this disorder usually meet the criteria for a major depression, yet it is difficult to untangle the physical from the psychological symptoms. Nevertheless, this condition is of great importance, for older people who have loss of vitality combined with depression are at great risk for dying and may actually be committing a type of slow suicide. The treatment strategies that have been devised for this particular type of depression are less effective with the elderly; nonetheless, a thorough evaluation and aggressive treatment are usually worthwhile.

Manic-Depressive Illness. About 10 percent of all mood disorders in older people are caused by *manic-depressive illness* (also called bipolar mood disorder). Manic symptoms involve a distinct period of abnormally elevated, or irritable mood with accompanying euphoria, decreased need for sleep, distractibility, pressure to keep talking, and racing thoughts. People with a history of these episodes may need to take medication to keep them from recurring. Treatment with medication for depression alone may actually cause an episode of mania. In late life, manic episodes are less frequent than in the earlier stages of life and may also change in the way they are experienced. For example, the older adult with mania is less likely to feel euphoric and is more likely to feel irritable, agitated, and have sleep disturbance.

When an older adult suffers from depression, one must consider as potential causes underlying medical illnesses, the side effects of medications, alcohol abuse, dementing illness, and other psychiatric conditions, such as hypochondriasis or a translation of anxiety into a physical symptom—a process known as a somatization disorder. While bodily complaints are often found in older people who suffer from depression, it is important to recognize that symptoms of depression often coincide with symptoms of physical illness. In addition, medications used to treat these illnesses can sometimes lead to depressive symptoms. In fact, many medical problems can lead to depressive symptoms. For example, stroke, congestive heart failure, and cancer can mimic a severe depression by causing weight loss, sleep disturbance, problems with concentrating, and low energy. People with Parkinson's disease may frequently have a number of symptoms suggestive of depression including lack of facial expression, slowed body movement, lack of spontaneity, decreased energy, and poor motivation. However, they may not report feeling depressed unless the Parkinson's disease has progressed to the middle or late stages. Abnormalities with the thyroid gland or other endocrine glands also produce depression. Changes in body chemistry, such as a low potassium in the blood, can also cause mood changes as well as disturbances in sleep, appetite, concentration, and energy. When these depressive symptoms result from physical illnesses, they are classified as "organic mood disorders." Other causes of organic mood disorders include nutritional deficiencies (such as vitamin B_{12} deficiency) and infections.

Depressive symptoms can also be prompted by prescribed medication. Drugs for high blood pressure head the list as the most frequent offenders. In addition, corticosteroids and other hormones such as estrogens can sometimes lead to depression. The medicines used to treat Parkinson's disease can also produce depression or manic symptoms. Any sedative medication can lead to depression.

Alcohol abuse (see elsewhere in this section), also linked to mood disorders, may go undetected in older people. It should be suspected in any older person who develops a shake or tremor, bleeding in the skin, heartburn, bleeding from the intestines, or symptoms of alcohol withdrawal, such as increases in temperature, heart rate, blood pressure, and sweating.

Other Causes of Depression in Later Life

Dementing illness is most frequently associated with depression in late life. Some people, however, who are diagnosed as having a dementing disorder may be primarily depressed (independent of the dementia), because symptoms such as apathy, thinking difficulties, and withdrawal occur with both dementing illness and depression. In addition, some depressed people without dementing illness may appear demented. Up to half of patients with Alzheimer's disease may show depressive symptoms, although only 10 to 20 percent may have severe depressive episodes.

Certain psychiatric conditions can resemble depression. Hypochondriasis is a preoccupation with the belief that one has a serious medical illness. It is quite different from the preoccupation with physical symptoms such as constipation, dizziness, and nausea that are sometimes noted in depressed older people. However, hypochondriasis may be difficult to distinguish from major depression; psychiatric consultation and evaluation may be the only means for distinguishing between these conditions. The person with hypochondriasis may be willing to entertain the fact she does not have a disease whereas a person with severe depression may have a psychotic delusion of a fixed and bizarre nature concerning the dread—but imaginary—disease. The person with depression also usually reports a history of depressive symptoms that have steadily gotten worse over time. The person with hypochondriasis usually has a history of other long-standing complaints that are not associated with any physical findings.

The condition called somatization disorder applies to someone who has had a long history of physical complaints that began before the age of 30 and include at least 13 different symptoms. The early-age onset, the multiple-organ systems that are imagined to be or actually are affected, and the lack of any associated other symptoms help to differentiate older people with this disorder from those with other major psychiatric conditions. Again, this is a condition best identified and treated by a psychiatrist.

Evaluation of Depression   The older person who feels depressed or appears to be suffering from depression should consult a physician or a psychiatrist in order to explore the background of the current symptoms or manifestations. Generally, major depression is a disorder that recurs many times. If the person has had a previous episode, it is also important to note what previous treatment approaches have been successful. Typically, recurrent episodes of depression in an older person last about the same length of time, exhibit the same symptoms, and respond to similar treatments. Further helpful information is the presence of any mood disorders in other family members, any thoughts of suicide, and any substance abuse in the immediate family members. Since the presence of manic symptoms may indicate that the person has a manic-depressive condition, the family history should incorporate a review of symptoms of mania. It is also important to know how a depressive episode starts and how long it lasts. It is particularly important to review the contribution of any stresses, any previous episodes of feeling depressed, and the presence of any other symptoms. Another factor is the person's level of cognitive function before the episode of depression began in order to determine whether this depression may be the early manifestation of dementing illness. Sometimes depressive symptoms occur in conjunction with a previously established decline in mental function.

It is usually helpful to watch for signs of depression while the person is responding to questions. For example, the person's speech may be slow and prolonged, he may have difficulty finding words, there may be a medical condition causing slurred speech, or some other speaking problem such as aphasia. It is also important to determine how the person's thoughts are organized to see if they make sense or reveal any unusual beliefs. Depressed people should also be asked whether they have had any thoughts of suicide. If they answer yes, supportive care should immediately be provided, including medical and psychiatric assistance.

People with dementing illness usually try to hide it in an effort to answer questions correctly. In contrast, people who are depressed are often unconcerned about their performance. They may make little effort to answer questions correctly or try to curtail the interview process with "I don't know" answers. There are a number of sophisticated neurologic and psychologic tests to clarify the picture. Generally, CT scans or MRIs are not necessary for people with mild or moderate depression. However, these imaging studies may be helpful if the person's depression is severe and if hospitalization is required. Another laboratory test for depression is the sleep electroencephalogram (EEG). This test is accurate and reliable in differentiating those people with very severe depression from those who have no evidence of it and in distinguishing depression from dementing illness. The sleep EEG test is most effective when the person has been off all medications from seven to ten days. It is generally not necessary for mild or moderate depression, but it may be helpful in the case of the severely depressed older adult who has profound sleep problems and who does not respond to medication.

Treatment of Depression

Depression can be treated with psychotherapy, medication, and electroconvulsive therapy. Often, a combination of psychotherapy and medication has the best results.

The branch of psychotherapy known as cognitive therapy emphasizes behavioral interventions such as daily or weekly activity schedules and graded task assignments that are designed to mold more adaptive levels of functioning. Negative statements such as "My life is not worth living" are examined and viewed as symptoms of the depressive process. Such statements are challenged and the depressed person is encouraged to adopt new ways of viewing life. Supportive psychotherapy is another approach to help the person deal with grief or feelings that might be contributing to the depression.

The decision to use antidepressant medications may depend as much upon the person's condition and preferences as on the physician's treatment preferences. People who have major as well as less severe depressions usually respond to these drugs. Because of this, the use of antidepressant medications is determined by weighing the benefits and the risks of the treatment.

All of the antidepressant drugs stay in the body a relatively long time (on the order of days to weeks), and therefore they tend to accumulate in the older person's body and can lead to side effects. Some of these medications may be stored in body fat. Since fat turnover in the body is slow, this means the elimination of antidepressants from the body may be even more prolonged. The risk of accumulation can be decreased by monitoring blood levels, but only a few antidepressants are able to be measured reliably in the blood. Desipramine and nortriptyline are two examples.

Table 19. Comparison of Side Effects in Antidepressant Drugs

	RELATIVE ANTICHOLINERGIC EFFECT	RELATIVE CAUSE OF ORTHOSTATIC HYPOTENSION	RELATIVE SEDATION
Amitriptyline	High	High	High
Amoxapine	Low	Moderate	Moderate
Bupropion	Low	Low	Low
Clomipramine	High	High	High
Desipramine	Low	Low	Low
Doxepin	Moderate-high	High	High
Fluoxetine	Low	Low	Low
Imipramine	Moderate	Moderate	Moderate
Maprotiline	Low	Low	High
Nortriptyline	Low	Low	Low
Trazodone	Low	Moderate	High
Trimipramine	Moderate	High	High

Source: Adapted from McDonald WM, Krishnan RR. Pharmacologic management of the symptoms of dementia. *American Family Physician.* 1990;42:126. Originally compiled from Pollack MH, Rosenbaum JF. Management of antidepressant-induced side effects; a practical guide for the clinician. *Journal of Clinical Psychiatry.* 1987;48:3–8, and Wise MG, Taylor SE. Anxiety and mood disorders in medically ill patients. *Journal of Clinical Psychiatry.* 1990;51(suppl):27–32. ©1987 and ©1990 by Physicians Postgraduate Press. Reprinted with permission.

The three major side effects of antidepressant medications result from their ability to block various receptors in the nervous system for acetylcholine, adrenaline, and histamine (see Table 19). Anticholinergic effects (the blocking of acetylcholine receptors) can include dry mouth, difficulty urinating, constipation, impaired vision, and memory loss and confusion. Orthostatic hypotension (the blocking of adrenaline receptors) causes a drop in blood pressure when a person changes position. This puts extra stress on the heart. Thus, if the person has underlying heart disease, serious problems can result. The primary effect of blocking a histamine receptor is sedation. The more sedating antidepressants may initially appear to be the more effective ones. Their initial effectiveness may not be due to the antidepressant effect, which may take two to six weeks of treatment, but rather the effect of eliminating the insomnia, which is a common symptom of depression. Other potential side effects include weight gain, trembling, and various effects upon sexual performance, such as impaired erections, inhibition of orgasms, and decreased sex drive. Physicians sometimes obtain an electrocardiogram before prescribing an antidepressant medication. This is because certain kinds of antidepressants should not be used with some types of heart abnormalities.

Antidepressants have become available with different range and degree of side effects. One medication called bupropion can cause nausea, insomnia, and agitation, but generally does not block acetylcholine, adrenaline, or histamine receptors. It can make a person more susceptible to having a seizure and must be used carefully by people with seizure disorders.

Another new antidepressant, fluoxetine, stays in the body a long time. For example, half of it may linger for two days in an older person, and active components of the drug may stay in the body for weeks. Such a lingering presence is particularly worrisome when the drug is given to very old people. It may also cause weight loss and agitation; nonetheless, it is a useful compound and offers a real advantage because it is not sedating and does not block the cholinergic receptors.

There are many other medication choices for people with depression. People with manic-depressive illness can be treated during a manic episode with lithium. In most cases, once the manic episode has resolved, people are put on lithium to keep new attacks from occurring. Blood levels of lithium can be measured.

Electroconvulsive therapy (ECT) may be a very effective treatment for depression especially in situations where medication is ineffective, when there are life-threatening consequences to the depression, or when other treatments have failed. A thorough medical evaluation is essential before ECT is administered. In the case of a person with a known brain tumor, treatment with ECT is out of the question. Older people generally respond well to ECT, and medication can be given to help reduce the rate of subsequent depressive episodes.

Frequently, family therapy is an effective addition to the treatment of the depressed older person. Families can unwittingly reinforce the depression because some family members may not recognize that their behavior is exacerbating the original depression of the older member. Moreover, a family's prejudice against mental illness may undermine the follow-up treatment by denying that the problem exists or that it is serious. The illness should be treated within a supportive and structured environment in which, for example, the older person is encouraged to eat, exercise, and engage in social activities. It is important to reemphasize that depression in elderly people is a devastating disorder with a high risk of suicide. Because of this, family and other caregivers need to join in a full supportive network as part of the treatment program. Family members, for example, need to be alerted to the possible side effects of medications, especially problems with falls, memory disturbances, and problems with driving. Older people suffering from depression should be carefully evaluated to determine their capacity to provide consent for various procedures.

Risk of Suicide

Whenever an older person suffers from a severe depressive disorder, the risk for suicide must be carefully evaluated. Among the risk factors to be considered are suicidal thoughts, a history of previous suicide attempts, whether the person has any other psychiatric disease, and most important, the severity of the depressive disorder. As mentioned earlier, suicide is more prevalent among white men who live alone. Alcohol abuse or drug dependency increases the suicide risk. Furthermore, when older adults suffer from long-term, painful, or potentially life-threatening medical conditions, the risk of their suicide increases. After assessing the risk of suicide, physicians generally determine whether hospitalization is necessary. If it is, every effort should be made to have the person admitted to the hospital for a period of observation and treatment despite the usual protests on the part of the individual. When family members, physicians, and any others involved in the situation are cooperative and honest in apprising each other of the potential risk of suicide, the older person will generally agree to the hospitalization. In extreme circumstances, however, some older people may need to be hospitalized against their will for a brief period.

If the physician determines that hospitalization is not necessary, everyone should be warned of the potential risk and means for committing suicide. Weapons in the home, for example, should be made inaccessible to the older adult. The older person who is suicidally depressed should be under constant supervision. However, the family members should not be placed under too great a burden of responsibility for preventing the suicide. If there is any question in this regard, hospitalization should be considered as the best preventive option.

Usually suicide is a risk for a relatively short period. Because of this, rapid intervention is often successful in alleviating the risk danger during that period. Afterward, successful treatment of the depression generally improves the outlook and lowers the risk of suicide. Nevertheless, in some cases the risk may be recurring and the older adult may continue to be at risk for suicide over months and even years. This prolonged risk is usually associated with a partially resolved depressive disorder or, more especially, with frequent recurrent episodes of depression.

Alcohol Abuse

Alcohol dependency is often thought to be a problem of young people, but community surveys suggest that about 5 percent of Americans over age 65 have significant drinking problems. Older men are four times more likely than women to abuse alcohol. About a decade ago, a large community survey of the prevalence of mental disorders in the United States revealed that alcohol abuse was the third most commonly diagnosed mental illness (after dementia and anxiety disorders) in men over age 65. Moreover, the survey found that abuse and dependence on alcohol or some other drug were the most common psychiatric diagnoses of men in their sixties. Other studies have found that alcohol plays a role in about a third of suicides in elderly people.

The terms "alcohol abuse" and "alcohol dependency" are frequently misinterpreted. Alcohol abuse includes a pattern of alcohol use that is demonstrated by at least one of the following: continued use of alcohol despite social, occupational, psychologic, or physical problems that are caused or worsened by continued use, and recurrent use in situations in which it is physically hazardous, such as driving. These problems must have been present for at least a month or have occurred repeatedly over a long period of time.

Alcohol dependency includes at least three of the following:

- The taking of alcohol in large amounts or over a longer period of time than intended
- The persistent desire or unsuccessful efforts to cut down
- A great deal of time spent in activities that are necessary for obtaining alcohol or for recovering from its effects
- Frequent intoxication or withdrawal symptoms when the user is expected to fulfill major role obligations or when alcohol use is physically hazardous
- The giving up or reduction of activities because of alcohol use
- Continued alcohol use despite social, psychologic, or physical problems caused or exacerbated by it
- Marked tolerance to alcohol
- Characteristic withdrawal symptoms
- The frequent taking of alcohol to relieve or avoid withdrawal symptoms

As with alcohol abuse, the symptoms must have persisted for at least a month or recurred repeatedly over a long period of time.

Alcohol and Aging

Although the chemical breakdown of alcohol in the body does not appear to change with aging, other changes that are associated with aging may increase the concentration of alcohol in the blood. These include changes in the liver, decreased lean muscle mass, and a decreased amount of body water. Decreased body water results in a higher concentration of alcohol for each amount consumed since alcohol quickly distributes in this water compartment. After drinking the same amount of alcohol, an average 60-year-old person's blood alcohol level is 20 percent higher than that of a 20-year-old, and a 90-year-old person's blood alcohol level is approximately 50 percent higher than that of a 20-year-old. The nervous system in older people also seems more sensitive to alcohol. In addition, people with dementia illnesses seem especially sensitive to the effects of alcohol.

**Signs and
Symptoms of
Alcoholism**

Alcoholism often goes undiscovered in older people. Medical problems, psychosocial problems, and the use of medications may obscure the signs of alcoholism. In addition, symptoms such as confusion, falls, and physical problems may be inappropriately attributed to aging. Some older people may have confusion or severe hearing impairment, making it difficult to question them about their alcohol abuse. The stigma associated with having an alcohol problem, especially in an older person, may prevent some health professionals from asking if such a problem exists.

Patterns of alcohol dependence in older people have generally been divided into the categories of "early onset," which occurs before the age of 60, and "late onset," which occurs after the age of 60. In one-half to three-quarters of older people with alcohol problems, the pattern is that of early onset; these people generally have a family history of alcoholism, are less well adjusted, and may have had alcohol-related legal problems. Late-onset alcohol abuse is thought by some to be due to the stresses and losses associated with aging. People in this category point to life events as the cause for their drinking more often than do those who have had an early onset of a drinking problem. However, early retirement, premature health problems, and other life stresses can be caused by alcohol abuse. People with late-onset alcohol dependence may respond more favorably to treatment.

Questionnaires and screening approaches increase the detection of alcohol-related problems. A doctor may ask four key questions: "Have you ever felt you ought to slow down on your drinking?" "Have you ever felt annoyed by criticism of your drinking?" "Have you ever felt guilty or bad about drinking?" "Have you ever felt the need for an eye-opener in the morning to steady your nerves?" Two or more positive answers should raise the suspicion of alcohol abuse. A positive response to even one question should prompt further inquiry.

Sleep problems can be a sign of alcohol misuse or abuse. With aging, the time that it takes to fall asleep increases, and alcohol may be used in an effort to induce sleep. Initially, alcohol may help one get to sleep, but overall it worsens sleep problems by decreasing the amount of restful sleep, which in turn increases anxiety and irritability. Alcohol abuse also decreases the deep levels of sleep and causes early awakenings, which can result in sluggishness and lethargy during the day.

Another major problem associated with alcoholism in older people is the increased likelihood and danger of drug-alcohol interactions. With age there is a decrease in the chemical processing of certain drugs in the liver, and this results in the drugs lasting for a longer time in the body. For some of these medicines the ingestion of alcohol increases this effect. On the other hand, there are some drugs whose effects are diminished in the person who abuses alcohol, such as drugs used for seizure disorders, anticoagulants (blood thinners), and some of the oral medications used to treat diabetes mellitus. Alcohol also unpredictably strengthens the effects of sedatives, which can compromise motor skills and alertness. Frequent use of alcohol can cause bleeding in the intestines; this risk can be especially increased if the person is taking arthritis medications or aspirin.

Drug Interactions with Alcohol

Alcohol can affect every part of the nervous system either directly or indirectly by depleting nutrients, especially B vitamins. Prolonged alcohol dependence can cause significant problems, including confusion, clumsiness, muscle problems, liver disease, coma, and degeneration of the brain and spinal cord. Some experts estimate that 5 to 10 percent of cases of dementia are caused by alcohol abuse.

Complications of Alcohol Abuse

People who abuse alcohol may have additional psychiatric problems such as anxiety disorders, depression, memory difficulties, and the abuse of medications. At times alcohol is used by older people for self-medication to ease both the emotional pain of psychiatric and physical illness. Tobacco dependence also tends to occur with alcohol abuse and dependence, further compromising the health of the alcoholic older adult. People who use sedatives or pain relievers seem especially predisposed to develop alcohol dependence.

Alcohol abuse can interfere with treatment for other problems. If a person with a physical illness does not respond to treatment, or if adverse drug reactions appear to be present, alcohol abuse or dependence should be considered as a possible contributing factor. On the other hand, the presence of a psychiatric condition or cognitive impairment does not seem to affect the chance of treating alcoholism.

Severe withdrawal symptoms occur as frequently in older people as in younger people. Approximately 5 percent of older alcoholic individuals experience withdrawal delirium also called delirium tremens, or DTs. This severe form of alcohol withdrawal is a medical emergency; older people have a higher risk of death than younger people and may take longer to complete the withdrawal process.

Treatment Principles of Alcoholism

Clearly prevention is the most effective treatment of alcohol abuse. The effectiveness of personal concern and advice and education on the effects of alcohol is well documented. People may be asked to keep a diary on their drinking patterns. In addition, they may respond to information on the particular effects of alcohol on their body's organs and systems. People with long-standing alcohol problems usually require more aggressive treatments.

Thankfully, it is not the case that older alcoholics must hit rock-bottom before they will agree to treatment. When an alcohol problem is identified, people important in the person's life need to be instructed by experienced counselors in ways to strengthen the person's motivation to begin treatment. Group confrontation can also be taught to air the problem of alcoholism. Older persons with alcohol problems who are confronted in a supportive way are more likely to enter into treatment programs and to remain abstinent for longer periods than those who are confronted antagonistically or not confronted at all. Family members can be given support and training by experienced counselors to help them deal with the alcohol abuser's behavior and to decrease behaviors of their own that might encourage and enable alcohol intake. Sometimes well-intended family members inadvertently find ways to allow and even ensure that the person's addiction to alcohol continues.

People with a long history of alcohol use should take multivitamins daily and a doctor may want to prescribe thiamine as soon as possible. People with very poor nutrition, mental impairment, or nervous system problems may need to have their vitamin B_{12} level checked to make sure they are not deficient in this critical nutrient. Occasionally, vitamin K supplementation may be necessary for people with bleeding problems.

Many people report symptoms of depression while they are off alcohol. Usually these symptoms get better after they have participated in treatment programs for three to four weeks. Antidepressant medications are sometimes useful and are given after about four weeks of abstinence.

The amount of time from the last drink to the onset of typical symptoms of alcohol withdrawal is similar across the life cycle, usually 24 to 36 hours. These withdrawal symptoms include shakiness, agitation, sweating, hallucinations, or seizures. Doctors use many types of medications to help address these withdrawal symptoms. Older people must be monitored continually for signs and symptoms of alcohol withdrawal as these medications are adjusted. Sometimes giving an older person magnesium can be helpful in treating withdrawal symptoms and in some cases allows for the decreased use of other medications. People with severe agitation, hallucinations, or paranoia may need stronger antipsychotic medication, usually haloperidol. It must be stressed that the treatment of alcohol withdrawal is a serious medical emergency and should not be undertaken without the supervision of a physician.

Treatment of Alcohol Withdrawal

The rehabilitation programs for alcohol and other drug dependence use many strategies. Individual therapy can help break down the person's denial that an alcohol problem exists and can focus on other specific problems, such as grief or difficulty in adapting to retirement. In addition, group therapy provides education on alcoholism, additional assistance in breaking down denial, and development of alternative coping mechanisms. Groups also provide emotional support and can give a person a sense of belonging and renewed self-respect.

Alcohol Rehabilitation

Involvement in Alcoholics Anonymous (AA), a worldwide group of recovering alcohol abusers who assist others in their recovery, is effective for many older people. About a third of the people in Alcoholics Anonymous are 50 and older. Family members or others who have unknowingly fostered the older person's alcohol abuse or at least denied that there was a problem, sometimes referred to as enablers, also need to be brought into the treatment process. Involvement in groups like Al-Anon (a companion group to Alcoholics Anonymous) can help these family members and others to recognize and change their harmful patterns of behavior. Al-Anon also offers relief and support to family members or others who have suffered with stress, strain, or victimization caused by a person with alcohol or drug dependency. Community resources such as senior citizens groups, visiting nurses, church groups, halfway houses, as well as opportunities for volunteer work should all be utilized. Some life care and retirement communities have developed support groups for people with alcohol problems.

The outlook for recovery from alcoholism in elderly people is generally good since older people who have this problem are more likely than younger people to remain in treatment and to maintain sobriety.

Drug Dependency

Drug abuse, which can be found in people of almost any age, gender, race, nationality, and socioeconomic class can be a major problem for elderly people. Those in this age group take on average 4 over-the-counter drugs daily; those who have a chronic disease may take 10 to 15 drugs daily. Those who are 65 and older are at increased risk for dangerous drug-alcohol interactions. Of the 100 drugs most frequently prescribed, over half interact with alcohol.

The frequency of drug addiction in older people is not known. Some people have a twofold diagnosis: a major psychiatric illness and drug addiction. Some older people may have lifelong histories of addictive behavior whereas others may have only recently developed a drug problem.

The drugs most likely abused by the older person are benzodiazepines, oral narcotics, and barbiturates. However, all other drugs, whether legal or illegal, have also been reportedly abused by older people including stimulants, cocaine, marijuana, hallucinogens, and intravenous narcotics.

Symptoms of Drug Abuse

Older people who are addicted to medication rarely complain about it. Instead, they may complain about anxiety (which may be related to tolerance or withdrawal symptoms), memory loss, depressed mood, agitation, falls, changes in blood pressure, pain in the upper abdomen, fatigue, sleep disturbance, appetite and weight loss, weakness, and confusion. Drug-seeking behavior is quite common among addictive individuals and some are quite clever at "doctor shopping"—a strategy that enables them to get several copies of the same prescriptions from different doctors and to fill the prescriptions at different pharmacies. Addiction to more than one drug is extremely common.

Several psychological symptoms are typical of drug addiction: denial, minimalization, rationalization, defocusing, and enabling. Generally, addicted individuals deny that they are addicted. Sometimes the denial is extreme to the degree that the person may not admit to taking any addictive drugs. In less extreme circumstances, the person might minimize the amount of drug taken or the effects of drug use on their behavior and life. In rationalization, addicted people try to find reasons other than the addiction for their use of the offending compounds. A common rationalization used by older adults addicted to prescription drugs involves blaming the physician for prescribing the medication. People with medication addiction also try to focus the discussion away from their addiction and onto anything else in their life such as marital conflicts or significant medical illness. Enabling relates to the families and others close to the addicted person. People who enable an addicted individual unconsciously support the addictive behavior. "Enabling persons" may also demonstrate the symptoms of denial and rationalization, and attempt to focus the discussion away from the addiction. (See also the section on alcohol abuse.)

Drug tolerance is a phenomenon to watch out for. Tolerance refers to the need of an increased dosage over time in order to maintain the same control of symptoms. The body adapts to each level of dosage and loses its sensitivity to the effects of the medication. The body can develop tolerance to many kinds of drugs, and some of these can become addicting. This is particularly true of antianxiety drugs and sleeping pills. When increasing dosage leads to addiction, any attempt at abrupt cessation of the medication will lead to withdrawal symptoms. While such symptoms vary with different drugs, they can be severe and can include tremor, sweating, hyperthermia, delirium, convulsions, and cardiac crises. Because of these potentially life-threatening dangers, drug withdrawal must always be monitored closely by a physician.

Treatment of Drug Addiction

Drug addiction is a disease and should be treated as such. Symptoms of other conditions need to be treated after the person is detoxified and frequently they diminish spontaneously. The two phases of treatment are detoxification and rehabilitation. Detoxification should begin the moment the decision is made to start treatment. This process usually requires an in-hospital stay where constant supervision can prevent the person from "sneaking" in drugs. Detoxification of the older adult can never proceed rapidly, and in some addicted individuals it may take eight to ten weeks to complete treatment. Rehabilitation should usually take place within the context of a program such as that of Alcoholics Anonymous (AA), even if the addiction is not related to alcohol. Addicts should start attending daily AA meetings as soon as their physical condition warrants it. As discussed in the section on alcohol addiction, family members should also be counseled regarding the process of addiction, and a discussion of their roles as enablers should be part of the treatment. Even if a person addicted to many drugs has not abused alcohol, attendance at an AA meeting is usually better than attendance at a Narcotics Anonymous (NA) meeting because the older person is more likely to be able to relate to people who attend AA than to the younger people who attend NA.

All addictive medicines must be stopped once detoxification is complete, regardless of the person's complaints of anxiety, inability to sleep, or pain. If the person experiences pain that is severe enough to warrant treatment with narcotics, such as after an acute injury or after surgery, narcotics are given under controlled circumstances and usually only in the hospital.

Once the inpatient treatment is complete, the older person with an addiction should always be considered to be recovering but never fully recovered. To prevent a relapse, it is necessary to attend AA meetings every day for one year and then to attend them frequently thereafter. Following all 12 steps of the AA program is important, from the first step in which people admit they are addicts and can explain why, to making contacts at AA meetings, to becoming a sponsor. All of the steps are integral parts of successful treatment.

CHAPTER 16

SKIN CONDITIONS

Overview
Symptoms
   Skin Dryness
   Skin Discoloration in Body Folds (Intertrigo)
   Skin Growths
   Itching
Conditions
   Allergic Skin Rash (Contact Dermatitis)
   Fungal Skin Infections
   Infestations
   Pressure Ulcers
   Psoriasis
   Shingles
   Skin Cancers
   Skin Changes Due to Poor Circulation (Stasis Dermatitis)
   Skin Infections

Significant skin problems affect about two-thirds of older people, but these conditions are often unrecognized or incorrectly labeled and treated.

   Obviously, our physical appearance has a powerful influence on how we interact with other people. Attractive skin has almost universal appeal. Appearance may be related to self-esteem, well-being, and possibly even overall health. In fact, one of the earliest

Overview

pieces of written history, the Sir Edwin Smith surgical papyrus (approximately 1500 B.C.) contains the prescription for a cream to reduce skin wrinkles. Interestingly, the book is entitled *How to Turn a Man of 70 into a Youth.*

Youth-oriented stereotypes of beauty and good looks can create considerable problems and anxieties for the aging person. The damaging nature of the stereotypes is that a person starts to believe that the changes represent a personal rather than a societal problem.

Skin conditions seen with aging result from either loss of elasticity, producing wrinkles and creases, or changes caused by sun damage. Characteristic skin changes are commonly seen in older people with medical illnesses such as diabetes mellitus, poor circulation, kidney disease, and thyroid problems.

There is a vast array of creams, lotions, cosmetics, and other options to help people deal with their skin concerns.

SYMPTOMS
Skin Dryness

Dry skin is a very common problem in older people and is characterized by rough, scaly skin that is worsened by low humidity. It is a difficulty that people frequently encounter in the winter because of low humidity and is worsened by frequent bathing because of the effects of soap. The legs are usually the most severely involved. The cause of this condition is not clear, but the dryness is not simply due to a lack of water or oil in the affected skin.

Treatment of Skin Dryness

It is important to minimize bathing (optimally every two or three days) to prevent soap and water from removing too much of the skin's natural oils. Emollients, or skin moisturizers, are the best treatment and should be applied immediately after the bath while the skin is still moist. Emollients should be used indefinitely to prevent recurrence.

Skin Discoloration in Body Folds (Intertrigo)

Complaints of discoloration, softening, and inflammation in skin folds are common in older people, especially in those who are obese. Intertrigo, the term used for this chronic condition, is characterized by skin folds that are painful and prone to develop cracks and redness. The affected area often smells and is usually accompanied by the presence of various skin bacteria or fungi.

When feasible, treatment consists of keeping the skin open to the air, which is best accomplished by removing the clothing and manually separating the skin folds. It is also useful to expose the areas to a fan, hair dryer, or other dry air source for at least 10 to 15 minutes several times a day. Liberal application of absorbent powders in the skin folds after bathing (and as needed to keep the area dry) is also helpful. Sometimes a physician will prescribe an antifungal cream if the affected area appears to harbor a fungal infection. Steroid preparations to the skin are usually not necessary and are best used only under the supervision of a physician or dermatologist because of the risk of added infection and skin atrophy.

Treatment of Skin Discoloration in Body Folds

Perhaps one of the best markers of skin aging are the benign skin growths that result from long-term sun exposure, and therefore depend upon the amount of sunlight exposure, clothing styles, and light versus dark complexion. On the other hand, skin tags, small reddish spots called cherry angiomas, and seborrheic keratoses (described below) appear regardless of the degree of sun exposure and whether or not the skin is protected from the sun. The major importance of these skin changes is the amount of distress that they cause people from a cosmetic standpoint, a distress that appears to result from a fear of changed body image due to aging.

Skin Growths

Small skin tags are commonly seen around the neck, under the arms, below the breasts, and in the groin. They are usually between 5 and 15 millimeters (¼ to ⅝ inch) in diameter and are generally flesh colored. Friction and hereditary factors appear to play a significant role in their development. Skin tags can be rapidly and painlessly removed by a physician. Cherry angiomas are smooth, dome-shaped red spots that are roughly the size of a match-head and commonly are seen on the trunk of the body. They also can be easily treated. Seborrheic keratoses are oily scaly patches, or plaques, that appear from brown to black and may become several centimeters in diameter. They appear to be stuck to the surface of the skin and have an irregular heaped-up appearance. This stuck-on or waxy appearance, as well as their coloration and smooth borders usually distinguish them from malignant growths. Seborrheic keratoses can be left alone or treated depending on a person's preference and a physician's advice. It is important to emphasize that any skin growth or discoloration that changes in appearance, has notched or irregular borders, bleeds easily, or contains a black coloration should be evaluated by a physician to exclude the possibility of a skin cancer.

Itching

Itching produces substantial discomfort for many older people. It sometimes severely compromises one's quality of life, especially by interfering with sleep.

Causes of Skin Itching

Commonly the itching is due to simple dryness that can be treated with frequent applications of moisturizing agents called emollients. For a very small number of elderly people (far less than 10 percent), the itching may be the sign of an underlying disease, which is more likely if the onset of itching appears suddenly and if it is extremely severe. Chronic kidney disease, diseases of the liver, gallstones, thyroid disease, and some malignant conditions (such as Hodgkin's disease) can produce itching.

Evaluation of Skin Itching

Because of the possibility of serious medical illness, the older person with a recent onset of itching needs to see a physician who will usually conduct a careful interview and physical examination to search for signs and symptoms of underlying diseases. Generally, extensive examination is not necessary.

Treatment of Skin Itching

Steroid creams are not usually recommended for the treatment of itching. They should only be used in the presence of a specific skin condition identified by a physician or other health worker. In addition, oral antihistamines should also be avoided, because they rarely help and may actually produce states of confusion in the older person. Aside from applying skin moisturizing agents, the best treatment of itching consists of attempting to improve any underlying disease.

CONDITIONS Allergic Skin Rash (Contact Dermatitis)

Contact dermatitis is probably underrecognized in older persons. It is an easily treated rash caused by skin exposure to substances that may be irritating or allergic in nature. Contact with poison ivy is a familiar example.

Finding the cause is important because effective treatment must include identification and avoidance of the offending irritant or allergen. Contact dermatitis can produce both immediate and longer-lasting changes to the skin, including redness; small, clear liquid-filled blisters called vesicles; and thickening and scaling of the skin. Because older skin often responds less vigorously and less rapidly than younger skin to an inflammatory stimulus, dermatitis may be subtle. As a result, the cause may be difficult to establish.

Symptoms of Contact Dermatitis

Until the cause is found and the symptoms resolved, doctors sometimes treat contact dermatitis with creams or lotions that contain corticosteroids. The severity and location of the dermatitis help the physician to know how strong and what type of preparation to prescribe. Medium- to high-potency steroids are used for initial treatment of the most symptomatic and severe cases and in areas where absorption from the skin is poor. Lower-potency preparations are used on the face, on the genitalia, in body folds, or in other areas where absorption is high. Creams or lotions are useful for cuts or skin breaks that weep fluid or for eruptions in areas that are covered by clothing. Ointments, which are greasier than creams or lotions, are often more soothing and effective for chronic dermatitis.

Treatment of Contact Dermatitis

Superficial skin infections caused by common fungi occur frequently, especially in warm climates. One fungus called tinea pedis (athlete's foot) may develop only in the space between the toes or can cause a scaliness over the entire sole of the foot. Fungal disease of the nail usually shows up by a thickened, crumbly, discolored nail but without other symptoms. Sometimes fungal conditions occur in the groin or on the hands.

Fungal Skin Infections

Beyond the itching and the unpleasant odor associated with fungus infections, these fungal infections can cause skin breaks and cracks that in turn predispose the tissue to bacterial infection beneath the skin. Such infections, known as bacterial cellulitis, are serious and require prompt treatment.

Symptoms of Fungal Skin Infections

Treatment of Fungal Skin Infections

In most circumstances, fungal infection is controlled by the daily application of some broad-spectrum antifungal cream or powder. Four to six weeks is generally required to eliminate a severe fungal infection of the foot, but this condition tends to recur very rapidly, and continued intermittent treatment is often necessary. Long-standing infections involving the nails are common and generally cannot be totally cured. Like fungal disease of the feet, the treatment for these areas consists of twice daily preparations of an anti-fungal cream. Treatment to prevent recurrence in the groin or hand is usually not necessary, however, because the long-term cure rates are much higher than they are for the feet.

Infestations

An infestation of mites affecting the skin, called scabies, is common among institutionalized people such as nursing home residents.

Symptoms of Infestations

Most people with scabies have severe itching that is really a kind of allergic reaction to the mite. Usually, signs of scratching are found on the hands, wrists, under the arms, on the abdomen, and around the groin. The head and neck are almost never involved. Physicians sometimes confirm the diagnosis by scraping the involved area and observing the mites under a microscope.

Treatment of Scabies

One highly effective treatment that is well tolerated by older people consists of applying 1 percent lindane cream to the entire body below the neck. The cream should stay on for 24 hours and then be washed off in a bath or shower. Because the mite eggs are resistant to this treatment, the treatment should be repeated a week later to kill any newly hatched mites. In the intervening week, all clothing, bedclothes, and towels should either be removed from human contact or thoroughly washed in hot water. Scabies mites can survive for several days away from the human host. This regimen will cure scabies for more than 90 percent of people, but it does not immediately decrease the itching. Skin moisteners, steroid creams, and a great deal of tender loving care usually improve the itching within a few days. Sometimes the skin remains easily irritated for weeks after successful treatment.

There are no firm guidelines for treating people who have had contact with a person with scabies. It seems reasonable that anyone who has similar itching areas or a history of intimacy with a person with the infestation should be given the same treatment as described above. Casual contacts, such as nursing home attendants, are infrequently affected.

Other Infestations

Body lice are far less common than scabies except in extremely impoverished people. These skin areas have moderate to severe itching and the areas tend to be grouped together. Treatment of body lice consists of dry cleaning or thorough washing and ironing of all clothes, blankets, sheets, and anything else that has come in contact with the person. Because the lice do not remain on the skin for very long, treatment of the individual is not effective.

Older people may also incur insect bites such as flea or spider bites. It is useful to keep this in mind when any itchy red areas appear on the skin. In these cases, the treatment consists of eradicating the insects or spiders from the person's environment. Topical ointments can relieve the itching.

If a person seems overly concerned about infestations and only has scratching, one must consider a delusion of being covered with parasites. On questioning people with this condition, they often vividly describe the movement of insects on or in their skin. They characteristically have a collection of scabs, dust, or other small particles that they have identified as the offending insects. This condition is a true psychosis and requires psychiatric management.

Pressure Ulcers

Pressure ulcers are localized areas of injured tissue in or below the skin that develop when these soft tissues are compressed between a bony prominence and another surface for a long time. These ulcers can appear as a red area that does not turn white when it is pushed; a crater formation indicating loss of soft tissue; a blister; or a large, dark area resembling a scab. Other terms for pressure ulcers include pressure sores, decubitus ulcers, or bed sores. Because pressure is mostly responsible for inducing the formation of these skin conditions, pressure ulcer has become the preferred term. The terms decubitus (meaning lying down) ulcer and bed sore imply that the ulcers occur only when one is lying down, but some of the most severe injuries to the skin caused by pressure may result from prolonged sitting.

Figure 13. Pressure Ulcers

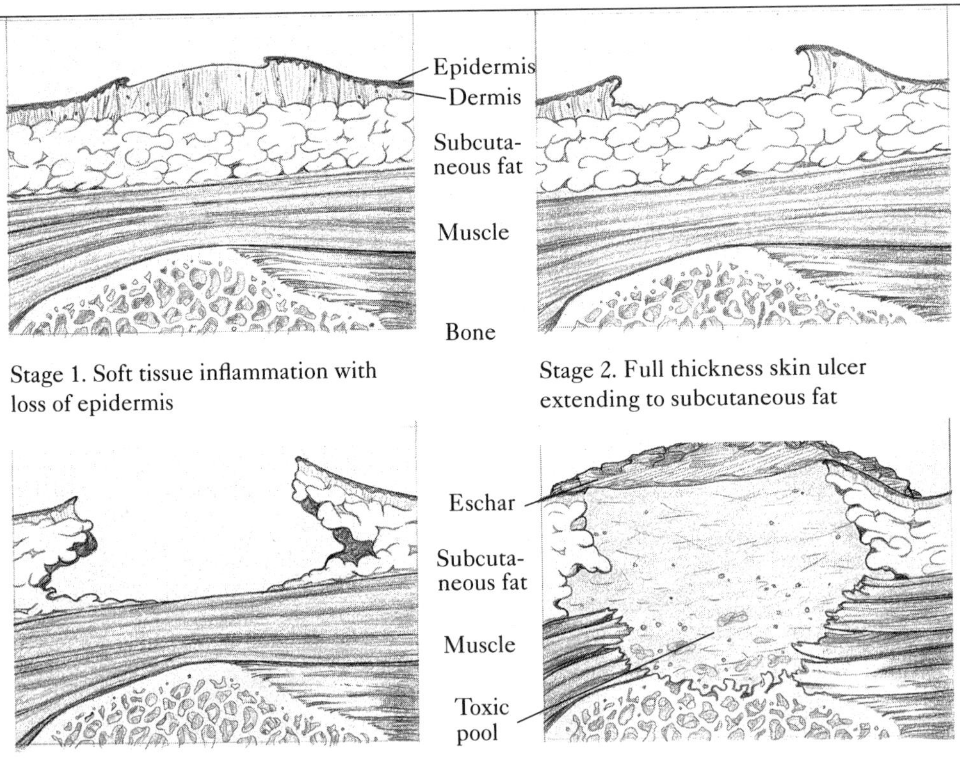

Epidermis
Dermis
Subcuta-
neous fat

Muscle

Bone

Stage 1. Soft tissue inflammation with loss of epidermis

Stage 2. Full thickness skin ulcer extending to subcutaneous fat

Eschar

Subcuta-
neous fat

Muscle

Toxic pool

Bone

Stage 3. Extension into subcutaneous fat with extensive skin undermining

Stage 4. Extension into muscle and bone. In some cases, a dark, crusty area (eschar) and a toxic pool may form.

The National Pressure Ulcer Advisory Panel has suggested the following system for classifying the extent and severity, or stages, of pressure ulcers (see Figure 13):

Stage 1: Skin redness that does not turn white with pressure

Stage 2: Loss of the outer skin layers

Stage 3: Loss of the full thickness of skin and some of the tissue below the skin

Stage 4: Deeper loss of the full thickness of skin and the tissue below, extending into muscle or bone

Pressure-induced blisters may occur on the heels and usually indicate stage 2 or stage 3 ulcers. Any injury manifested by eschar

Figure 14. Common Locations of Pressure Ulcers

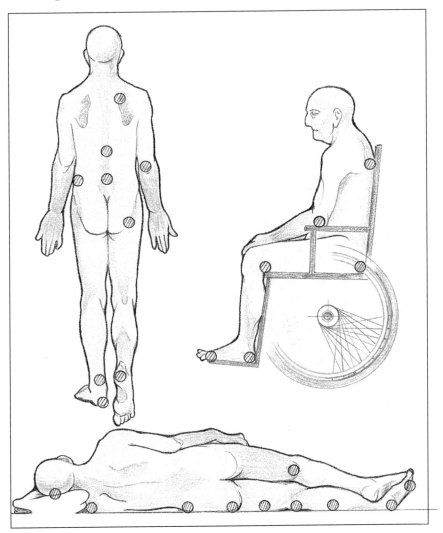

formation, that is, a large, dark crusty area covering raw tissue, is at least a stage 3 ulcer.

More than 50 percent of people with pressure ulcers are 70 years of age and older. This highlights the fact that pressure ulcers are a common problem for older people who are less mobile and less active than younger people. Nearly two-thirds of pressure ulcers

Incidence of Pressure Ulcers

first develop in the hospital. About 70 percent of these ulcers occur within the first two weeks of hospitalization. In addition to these, approximately 18 percent of all ulcers occur in the community and about 18 percent in nursing homes.

Pressure Ulcers and Mortality

Hospital patients who develop pressure ulcers have about a fourfold increased risk of death. A similar increase in death rate over a six-month follow-up period has been observed in nursing home individuals who develop pressure ulcers. In addition, nursing home individuals who have a pressure ulcer that fails to heal within six months have a nearly sixfold increase in their death rate. The mortality rate for people discharged from the hospital with a diagnosis of pressure ulcers is about 15 percent, which is over two times higher than the average of about 7 percent for all hospitalized Medicare patients. However, since most of these deaths occur in people with very severe, underlying illnesses, the specific contribution of the pressure ulcers to these deaths is difficult to define.

Risk Factors Leading to Pressure Ulcers

It is clear that pressure ulcers occur most frequently when a person is very limited in mobility and activity. Older people with a reduced number of spontaneous movements during sleep (fewer than 20 movements) have an increased risk of developing pressure ulcers. A low level of albumin in the blood, loss of bowel control, and the presence of a fracture may identify bed- and chair-bound individuals who are at a particularly high risk for pressure ulcers in the hospital. These three characteristics may not be as important in bed- or chair-bound nursing home individuals for whom a stroke or impaired capacity for eating appears to be the important risk factor. For people who live in the community, older age, reduced activity, cigarette smoking, dry scaling skin, and poor self-assessment of health appear to be the risk factors related to the development of pressure ulcers over a ten-year period.

Some additional factors that may predispose a person to develop pressure ulcers include aging changes in the skin and malnutrition. Several simple scales have been developed to assess and identify older people who are at risk for pressure ulcers. Among them, the Braden Scale (see Table 20 for a modified version) is the most reliable and valid.

Table 20. Braden Scale for Predicting Pressure Sore Risk

PATIENT'S NAME _____	EVALUATOR'S NAME _____		DATE OF ASSESSMENT
SENSORY PERCEPTION Ability to respond meaningfully to pressure-related discomfort	1. Completely limited: unresponsive to painful stimuli OR limited ability to feel pain over most of body surface	2. Very limited: responds only to painful stimuli; cannot communicate discomfort OR has a sensory impairment that limits the ability to feel pain or discomfort over 1/2 of body	3. Slightly limited: responds to verbal commands OR has some sensory impairment that limits ability to feel pain or discomfort in 1 or 2 extremities	4. No impairment
SKIN EXPOSURE TO MOISTURE	1. Constantly moist due to perspiration, urine, etc.	2. Very moist: skin is often, but not always moist	3. Occasionally moist	4. Rarely moist
DEGREE OF PHYSICAL ACTIVITY	1. Bedfast: confined to bed	2. Chairfast	3. Walks occasionally	4. Walks frequently
ABILITY TO CHANGE BODY POSITION	1. Completely immobile	2. Very limited: makes occasional slight changes in body positions	3. Slightly limited: makes frequent, slight changes in body position	4. No limitations
NUTRITION Usual food intake pattern	1. Very poor OR takes nothing by mouth or is maintained on clear liquids or IVs for more than 5 days	2. Probably inadequate OR receives less than optimum amount of liquid diet or tube feeding	3. Adequate OR is on a tube feeding, which probably meets most of nutritional needs	4. Excellent
FRICTION AND SHEAR	1. Problem: requires moderate to maximum assistance in moving; complete lifting is impossible; frequent repositioning with maximum assistance	2. Potential problem: skin probably slides to some extent against sheets, chair, restraints, or other surfaces, but occasionally slides down in bed	3. No apparent problem: maintains good position in bed or chair at all times	4. N/A

The Causes of Pressure Ulcers

Four factors contribute to the development of pressure ulcers: pressure, shearing forces (the stretching of tissue layers in opposite directions), friction, and moisture. Muscles and soft tissues below the skin are more sensitive than the skin to pressure-induced injury (see Figure 14). When a person is lying on a regular hospital mattress, the pressure measured under bony prominence such as the lower back can be high enough to decrease the oxygen tension to nearly zero. Such pressures can cause full-skin-thickness ulcers. For people who are seated for long periods, pressure under the buttocks may be even higher.

When repeated exposure to high pressures has caused a progressive and unnoticed injury deep in the skin tissues, it does not take much ongoing additional pressure or additional time for a full-thickness injury to occur. Shearing forces, which can also disrupt the blood flow in vessels near or in the skin tissues, occur when a seated person slides toward the floor. This can also happen when the head of the bed is elevated and the person slides toward the foot of the bed. The skin surface along the back remains stationary, being temporarily stuck to the sheets, while the blood vessels and soft tissues beneath the skin become stretched and pulled. These shearing forces are three times more destructive in older persons than they are in younger people, probably because of age-related loss of tissue in the skin.

Friction causes blisters that, when they open, lead to superficial pressure ulcers. This is the kind of injury that can occur when a person is pulled across a sheet or when repeated movements expose a bony area to the forces of friction. Moisture may increase the amount of friction produced between the person and the support surface, and skin moisture may by itself lead to skin injury. In one study, pressure ulcers were 5½ times more likely to occur in incontinent people, presumably because of the extra moisture. Because of the toxins and bacteria in stool, loss of bowel control may cause more skin breakdown than loss of bladder control.

Pressure ulcers within the tissues that overlie the bones are more likely caused by loss of blood flow and the loss of the ability to drain tissue fluid than to mechanical injury caused by friction. Shearing forces may cause direct injury to the soft tissues below the skin and also to muscle. Typically, the injury due to pressure alone begins in the very deepest tissues and spreads toward the skin surface. If the pressure is relieved, the normal response is a redness, but if it persists, the resulting pressure-induced injury leads to swelling of and leakage from the blood vessels. As fluid leaks into the space around the blood vessels, the skin and blood vessels stretch apart, which ultimately causes bleeding, leading to a stage 1 pressure ulcer (in which the redness of the skin does not turn white when it is pushed on).

Bacteria in the blood become deposited at sites of deep pressure-induced injury, where they develop into an abscess. This observation may explain why people with deep pressure ulcers may have significant problems even though the skin overlying the ulcer initially appears to be intact. The accumulation of fluid, blood, inflammatory cells, toxic waste products, and possibly bacteria, all combined with the loss of blood flow, ultimately and progressively leads to the death of muscle and the surrounding soft tissue. Eventually, the skin is affected as well.

Complications of Pressure Ulcers

Blood poisoning (septicemia) is the most serious complication of pressure ulcers. In a study of pressure ulcers associated with bacteria in the blood, the mortality rate was nearly 100 percent in people aged 60 and older. About half of people who have pressure ulcers that require significant cleaning (debridement) may have temporary bacteremia (bacteria in the blood) that usually resolves itself without further treatment, other than keeping the ulcer clean.

Besides blood poisoning, the other infectious complications of pressure ulcers include local infections, skin infections, and bone infections. For about 25 percent of people with nonhealing pressure ulcers, the underlying bone is involved in the infection. More rarely, the infected ulcers may lead to infection of a joint or of the abdominal cavity. Pressure ulcers can also serve as reservoirs for significant infections involving bacteria that are resistant to normal antibiotics.

Prevention of Pressure Ulcers

When a person is identified as being at risk, either because of the presence of multiple risk factors or by other means such as the Braden Scale, preventive measures should be immediately taken. The traditional approach to prevention is to intermittently reposition the person to relieve pressure over the bony prominence. The standard recommendation is to reposition the person every two hours to help prevent these injuries. The frequency of repositioning depends upon whether the support surface decreases the pressure on the bony prominence.

People who are highly susceptible to pressure ulcers should be repositioned alternately from the back to the right side or to the left side, in such a way that the person's back is at a 30-degree angle to the support surface. This regimen avoids direct pressure on the bony prominence of the lower back, hips, heels, and ankles. These sites account for 80 percent of all pressure ulcers. In contrast, lying with the back at a 90-degree angle to the support surfaces exposes the lower back and ankles to significant pressure. Pillows placed between the legs, behind the back, and supporting the arms can help in maintaining good positioning.

Although one should not rely on a pressure-relieving device such as a low-pressure mattress or support surface as a substitute for good care, these devices are certainly recommended for all who are at high risk for pressure ulcers. These devices can also reduce the frequency of required repositioning. Even when a device to reduce pressure is used, the skin over a bony prominence should be observed every two to four hours, and at the first sign of redness that does not turn white to pressure, more frequent repositioning or an alternative device should be considered.

There are a number of products and devices marketed in the United States for the prevention and treatment of pressure ulcers. These include sheepskins, foam pads, air mattresses, water- or gel-filled mattresses, and heel and elbow protectors. Doughnut-type cushions should not be used because they decrease the blood flow to the skin in the center of the cushion.

The Assessment of Pressure Ulcers   The appropriate management of a person with pressure ulcers requires assessment and treatment of underlying conditions that may be contributing to immobility, impaired nutritional status, and incontinence. The size, number, location, and stage of pressure ulcers should be recorded, and any evidence of infection such as a milky drainage, fever, foul odor, or surrounding redness of the skin should be noted. The doctor's and nurse's assessment often includes determining the deepness of the ulcers by gently pushing around the edge and probing with a clean cotton swab.

Underlying bone infection may also lead to a nonhealing pressure ulcer, but identifying this disorder beneath a pressure ulcer can be difficult. There is no foolproof way other than bone biopsy to determine this condition. Other procedures such as X rays, bone scans, and blood tests are less reliable by themselves. If the white blood cell count is elevated in association with an elevated erythrocyte sedimentation rate (a blood test of inflammation) or an unusual X ray, an underlying bone infection is a strong possibility. If none of these tests is abnormal, an underlying bone infection is highly unlikely.

Treatment of Pressure Ulcers

Attention to the person's nutritional status is especially important in managing pressure ulcers. Protein intake is one of the most important predictors of pressure ulcer healing. The adequate intake of vitamins and minerals, especially zinc and vitamin C, also appears to be an important factor in the healing process. Antibiotics given under a doctor's supervision are required for people with blood poisoning, infections in the skin or of the underlying bone. Antibiotics are also given to prevent the infection of diseased heart valves or in cases that require surgical removal of dead tissue around the ulcer. It is very important that a person use gloves in handling any infected material from the ulcer because of the potential for transmitting infectious organisms from the pressure ulcer.

Because people with pressure ulcers are at high risk for additional skin breakdown, the relief of pressure at the site of skin ulceration is absolutely essential. Attention to all the preventive measures listed earlier is also particularly important. This approach should help resolve early stage 1 pressure ulcers. The goal of local care for stages 2 through 4 pressure ulcers is to lower the number of bacteria so that healing can take place. Some people have reported dramatic results when granulated sugar is applied to the ulcer. Other ways to remove infected material include irrigating the wounds with whirlpool-type treatments or by means of dental-type irrigation devices.

As soon as the ulcer is clean and healing begins, a moist environment should be maintained without disturbing the healing tissue. Stage 2 ulcers generally heal by migration of cells from the borders of the ulcer while deeper stages 3 and 4 ulcers heal as tissue fills the base of the ulcer. Various dressings allow vapors to escape and to permit the accumulation of body fluid on top of the wound. To avoid hurting normal tissues, the moist dressing should be kept off the surrounding intact skin.

The Use of Special Beds and Mattresses

The air or foam mattresses used to prevent pressure ulcers should also be used for most people who have pressure ulcers. Some people may require a more expensive special bed such as an air-fluidized one. These beds contain small particles that are suspended in warm, pressurized air so that they take on the characteristics of a fluid. As the person floats on these particles, the pressures underneath a bony prominence are reduced. It is uncommon to achieve complete healing of pressure ulcers with this therapy. These beds can be expensive to buy or rent. There are some special beds available that automatically reposition immobilized people. These tend to be even more expensive than air-fluidized beds.

Surgery for Pressure Ulcers

There are many surgical procedures for the treatment of pressure ulcers, including closing of the ulcer margins, skin grafts, and flaps. The person's ability to tolerate rehabilitation and the surgical procedure should be carefully assessed before considering these procedures.

A number of experimental treatments have been advocated including high-pressure oxygen and electrical stimulation of the wound margins. In addition, a number of growth factors and nutrient solutions are being developed to stimulate wound healing. Lasers may facilitate removal of dead tissue in or around the ulcer. Despite the potential effectiveness of these treatments, prevention of the pressure ulcer remains the best approach to the problem.

Psoriasis

Psoriasis, a skin condition producing a red patch covered with a silvery scale, affects between 1 and 3 percent of the entire population and probably has a similar incidence rate in older people. The basic problem in psoriasis is that the skin growth is too rapid.

The first patches of psoriasis may appear at any age, but once they are present, psoriasis usually persists indefinitely with a course that tends to wax and wane. The extent and severity of the disease varies widely among older people. Fortunately, for most people the disease is relatively limited and typically consists of a well-defined scaly red plaque on the elbows or knees. Sometimes this is accompanied by scaling of the scalp or pitting of the fingernails. These pits are small depressions that look as though the nail had been pricked with a pin. Sometimes the areas of psoriasis appear on skin injured several days earlier (for example, on the site of a burn or a surgical scar). This is called Kobner's phenomenon (for the 19th-century German dermatologist, who first described it). In older people, psoriasis commonly develops in body folds such as the buttocks, with or without cracking, and especially in those who are overweight. Such areas can be painful. For some people the plaques of psoriasis are itchy but for most people this is not the case. Extensive disease is marked by the rapid loss and replacement of skin surface layers, which involves a constant shedding of the protein-rich scales from the skin's surface. This can create a substantial increase in the person's dietary protein requirements. The whole body surface may become covered with psoriasis, causing severe chills because the body is no longer able to regulate its temperature. In people with heart disease, congestive heart failure can occur.

Symptoms of Psoriasis

Treatment for psoriasis must be individualized and is based on the location and extent of the disease. An additional factor is the person's willingness and ability to comply with the treatment. In limited psoriasis with only a few plaques, topical corticosteroid creams or ointments rapidly decrease the scaling and often provide marked improvement. Usually potent corticosteroids are required for patches on the trunk of the body and the limbs, but nothing stronger than hydrocortisone should be used for areas on the face or body folds. A wide variety of other products derived from tar and anthralin are available. Physician-supervised phototherapy (exposure to artificial light containing ultraviolet and infrared rays) or even casual sun exposure is helpful and avoids the need for applying medication to individual plaques. For very extensive psoriasis, more aggressive therapy is warranted.

Treatment of Psoriasis

Figure 15. Skin Areas Supplied by the Spinal Nerves, or Dermatones

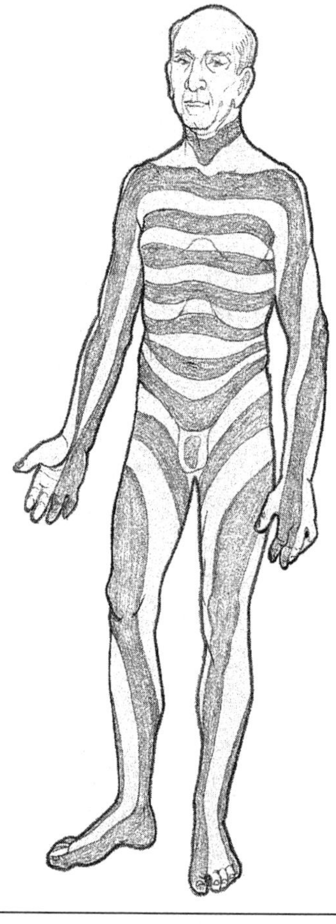

Shingles align along a dermatone, a skin area supplied by a single spinal nerve

Shingles

Shingles is a specific type of painful skin rash caused by the reactivation of the herpes zoster (chickenpox) virus. The rash is most commonly seen in older people or in people with impaired functioning of the immune system.

Symptoms of Shingles

The first signs on the skin are little grouped blisters, called vesicles, that sit (like dewdrops on a rose petal) on a linear patch of reddened skin. After several days, the vesicles begin to form scabs and dry out. These areas begin to heal after about four weeks. Sometimes shingles can be suspected before the skin blisters appear because a person will feel a burning pain or a sense of heightened skin sensitivity that feels as if it follows a thin line along one side of the body. This is, in fact, a line following the distribution of spinal nerves and is called a dermatome (see Figure 15). Shingles usually gets better on its own in older people who otherwise have normal immune function. Significant pain after the skin rash resolves, however, is experienced by many people following an acute attack.

Soaking these areas with various solutions will help treat the vesicles. Until crusting occurs, a soft cloth dampened with a solution such as Domeboro should be placed over the scabs and vesicles for 10 to 15 minutes several times a day. The area should be carefully observed for evidence of bacterial infection, which requires treatment with antibiotics should it occur.

Treatment of Shingles

Drug therapy for shingles remains controversial, although some experts recommend high doses of corticosteroids. Corticosteroids can help reduce the facial swelling around the eye that is associated with shingles that involves the optic nerve. While the complications of corticosteroids appear to be uncommon, corticosteroid therapy must always be used cautiously in older people. Several studies suggest that acyclovir, a well-tolerated but expensive antiviral drug, can reduce the pain and hasten the healing of shingles. Older people with known problems of their immune system clearly benefit from this treatment.

The treatment of the residual pain that can linger after a bout of shingles is problematic. Many approaches have been tried, ranging from the use of oral antidepressants to spinal nerve blocks, acupuncture, and capsaicin (a cream derived from red chili peppers), but none has gained wide acceptance.

Skin Cancers

More than 600,000 cases of skin cancers are reported each year in the United States and many more are probably treated without being documented.

Cause of Skin Cancers

Most of these skin cancers appear to be caused by exposure to sun. There is compelling evidence that more than 90 percent of basal cell cancers, about three-quarters of squamous cell cancers, and a large proportion of melanomas are sun-induced. In parts of the South and Southwest, the annual individual risk for developing skin cancer exceeds 3 percent among white individuals over the age of 65. The likelihood of having a skin cancer increases at least through the age of 80. The rapid and continuing increase of all forms of skin cancer, especially melanoma, is attributed to the increased total lifetime sun exposure by a large portion of the population. This probably results from such factors as more revealing bathing suits and winter vacations in sunny climates. This situation could be compounded by a decrease in the earth's ozone layer, which is responsible for absorbing the ultraviolet radiation in sunlight that can cause skin cancer.

Prevention of Skin Cancers

Because of this increase in sun-induced skin cancer, its prevention is a major public health issue. Ideally, protection from the sun should begin in childhood. Since disability and mortality are directly related to the size and depth of a malignancy, early detection is the second most important goal. The entire skin surface should be regularly examined for darkened lesions that are larger than 5 millimeters (¼ inch) in diameter, having variable color such as red, white, blue, and shades of brown, or having an irregular (notched) contour or surface. Ulcers and bleeding are signs of serious disease. Any suspicious-looking areas should be biopsied. Clearly, a dermatologist or a physician experienced in melanoma diagnosis should be involved. Complete removal constitutes the treatment for potentially curable lesions with the character and location of the melanoma determining the width of the margin.

Types of Skin Cancer

Basal Cell Carcinoma. Basal cell carcinoma, by far the most common human malignancy, is generally found on the body surfaces that have received the most sun. It looks like a pearly dome-shaped growth with prominent small blood vessels. As the tumor enlarges, a central ulcer may occur. This tumor grows by direct extension and hardly ever spreads to distant sites. However, untreated tumors can cause extensive destruction of the surrounding tissues. The treatments are tailored to the site and the cell type. Cure rates exceed 95 percent for most treatments.

Squamous Cell Carcinoma. Squamous cell carcinomas can occur in sites of chronic ulceration and radiation damage, but the vast majority are related to sunlight exposure. These skin cancers show far less tendency to metastasize than those attributed to other causes. Squamous cell cancers may show themselves as a scaly red bump, a plaque, or a nonhealing ulcer. For tumors that have not metastasized, the treatment and outlook are similar to that of basal cell cancers.

Melanoma. Melanoma is the most dangerous form of skin cancer and its prognosis depends strongly upon the depth of invasion. A five-year survival for a melanoma entering but not filling the full skin layer is better than 95 percent. Among people in whom the melanoma has entered the body fat, 40 percent have a five-year survival rate. Melanoma that has metastasized is rarely cured, and the survival rate depends upon the type of melanoma involved. Most melanomas are found in middle-aged people, but the incidence of the disease continues to increase until about the age of 90. As in all age groups, the superficial spreading melanoma is the most common type of melanoma in elderly people. Overall, after correcting for the type of melanoma and the depth of invasions at the time of diagnosis, the prognosis for melanoma does not appear to depend on the person's age.

A change in the skin due to poor circulation is called stasis dermatitis. This condition is due to a deterioration in the veins resulting in increased venous pressure.

Skin Changes Due to Poor Circulation (Stasis Dermatitis)

Symptoms of Stasis Dermatitis

Stasis dermatitis affects the lower legs, and in the early stages the skin has very itchy, small purple dots about the size of a pinhead. These areas represent points where blood has leaked from the capillaries because of the increased pressure in the veins. Over the course of time, the skin surface of the lower legs develops a red-brown color and may become shiny and feel bound down. The legs may swell with fluid, although this is not always the case. The presence of fluid can be detected by pressing a finger onto the skin over the ankle. If a deep fingerprint is left when the finger is taken away, then fluid is present. Sometimes minimal trauma to these skin areas can produce ulcers that do not heal well because of the impaired circulation.

Treatment of Stasis Dermatitis

The ideal treatment of stasis dermatitis would be to correct the increased pressure in the veins, although this is rarely possible. The immediate goal of treatment is to help reduce the pressure in the veins. This is sometimes accomplished by using support stockings or other forms of external pressure to help push the fluid back into the vessels. Raising the legs above the level of the heart intermittently is also helpful. Physicians sometimes prescribe hydrocortisone ointments to improve the itching and the irritation. Using these ointments over a long period of time can actually cause the skin to thin; therefore, their use should be minimized. It is very important to prevent injury to the lower legs to avoid ulcer formation. People who have stasis dermatitis should see their doctors right away for even apparently small ulcers. Treatment of an ulcer in the lower leg is best managed by a physician; home remedies or neglecting these ulcers can lead to rapid enlargement and significant complications.

Skin Infections

Any of the common skin infections that may be seen in the general population, such as boils or fungal disease, may also be seen in elderly people. However, two particular skin infections are especially relevant in the older person. These are erysipelas and cellulitis. (See also Infections in Chapter 26.)

Erysipelas

Erysipelas (from the Greek, meaning "red skin," also known as St. Anthony's fire) occurs usually in very young and very old debilitated people. In older people the infection is especially severe because it usually involves the face. This skin infection can be complicated by significant eye problems, blood clots within the head, or blood poisoning (septicemia). The infection is characterized by a red, warm, tender area that has a raised, swollen, well-defined border. Occasionally, small blisters may be seen. Generally, older people are very ill with fever, chills, headache, and general distress.

The diagnosis of erysipelas is normally made by a physician recognizing the characteristic appearance of the skin. Blood cultures are often obtained to determine if the infection has spread to the bloodstream. Intravenous antibiotics are immediately given until the results of these cultures are known. Like other infections in older people, this is a serious problem and a physician's supervision is urgently needed.

Cellulitis is a sudden, red skin rash that initially involves the uppermost layers of the skin. Eventually, it can spread to the deeper structures below the skin. It's found anywhere on the body but is most frequently seen on the legs of older people, usually as the result of trauma, poor circulation, diabetes mellitus, or edema. The source of the infection in the legs is most often a crack in the skin between the toes. It is also a common complication of infected pressure ulcers, bites, scrapes and scratches, puncture wounds, and surgery. Typically, the rash appears red, tender, warm, and swollen, but with no elevation or distinct borders.

Cellulitis

Cellulitis is caused by any number of microorganisms that vary according to circumstances—that is, whether the disorder is associated with pressure ulcers, diabetic foot ulcers, human bites, or surgery. People with very poor immune systems are also at risk for cellulitis.

A physician will diagnose cellulitis based on the clinical appearance of the involved skin. Blood cultures are warranted in persons sick enough to require hospitalization and intravenous antibiotics. Older persons with cellulitis who are otherwise generally well and do not have involvement of the face, can sometimes be treated without hospitalization. In these cases oral antibiotics are generally given.

CHAPTER 17

JOINTS, MUSCLES, AND BONES

Overview   Joint problems are extremely common and are the number-one cause of reduced activity as we get older. At least half of us will have joint conditions, but most of us are not bothered by our symptoms.

Joint problems in older people are more difficult to identify and treat than they are in younger people. The X rays and blood tests used to diagnose joint problems often show joint narrowing, bony changes, and other abnormalities that are unrelated to any symptoms. In addition, there may be more than one joint condition: osteoarthritis and rheumatoid arthritis, for example. Obviously, the presence of two or more forms of arthritis increases the chance of disability. Older people experience different types of joint problems, and conditions such as bursitis or tendinitis take longer to heal. Although there is less disk disease in older people, they experience more back pain caused by compression fractures (due to osteoporosis), unstable vertebrae, and cancer. Most people do not realize that rheumatoid arthritis occurs at a high rate among older people (about 3 in 100 women and 1 in 100 men). Moreover, rheumatoid arthritis involves different joints, has a different course, and requires different treatment in older people as compared with younger individuals. Other muscle and joint conditions such as polymyalgia rheumatica and pseudogout are seen primarily in older people. Each of these conditions is addressed later in this chapter.

Joint conditions are generally more difficult to manage in older people because of increased medicinal and surgical complications. However, despite these concerns, skillful professional care can substantially reduce the burden of disability that joint problems often cause for older people.

Generally, joint problems fall into one of five categories (shown in Figure 16):

Causes of Joint, Muscle, and Bone Problems

- Problems around the joint
- Mechanical problems with the joint
- Sudden inflammatory arthritis
- Smoldering inflammatory arthritis
- Wear-and-tear arthritis, called osteoarthritis

The symptoms of conditions involving structures around the joints, such as tendons or bursae, usually consist of pain brought on by some movements but not others. Pain that worsens at night and pain that occurs only in certain body positions suggests problems around the joint. Conditions around the joint do not show more stiffness in

Problems Around the Joint

237

Figure 16. Types of Joint Problems

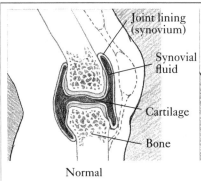

Normal

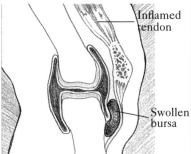

Problems around the joint

Pain increases with movement, though not with all maneuvers; pain is worse at night; no joint abnormalities or swelling

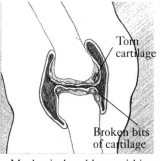

Mechanical problems within joint

Recurrent joint swelling; joints lock or give way; intermittent pain and pain-free intervals; limited flexion extension of joint; in the case of the knee, combined rotation and extension causes pain

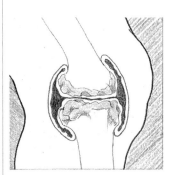

Wear and tear

Gradual progression of pain; pain increases with weight bearing; enlargement of joints; affects the finger and thumb joints, the hips and knees; does not affect the wrists, elbows, ankles or finger knuckles

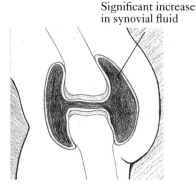

Sudden inflammatory arthritis

Develops abruptly and peaks in 12 to 48 hours; pain at night; fever, chills; marked redness, warmth, and swelling of the joint; sometimes associated with rash and heart murmur

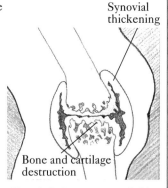

Chronic inflammatory arthritis

Develops unnoticeably over time; morning stiffness of an hour or more; can be associated with skin rash, fever, and weight loss; affects the knuckles, wrists, elbows, ankles; fingers become deformed; wrists and elbows lose range of motion

the morning and are not accompanied by symptoms such as fever, chills, weight loss, or change in appetite. Generally, people with problems around the joint (usually tendinitis or bursitis) have pain that is felt not at the joint but beyond it (toward the extremities) when the joint is in motion. These conditions can also limit the movement of the joint. The physician will attempt to reproduce the pain of tendinitis by applying resistance during the active range of motion of the affected muscle. For example, pressing down on the arm as the person attempts to lift it may reproduce the pain associated with tendinitis around the shoulder.

Mechanical Problems with the Joint

Mechanical problems may be caused by trauma that tears a joint's cartilage (a little pad that cushions the joint) or ligament (a fibrous band that connects bones) or changes in the underlying bone. People with these mechanical joint conditions generally have pain-free intervals with intermittent pain and dysfunction. The pain often occurs abruptly and the joints may frequently "give way" or "lock." There are no additional symptoms such as fever, weight loss, or change in appetite. People who have mechanical problems inside the joint generally have swelling around the joint and have pain with specific movements. For example, a torn cartilage in the knee may produce pain when the leg is straightened and slightly twisted.

Sudden Inflammatory Arthritis

With arthritis that occurs suddenly, people have an abrupt onset of joint pain and swelling, usually at its worst within 12 to 48 hours, accompanied by additional symptoms such as fever and chills. People usually cannot rest because of the pain, and will have a lot of fluid around the joint. These joints are not always warm, because active inflammation does not always produce an increase in skin temperature. People with this kind of active arthritis need to be evaluated immediately by a physician to check for infectious diseases, skin rashes, heart murmurs, and other evidence of underlying disease.

Chronic Inflammatory Arthritis

People with a chronic inflammatory arthritis such as rheumatoid arthritis have a slower onset of joint pain. Morning stiffness generally lasts more than an hour and involves the small joints such as the hands, wrists, ankles, and feet. This form of arthritis may be associated with weight loss, chest and abdominal pains, and skin rashes.

A careful physical examination provides the best way to determine the forms of chronic inflammatory arthritis. An older person may have painless loss of motion of the wrists or elbows and there may be early signs of thickening around the joint because of an increase in the synovium tissue that makes joint fluid. This synovium thickening may be seen along the knuckles of the hand, the wrists, the elbows, knees, and along the ball of the foot. Lymph gland enlargement in the armpit sometimes indicates joint inflammation in the arm. Severe deforming changes in the fingers can be seen in some forms of rheumatoid arthritis.

Osteoarthritis People with osteoarthritis have a gradual progression of pain, pain that worsens with the use of the joint, and stiffness in the morning that lasts less than a half hour. People with osteoarthritis may have bony enlargements of the joints and deformities of their fingers or legs caused by an asymmetric loss of the cartilage. In the usual form of osteoarthritis the characteristic joints involved are the very end joints of the fingers, the thumb, the hips, knees, and the base of the big toe.

The physician's examination of a joint, muscle, or bone problem focuses on joint swelling, stability, and range of movement. A search for any difficulty in walking and getting in and out of a chair is usually undertaken if the hips or legs are involved.

The most helpful test for diagnosing these various joint conditions is an examination of the joint fluid. This test is absolutely essential in people with sudden-onset arthritis to look for infection and for crystals that would indicate gout or pseudogout. Normal joint fluid is a clear viscous fluid that looks like motor oil and contains up to 200 white blood cells per microliter. The number of white blood cells helps the physician identify the cause of the joint condition. White blood cell counts between 200 and 2,000 are generally seen in osteoarthritis; and counts above 5,000 prove there is joint inflammation. People with white blood cell counts in joint fluid of more than 50,000 generally have cloudy joint fluid caused by either an infection, gout, or pseudogout.

Based on the joints involved, the nature of the discomfort, the results of the physical examination, and the examination of the joint fluid, the physician may order other laboratory tests to determine the cause of the arthritis more precisely. X rays may be difficult to interpret in older people with joint complaints because most older people have joint abnormalities on X rays. But, there is very little relationship between the appearance of X rays and the presence of pain. Consequently, before recommending treatment most physicians make sure that the symptoms and physical features of the person's condition are consistent with the results of diagnostic X ray studies.

Neck discomfort is very common, and the most frequent source is tension in the neck muscles. This discomfort usually improves on its own, but any pain that lasts more than a few weeks should be evaluated by a physician. Other warning symptoms are fever, arm weakness or numbness, and neck pain after a fall.

SYMPTOMS
Neck Pain

Changes in the neck (cervical spine) due to normal wear and tear are seen on neck X rays in virtually everyone over the age of 65. Three conditions that can cause neck pain are the following (see Figure 17):

Causes of Neck Problems

- Compression of the spinal cord
- Compression of a nerve root
- Pressure from a slipped disk

Compression of the Spinal Cord in the Neck. Compression of the spinal cord in the neck by bony growths called osteophytes (see Osteoarthritis, later in this chapter) can produce weakness in the legs and an urgent and frequent need to urinate (see Figure 17). Because the course of this condition is variable, specific recommendations for management are difficult to make. Many people have a slow progression or even a stable course despite significant changes in the weak structures on X rays. Aggressive surgery is risky and the results are inconsistent. About half of the people undergoing surgery experience significant improvement. The decision to operate, therefore, depends greatly on the progression of symptoms and on the severity of impairment in the nervous system.

Figure 17. Slipped, or Herniated, Disk

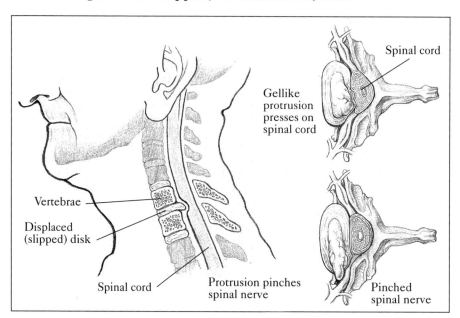

Compression of a Nerve Root. Pressure on a nerve root—causing a pinched nerve—in the neck can be caused by many things. There may be bony growths, osteophytes, pressing against the nerves where they exit from the spinal column or the nerve may be compressed by a slipped disk. Symptoms of a pinched nerve consist of pain, sometimes numbness and tingling, and sometimes changes of sensation occurring in bands (called dermatomes) along the neck, shoulders, upper chest, and arms. An illustration of dermatomes is shown in Figure 18. There may be weakness in the arms, hands, or fingers. These symptoms often resolve on their own in three to six weeks. If there is persistent or progressive arm weakness, one should seek medical attention.

Pressure from a Cervical Disk. Pressure from a ruptured disk in the neck (a cervical disk) produces pain in the neck, shoulder blades, and upper shoulders. The condition is sometimes confused with a muscle spasm. People with this condition have pain and limited motion on some, but not all neck movements. Cervical disk displacement can

Figure 18. Radiation of Pain from a Slipped Disk Along a Dermatone

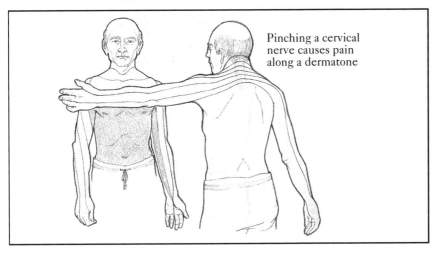

Pinching a cervical nerve causes pain along a dermatone

affect nerve roots, which in turn may affect the muscles associated with these nerves. A physician will examine carefully for such muscle involvement. Treatment of cervical disk displacement by immobilizing the neck with a soft foam rubber collar combined with intermittent cervical traction is a more logical approach than resorting to more aggressive neck braces and injections to the muscles. If left untreated, cervical disk displacement usually resolves itself in one to four weeks. If muscle weakness continues beyond four weeks, one should seek further, more extensive evaluation and treatment.

Shoulder Pain

Shoulder problems are quite common in older people. The shoulder structures are complex, consisting of three interrelated joints. A series of tendons and muscles around one of the joints form the rotator cuff, which reinforces the position of the upper arm to the shoulder blade. The muscles of the rotator cuff assist in moving the arm away from the body and reinforce the upper arm to hold the top portion of it in proper alignment with the other shoulder structures when the arm is lifted. The shoulder joint allows the arm to move more than any other body part. The shoulder is surrounded by many bursae, which are small pillowlike sacs that permit an easy gliding motion throughout joint movement.

Figure 19. The Shoulder

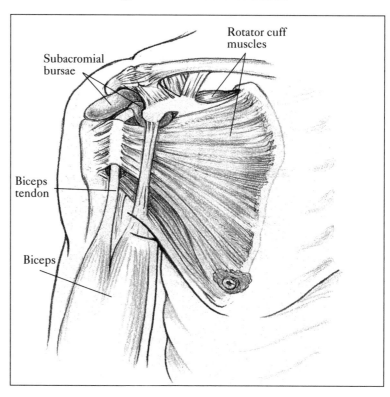

Causes of Shoulder Problems

The most vulnerable structures in the shoulder (see Figure 19) are these:

- Rotator cuff tendons
- The tendon that attaches the biceps muscle to the shoulder blade
- A large subacromial bursa that is between the large shoulder muscles and the upper part of the arm
- The joint between the collar bone and the shoulder blade

Any mechanical problem with these structures causes pain, usually felt in the upper part of the arm. This type of pain often increases after exercise and worsens at night. Medical attention should be obtained for shoulder pain with fever, severe shoulder pain with no movement, or if the arm cannot be lifted straight out to the side. Shoulder injuries can cause the shoulder to stiffen, but specific exercises and treatments can help maintain and restore function.

The rotator cuff tendons lie next to a large bursa called the subacromial bursa. Inflammation of either the rotator cuff tendons or the subacromial bursa produces similar pain. Because the treatment of rotator cuff tendinitis and subacromial bursitis is the same, we will consider them together.

Rotator Cuff Tendinitis and Bursitis

At the very end of the rotator cuff tendons on the upper arm the blood supply is limited. As a result, this region is subject to inflammation, reduced delivery of oxygen and nutrients to the tissues, and small tears of the tendons. These factors appear to cause rotator cuff tendinitis and bursitis. Usually this discomfort begins with a dull ache that extends from the shoulder into the upper arm and worsens at night. The pain is made more severe by such movements as reaching over one's head or putting on a coat.

Evaluation of Rotator Cuff Tendinitis and Bursitis. The physician can usually tell the difference between rotator cuff tendinitis and subacromial bursitis by pushing against the arm to resist the range of motion. Pain with resistance is typical of tendinitis. If the pain does not increase when resistance is applied, then the condition is probably bursitis.

Treatment of Rotator Cuff Tendinitis and Bursitis. As mentioned earlier, small tears of the tendons are a predominant cause of rotator cuff tendinitis. These take longer to heal in older people; an 80-year-old suffering from such small tears might need from three to four months for full recovery. A 20-year-old by contrast usually heals in two or three weeks. Therapy consists of either anti-inflammatory drugs or injections of corticosteroids into the painful area. It is also important to gently exercise the shoulder per a doctor's directions to help maintain movement and prevent scarring of the shoulder capsule.

Rotator cuff tears are muscle or tendon injuries that usually occur in people over the age of 50. Those who are being treated with

Rotator Cuff Tears

corticosteroids or who are receiving treatment for kidney failure tend to develop this problem.

Causes of Rotator Cuff Tears. Most people with rotator cuff tears resulting from these treatments have symptoms similar to those of rotator cuff tendinitis described above. In other cases, a tear may occur after a strain, collision, or fall.

Evaluation of Rotator Cuff Tears. A rotator cuff tear is identified during a physical examination by a physician. A person's inability to move the shoulder in the direction of the affected muscles (or tendons) indicates which muscle or tendon is torn. The confirmation of a suspected rotator cuff tear is often accomplished by special X ray studies.

Treatment of Rotator Cuff Tears. Treatment for complete rotator cuff tears is problematic. The only effective therapy is surgery to repair the torn muscle or tendon, but this goal is difficult to achieve in elderly people. Surgery should be carefully considered when a complete rupture prevents effective functioning.

Tendinitis of the Biceps Tendon

The tendon attached to the shoulder blade from the biceps muscle in the upper arm is frequently inflamed. When such inflammation occurs, pain is felt along the side of the shoulder. Sometimes, a portion of the biceps muscle fibers tears or ruptures, producing a large bulge near the elbow and a hollow space in the middle of the arm where the biceps muscle usually is. Fortunately, this condition does not significantly affect arm or shoulder function, and it often requires no therapy.

Frozen Shoulder

Frozen shoulder is a chronic condition characterized by a gradually progressive, painful restriction of shoulder movement. The cause of frozen shoulder is unknown. There is often a slow recovery in shoulder motion over a period ranging from months to years. In about 15 percent of people, both shoulders are involved.

People with a frozen shoulder experience aching in the shoulder region that often radiates to the upper arm. The pain is often worse at night and is aggravated by moving the affected arm. Although frozen shoulder sometimes follows an injury, it usually occurs without any clear precipitating event.

Evaluation of Frozen Shoulder. People with frozen shoulders lose shoulder motion in every direction, with the least ability to move the arm away from the body. Even though a frozen shoulder usually does not produce changes on an X ray of the shoulder, a physician may order an X ray to look for other possible causes, such as rheumatoid arthritis, bone deterioration caused by poor blood supply, and fractures of the upper arm.

Treatment of Frozen Shoulder. The natural untreated course of a frozen shoulder is an important consideration. Usually the painful phase lasts 2 to 4 months and is followed by a relatively stable period of immobility lasting 4 to 6 months. The full range of motion then gradually returns during the next 6 to 12 months. Regardless of the type (or lack) of treatment, the chance of a complete return of function is excellent. However, return of function may take up to two years.

A sensible approach to treatment, therefore, entails first understanding that the problem usually goes away without treatment or therapy. During the two to four months when there is shoulder pain, steroid injections or nonsteroidal anti-inflammatory drugs may provide relief. Once the pain has resolved, an active stretching program supervised by a physical therapist may be helpful, but it should be discontinued if it causes a recurrence or worsening of the pain. Active stretching programs usually yield the most improvement within the first three to four weeks of treatment. Aggressive therapies such as manipulation of the shoulder under anesthesia are not necessary.

Back Pain

Most of us will experience back pain—it is a chronic illness with a high likelihood of both recovery and recurrence. As with a number of other musculoskeletal or joint conditions, the cause, course, and evaluation of back pain in older people is quite different than in younger people. Changes in the lower back due to wear and tear constitute a normal feature of aging, and interestingly these changes by themselves do not cause back pain. In younger people, distortion of the gellike disks sandwiched between the vertebrae in the lower back is a common cause of back pain, but these disks lose much of their water content with age and are much less likely to become distorted (see Figure 17, page 242).

Causes of Back Pain

In older people, back pain can be produced by movement, disk compression of an already narrowed spinal canal with a displaced disk, and instability of the lower back vertebrae.

The range of causes in older people also includes an increased possibility of malignancy, infections, and abdominal aortic aneurysm (ballooning of a blood vessel wall described in more detail in Chapter 19).

Changes at one disk space in the lower back out of proportion to the rest of the spine can result in an unstable lower back spine. This instability sometimes pushes some of the vertebrae forward, which in turn pinch spinal nerves and cause severe pain in the back or down the back of the leg. This pain comes on suddenly, lasts a short period of time, and often recurs. It is frequently brought on by sudden movements. The person moves very carefully and has pain when moving from a flat to a sitting-up position. Sometimes a special corset with metal supports or abdominal-muscle strengthening exercises can help.

A backache caused by underlying diseases such as infections, aneurysms, and tumors usually has a distinct course that calls for prompt and vigorous investigation. Pain from a backache caused by an underlying disease gets steadily worse during a course of several days to weeks. The pain is not usually related to the person's position (lying or sitting) as it becomes more severe and persistent. Urgent warning signals that require immediate evaluation by a physician are pain in the upper to midback, fever, pain going down below the knee, difficulty walking, significant pain after a fall, and loss of bowel or bladder control. Because of the risk of spinal cord compression, a person with a known malignancy who experiences back pain should receive an emergency evaluation.

Evaluation of Back Pain

To determine the cause of most back pain, a physician needs to know how the condition started and its progress, the results of a physical examination, and a knowledge of applied anatomy.

Sophisticated X ray imaging usually does not reveal the cause of a person's back pain.

In older people, back pain is less likely to resolve without treatment and is more likely to require aggressive evaluation and treatment.

Treatment of Back Pain

Because low back pain usually produces muscle spasms, the basic treatment consists of rest and pain relievers. Generally the pain resolves in a week; persistent pain should prompt additional medical evaluation. Surgery may be considered for severely pinched nerves, but it is not always helpful and failures are common. Backache produced by infections, tumors, or aneurysms is treated by addressing the specific cause.

The hip joint is formed by the knob-shaped end of the femur (the thigh bone) and a socket made of bones in the pelvis (see Figure 20). The joint is located deep in the body and is protected by the large upper leg muscles. Because of its deep location, hip pain can be felt in many locations such as the groin, outer thigh, or even down the leg to the knee.

Hip Problems

Any of the common joint diseases mentioned in the introductory section on joint problems and specific conditions discussed later in

Causes of Hip Problems

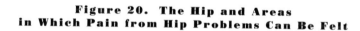

**Figure 20. The Hip and Areas
in Which Pain from Hip Problems Can Be Felt**

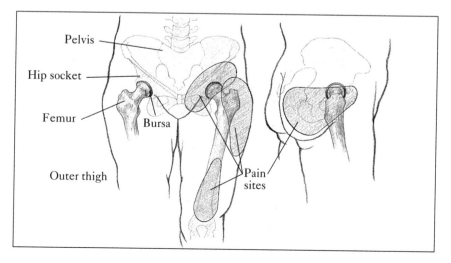

this section can affect the hip, including osteoarthritis, rheumatoid arthritis, and gout. Structures around the hip such as bursae can become inflamed. In addition, if blood supply to the knob-shaped end of the femur is reduced, the bone will wither. The femur can break relatively easily if the older person falls or has extensive osteoporosis (these conditions are discussed later in this chapter).

Evaluation of Hip Problems

Hip pain usually requires a medical evaluation. Medical attention should be sought immediately if there is fever, recent injury, walking difficulty, pain with bearing weight, or severe pain with no movement or weight bearing. The physician will probably order X rays.

Treatment of Hip Problems

The treatment of hip pain depends on the results of the physician's evaluation. Surgery may be helpful in some circumstances to reduce pain and improve ambulation.

Osteoarthritis of the Hip

Osteoarthritis of the hip is characterized by the gradual development of pain in either the buttock, groin, thigh, or front of the knee.

Cause of Osteoarthritis of the Hip. The pain is directly related to bearing the weight of the body, thus it is relieved when the person sits or lies down. People find that going up stairs is difficult because this activity requires the hip to bend. They also have difficulty in moving from a sitting to a standing position, and they walk with a gait that appears painful, which is often characterized by a short stride and extended buttock.

Evaluation of Osteoarthritis of the Hip. The inability to cross legs, tie shoes, or bend at the waist is an early sign of osteoarthritis of the hip. Because hip disease sometimes produces pain in the back or the knee, the hip must be carefully examined when either back or knee complaints occur. A physician usually checks the movement of the hip with the person lying flat (first on the back, then lying prone). The leg is moved up and down and from side to side to check the hip movements.

Treatment of Osteoarthritis of the Hip. Treatment of osteoarthritis of the hip involves pain relievers, weight loss, limitation of weight-bearing activities, an exercise program, and the use of supportive devices such as a cane (see Chapter 8). The cane should be used on the person's good side so that the cane and the weak hip form an arch. When walking, the weight is borne by the shoulder, arm, and cane and is shifted away from the painful leg. When done appropriately, as much as 40 percent of the weight can be shifted off a painful hip.

For the person with osteoarthritis of the hip, activities that produce the pain should be avoided and exercise begun cautiously. Usually severe pain at night indicates that there has been too much activity during the day. Extensive inappropriate weight-bearing activity may speed up the need for joint replacement surgery. Because of this, prolonged standing and walking should be avoided. On the other hand, too much sitting or use of a wheelchair can produce a stiff joint, so a balance between sitting, lying, and standing must be achieved to maximize function.

An exercise program usually performed under the supervision of a physical therapist can help to maintain the strength of the muscles around the joint to prevent deformity and maintain function. Exercises that stretch the joint or increase the range of motion are not likely to be helpful because the loss of range of motion is caused by loss of cartilage. Rather, a person with osteoarthritis should follow a regimen of exercises done while lying on the stomach and designed to prevent hip contractures. A swimming program to maintain the muscles around the joint without irritating the joint is also likely to help.

A decision to replace a hip joint destroyed by osteoarthritis is a major one. The primary reason for a hip replacement is the relief of pain. Surgery should be considered if the person has pain that makes transferring weight from side to side and short walks difficult, has significant pain at night, or pain that has a disabling impact on the person's lifestyle.

Knee Problems

Knee problems are very common, affecting about 5 percent of elderly people. Knee disorders can produce considerable disability, especially in walking or using stairs because there are few ways to compensate for impaired knee function.

The knee joint is a hinge that can move a little over 120 degrees. Normally the knee locks into position when fully straightened.

Figure 21. The Knee

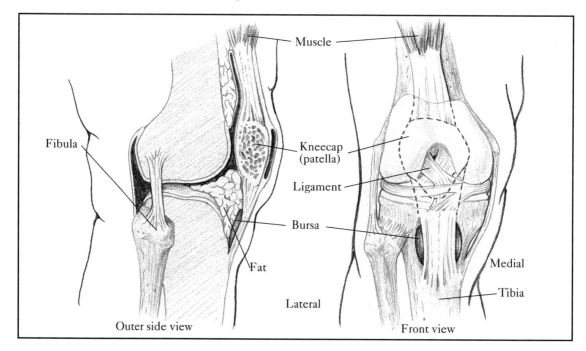

Outer side view

Muscle

Fibula

Kneecap (patella)

Ligament

Bursa

Fat

Lateral

Medial

Tibia

Front view

Horses take advantage of this and are able to sleep while standing. Stability of the knee depends on the strength of the bones, muscles, and ligaments as well as the cartilage pad that sits in the joint.

Causes of Knee Problems

Any of the common joint diseases can affect the knee. Osteoarthritis is the most common and produces pain on standing (see page 253). Serious conditions such as infection and gout can also frequently produce swelling and knee pain.

Evaluation of Knee Problems

Because knee problems can result in significant walking difficulty, most people should seek medical attention if they notice swelling, severe knee pain, or any knee instability. Medical attention should be immediately sought if there is fever or if the person cannot walk.

Treatment of Knee Problems

The treatment of knee problems depends on the results of the physician's examination. Medications and physical therapy are often prescribed, and surgery may be appropriate for torn cartilages or severe deformity.

Osteoarthritis of the knee can involve three components of the knee: the kneecap, the inner (medial) portion of the knee, and the outer (lateral) portion (see Figure 21). Usually, a narrowing of the medial joint space, resulting in bowleggedness, is the earliest feature of the condition.

Osteoarthritis of the Knee

The pain produced by problems of the kneecap commonly occurs over the top surface of the knee and radiates down into the lower leg. Since bending the knee while bearing weight stretches this compartment, going down stairs often creates the pain. Many people compensate for this by going down stairs sideways or even backward. The strain on tissues attached to the kneecap is made worse by atrophy of the large muscles in the thigh. Osteoarthritis involving the kneecap can produce crepitus, a crackling and popping sound that can be produced by placing the hand on the kneecap as the person straightens the knee.

The medial component of the knee is the most commonly affected portion of the osteoarthritic knee—bending the knee will produce pain. The loss of the ability to straighten the knee makes the transfer of weight from one position to another difficult; there is also a strain on the hip and back during walking. A reasonable exercise program has three goals: strengthening the large thigh muscles as much as possible, avoiding any further irritation around the kneecap, and preventing knee stiffness and resistance to movement, called contractures. These aims can be achieved by sitting on the edge of a high chair or table and gently kicking one leg out as straight as possible, then holding the leg straight out without support for a count of five. This exercise can be built into the daily routine and done, for example, while watching television. One leg can be raised and held straight out for the duration of a television commercial then the opposite leg raised and held out for the duration of the next commercial and so on.

Foot disorders almost always cause walking problems in older people. Close inspection of the feet often provides useful clues to the overall hygiene and health status of the individual. People with alcohol problems, for example, will often have feet that are not well cared for and that perspire freely.

Foot Problems

Table 21. Causes of Foot Pain

Big toe deformities

Blood vessel disease

Congenital causes

Gout

Ill-fitting shoes

Neurologic disease

Plantar warts

Rheumatoid arthritis

Stress fractures

Trauma

Tumors

Figure 22. Foot Problems

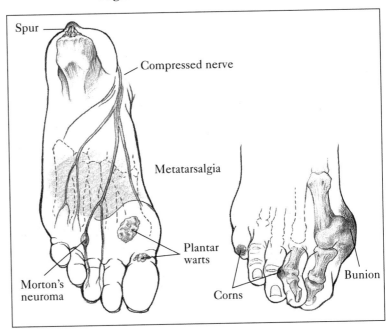

Causes of Foot Problems

A lifetime of habitual foot activity and the use of ill-fitting footwear can produce a number of foot deformities including bony growths called exostoses. These bone growths may lead to foot distortions, swelling over the exostoses, skin growth over the protuberance (commonly called a corn), and a need for therapeutically designed footwear. Foot pain can result from a variety of conditions, as listed in Table 21.

Treatment of Foot Problems

The first step in treatment involves modifying the footwear to accommodate the changes in the foot. This may mean stretching the current shoes, buying new shoes, or having specially designed shoes made to accommodate the foot abnormality. Treatment of corns with corn plasters may reduce the pressure on the affected area. Sometimes weight-bearing activities must be stopped for a few days to control the symptoms. Nonweight-bearing exercises should be done during this time to maintain strength and movement. Non-steroidal anti-inflammatory drugs may provide some pain relief, especially when minor swelling and redness are present. When the symptoms of foot disorders limit one's activity and do not get better, a visit to the physician or a podiatrist is in order.

While surgical procedures to correct foot problems are sometimes successful, these procedures involve substantial discomfort and limit standing and walking for weeks to months. People recovering from foot surgery must be sure to maintain their muscle strength during convalescence.

Pain in the ball of the foot (called metatarsalgia) is one of the most common foot problems seen in older people.

Pain in the Ball of the Foot

Causes of Pain in the Ball of the Foot. The condition appears to be more common in women than in men and may be caused by wearing pointed-toe shoes and by a number of disorders that distort the metatarsal joints.

A bunion, sometimes called hallux valgus, is a condition in which the big toe turns sideways, almost pointing directly toward the little toe on the same foot (see Figure 22). This produces a protrusion and sometimes bony growth at the joint at the base of the large toe. A bunion can also be a consequence of rheumatoid arthritis or osteoarthritis. As the large toe turns to the side, the second toe may overlap it and develop corns on its top surface caused by friction with the shoe. Occasionally, small branches of the nerves in the foot are compressed, producing tenderness and tingling in the areas around the toes and just behind the toes.

Morton's neuroma, a benign small nerve growth, can form on any of the small nerves of the foot but usually involves the third toe. Early on, the growth produces a mild ache in the area of the ball of the foot that is sometimes accompanied by a mild burning sensation. The pain can be reproduced by pushing on the space at the base of the third or fourth toe.

Causalgia, a type of reflex in the nervous system that follows an injury to a large (trunk) nerve, produces a severe burning pain in the foot.

Tarsal tunnel syndrome is caused by trauma (especially a fracture), foot deformity, or excessive movement in the foot and ankle. The nerve supplying sensation to the foot, called the posterior tibial nerve, is compressed near the ankle, resulting in numbness, tingling, burning pain, and other changes of sensation in the toes and soles of the feet. Sometimes the person cannot feel the prick of a pin in these areas. Ankle, foot, and leg movements may relieve the pain in tarsal tunnel syndrome. The condition is similar to the carpal tunnel syndrome that can involve the hands.

Plantar warts resemble corns and callouses and are flat and surrounded by extra skin growth. They can be extremely tender and may appear anywhere on the sole of the foot.

Treatment of Pain in the Ball of the Foot. Usually, the initial treatment for metatarsalgia is conservative, consisting of weight loss for people who are overweight and choosing appropriate footwear. Physical therapy and anti-inflammatory medication are often helpful. Custom-made shoes are usually not necessary and most people can be treated initially with simple soft pads in their shoes designed to transfer weight-bearing to areas of the foot that are not painful. If such adaptations of footwear do not work, then it may be necessary to obtain special devices. As mentioned earlier, surgery should be considered only when less invasive measures for correcting foot problems have failed.

Heel Pain
Older people frequently have heel pain that begins immediately upon walking and lessens as walking continues. In most situations, however, the pain is felt at the base of the heel most when the person is standing.

The most common cause of such heel pain is a bone spur that presses into the heel area. Placing a pad or special insert into the person's shoe to decrease weight on the heel may relieve the pain. Footwear that provides maximum cushioning such as shoes with rubber soles is helpful. Sometimes it is necessary for a physician to inject the area with a corticosteroid, which often provides relief for many weeks. Surgical treatment is rarely necessary.

Haglund's deformity (sometimes known as the "pump bump") appears to arise from pressure on the back of the heel where a bursa may become irritated by pressure from a shoe. This condition may respond to NSAIDs or a corticosteroid injection. Heel lifts that raise the heel above the shoe top can also help in reducing pain and discomfort. If these efforts do not work, surgical removal of the bursa may be necessary.

Itching of the feet is common in older people and may simply be due to dry, scaly skin. Contact dermatitis and fungal disease such as athlete's foot are also common causes of itching. A moisturizing cream may help reduce the itching problem. For seriously irritated feet, it may be necessary to apply a cream or lotion containing a small amount of corticosteroids. A skin condition called contact dermatitis can result from an allergic reaction to shoes or other footwear. Sometimes a change in footwear relieves this condition. Athlete's foot is identified by the presence of small blisters, cracks, or fissures in the skin. The most common site for these conditions is between the toes. Older people may be predisposed to develop other complications, especially if they have poor circulation to the feet. Treatment of athlete's foot includes soaking the feet with Epsom salts and applying topical antifungal creams. Close examination of the area between the toes is especially important in any older person since this is one of the most common sites from which serious infection (such as cellulitis) can spread to the legs.

Corns and calluses result from friction around bony prominences and are particularly associated with shoes that do not fit correctly. Corns are especially common over bunions or other abnormalities in the feet. If corns and calluses are causing problems a physician or nurse can trim them or provide padding to the shoe to relieve pressure and to reduce friction.

Miscellaneous Foot Disorders

Although gout most frequently develops in middle-aged men, it can occur at any age. In women, gout most often appears after menopause. Development of a sudden painful large joint in the foot or lower leg suggests the condition.

CONDITIONS
Gout

Gout is a disease usually associated with a high uric acid level in the blood and the deposition of uric acid crystals in body tissue. Uric acid comes from the chemical breakdown of purines—one of the building blocks of DNA. Alcohol use may increase the chance of getting gout. People taking diuretic medication, alcohol, or who

Causes of Gout

257

have recently had a serious illness or surgery also have an increased likelihood for gout. Gout tends to be episodic and recurring.

Evaluation of Gout

Although elevated uric acid in the blood is often present, a doctor usually bases a diagnosis of gout on the results of a microscopic examination of fluid drawn from the affected joint with a needle. Characteristically, the examination will reveal needle-shaped uric acid crystals.

Treatment of Gout

There are many effective methods of treating acute gout. High doses of nonsteroidal anti-inflammatory drugs (NSAIDs) are effective in most cases. Colchicine, a drug that can be given intravenously, is also an effective medication for flare-ups. Oral colchicine once or twice a day can also act as an effective preventative measure against recurrent attacks of gout. The high oral doses of colchicine required for treating an acute attack almost always cause diarrhea and do not appear to be as effective as NSAIDs or intravenous colchicine.

A high uric acid itself does not need to be treated unless the person is having recurrent symptoms of gout, or has kidney stones caused by high uric acid. Some people undergoing cancer treatment by chemotherapy receive treatment to lower uric acid because chemotherapy can produce extremely elevated uric acid levels in the blood. The use of uric acid–lowering drugs has no role in the management of a sudden gout attack, but can be useful in some people to prevent attacks.

Pseudogout

Pseudogout, also known as calcium pyrophosphate deposition disease (CPPD), is a common cause of joint pain in older people. The average age of onset is the late fifties. It is called pseudogout because it resembles acute attacks of gout and may be difficult to distinguish clinically.

Cause of Pseudogout

Pseudogout is characterized by calcium deposits in the joints and the presence of crystals of calcium pyrophosphate in the joint fluid seen under a microscope.

Evaluation of Pseudogout

There are many forms of pseudogout and any joint can be affected, although it most often involves the knees and wrists. In addition, as in authentic gout, pseudogout can be provoked by severe illness, injury, or surgery; attacks are often accompanied by fever.

One form of pseudogout resembles rheumatoid arthritis. People with this form have chronic discomfort that lasts from weeks to months, and may have very stiff joints in the morning. A useful clue is wrist and knee involvement without the involvement of any other small or large joints. Some people experience a progressive destruction of many joints with pseudogout, which may indicate another underlying problem. Although X ray evidence of calcium in the joint can help a physician diagnose pseudogout, this finding by itself does not indicate the cause of pain, because over 25 percent of older people (most of them pain-free) have calcium in their joints.

Treatment of Pseudogout

Usually the treatment of pseudogout consists of NSAIDs for abrupt attacks, although low-dose colchicine may also decrease the frequency of attacks. In people with only one affected joint, draining the inflamed fluid from the joint and injecting corticosteroids can be helpful.

Osteoarthritis

Osteoarthritis is a slowly progressive disorder principally affecting the hands, hips, and knees. (See the sections on hip and knee problems for more information.)

Cause of Osteoarthritis

Loss of cartilage, the normal cushion of the joint, is the main feature of osteoarthritis. This loss causes bone changes: formation of bony growths called osteophytes, small holes (cysts) in the bone near the joints, and changes below the cartilage in the bone that supports the joint. Normal cartilage is made of chemical building blocks that have water-absorbing and elastic properties. The earliest signs of osteoarthritis are changes in some of these building blocks, resulting in less water absorption and reduced elasticity within the cartilage. Pain and dysfunction are the major problems associated with osteoarthritis. The pain itself is probably not due to the changes in the cartilage (cartilage does not contain nerve fibers), but most likely results from small fractures around the joint, stretching of the joint lining, or irritation of nerves that accompany the blood vessels below the cartilage. These mechanical problems can cause pain and swelling in the joints.

X rays show a characteristic, asymmetric joint space narrowing, reflecting loss of cartilage. X rays also reveal bone cysts and extra bone growth where two bony surfaces touch or rub each other. Osteoarthritis can also result as a by-product of fractures, repeated trauma, diseases such as gout and pseudogout, bleeding in the joint, and inadequate blood supply to the bones that make up the joint.

Evaluation of Osteoarthritis

The most common form of osteoarthritis is seen in postmenopausal women. The first clue is usually a bony enlargement of the end joints of the fingers; however, other finger joints and the base of the thumb can be affected. Other joints frequently involved include the hips, knees, and the base of the big toe. Lack of involvement in the wrist, elbow, and ankle helps to differentiate this condition from arthritis caused by gout, pseudogout, and other inflammatory conditions. People who have bony enlargement of the joints generally maintain complete functioning of these joints. Stiffness and aching, however, can develop in the early years of the condition. Even so, most people with osteoarthritis can use their hands with little discomfort over long periods of time.

Treatment for Osteoarthritis

Ice packs applied once or twice a day can be quite helpful for reducing the pain around an osteoarthritic joint. Injection of corticosteroids into irritated bursae or ligaments can often relieve discomfort. Generally, for additional pain relief acetaminophen should be tried first. If this is not effective, a trial of low-dose aspirin (4 to 6 tablets per day) is often recommended as the next best medication for people who can take aspirin. If these two simple regimens do not work, a physician should be seen for additional evaluation and guidance.

Rheumatoid Arthritis

Rheumatoid arthritis is a chronic systemic disease characterized by inflammation of small joints, usually symmetrically (on both sides of the body). Other body organs such as the blood vessels, heart, lungs, and nerves can be involved.

Cause of Rheumatoid Arthritis

The cause of rheumatoid arthritis is not known. The joint lining (synovium) grows and thickens, which starts an inflammatory reaction that chemically destroys the cartilage, ligaments, tendons, and bones, ultimately affecting the joints. Rheumatoid arthritis occurs in about 3 percent of elderly women and 1 percent of elderly men. While the peak onset of rheumatoid arthritis is usually in the thirties or forties, it starts after the age of 60 in at least 10 percent of people. Women, whether young or old, are more commonly affected. Many elderly people with rheumatoid arthritis have antibodies in their blood called rheumatoid factors.

The classical features of rheumatoid arthritis include stiffness, swelling, and pain of the small joints of both hands, both wrists, both feet, and both ankles. The course of the illness is often progressive and destructive. This classical pattern is seen in older as well as younger people.

A second pattern of the disease is more characteristically seen in people who develop rheumatoid arthritis at an older age. Typically there is an abrupt onset of the disease, with involvement of large joints such as the shoulder, hip, and knee. More men have this type than women and rheumatoid factors are often not elevated in the blood. There is a reasonable chance of spontaneous remission within a year. The large joint involvement often makes this condition difficult to distinguish from other arthritis.

Evaluation of Rheumatoid Arthritis

Rheumatoid arthritis is usually diagnosed through a physical examination. The presence of swelling of the joints in the hands, ankles, and elbows as well as loss of motion of the wrist, shoulders, and hips points to inflammatory arthritis. Laboratory tests have a limited role in making the diagnosis because an abnormal result is not very specific for rheumatoid arthritis. A key to the identification of this condition in older people is the presence of joint inflammation in joints not involved with general wear-and-tear osteoarthritis. An increased number of white blood cells in the joint fluid is a good indicator of an inflammatory arthritis.

Treatment of Rheumatoid Arthritis

Nonsteroidal anti-inflammatory drugs are used cautiously in treating rheumatoid arthritis because of the potential gastrointestinal, kidney, heart, and other complications. Short courses of low doses of corticosteroids can be helpful in some older people (for example, 10 milligrams of prednisone a day). Long-term use of high doses (more than 10 milligrams of prednisone a day) can produce devastating side effects such as bone fractures, tendon ruptures, infections, and skin

Figure 23. Osteoporosis and Osteomalacia

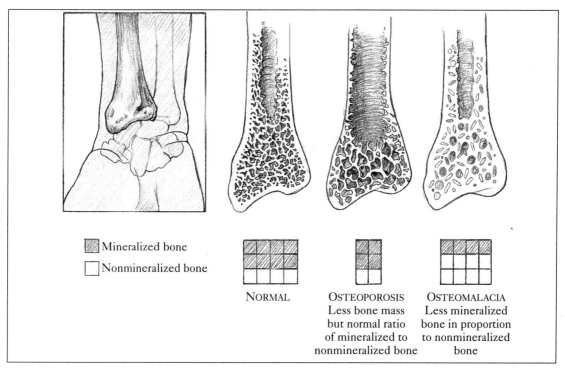

Mineralized bone

Nonmineralized bone

NORMAL

OSTEOPOROSIS
Less bone mass
but normal ratio
of mineralized to
nonmineralized bone

OSTEOMALACIA
Less mineralized
bone in proportion
to nonmineralized
bone

breakdown. High doses of corticosteroids are used only if the disease is not responding to other measures.

Osteoporosis and Osteomalacia

Osteoporosis and osteomalacia are both diseases producing a lack of bone. However, osteoporosis and osteomalacia differ: In osteoporosis the bone is normal in its mineral composition but is decreased in amount, whereas osteomalacia is characterized by having decreased bone mineralization (see Figure 23).

Osteoporosis

Under the microscope, osteoporosis is defined as a decrease in the amount of bone, with the remaining bone appearing normal. A useful, clinical definition of osteoporosis is less clear. A panel of experts convened by the National Institutes of Health defined osteoporosis as "an age-related disorder characterized by decreased bone mass and increased susceptibility to fracture in the absence of other recognizable causes of bone loss." To some extent osteoporosis is part of normal aging. The challenging task is distinguishing between the amount of bone loss that is normal for a person's age and that which should be considered abnormal. It seems clear that with decreasing amounts of bone that the likelihood of fractures goes up, but even at the lowest levels of bone density, some people do not experience fractures.

For white women over the age of 65 the lifetime risk of hip fracture is about 15 percent, vertebral fracture 30 percent, and forearm fracture 10 percent. African-American women have about one-third the risk of fracture of white women. White men have a 6 percent risk of hip fracture compared with a 3 percent risk in African-American men. The lifetime risk of hip fracture remains stable from the ages of 60 to 90. The estimates for vertebral crush fractures are more difficult to determine because many do not cause symptoms. Most fractures occurring in vertebrae happen in the middle and lower back. The principal problems include decreased height, stooped posture, possible back pain, and a significant amount of psychologic distress. Wrist fractures, the third most common type of fracture associated with osteoporosis, are relatively benign but cause significant transient disability.

Causes of Osteoporosis. The fundamental causes of osteoporosis are considered to be related to the menopause and to age. For other causes the mechanisms appear to be complex and are not well understood. A simple classification is shown in Table 22.

Because women have so many more fractures of the hip, wrist,

Table 22. Causes of Osteoporosis

Aging

Alcohol

Cigarettes

Disuse (immobilization)

Drugs

Hormone changes (estrogen, diabetes mellitus, thyroid disease, others)

Malignancy (multiple myeloma, leukemia, lymphoma)

and vertebrae than men, estrogen deficiency is thought to be a cause of osteoporosis. Women who take estrogen have about half the number of hip fractures than women not taking estrogen have. Estrogen replacement corrects poor absorption of dietary calcium in postmenopausal women. Bone density is maintained in women treated with estrogens as compared with women not so treated. Estrogen also has an effect on vitamin D and parathyroid hormone levels, two compounds intimately related to bone growth and bone loss.

A relative deficiency of calcium has also been suggested as a cause of both postmenopausal and age-related osteoporosis. The age-related decrease in calcium absorption by the intestine may be due to problems with vitamin D activation by the kidney. Another factor is that lack of exercise or activity may cause the bones to release calcium.

Additional evidence for calcium's role in the development of osteoporosis comes from studies looking at the amount of calcium in the diet. Studies suggest that a high level of calcium intake through life may decrease the risk of fracture and help maintain overall bone density. Other studies have suggested that people with osteoporosis have had lower calcium intake than people who do not have osteoporosis.

Decreased calcium absorption from the intestine is at least partially responsible for the calcium loss that occurs when someone is completely immobilized in bed, and conversely, calcium absorption increases with physical activity. These changes are consistent with the observations that immobility causes bone loss while exercise may have a protective effect against osteoporosis. Exercise may also have a beneficial effect in preventing osteoporosis by directly increasing bone density.

Symptoms and Manifestations of Osteoporosis. A fracture due to little or no apparent trauma may be the first indication of osteoporosis. Sometimes incidental fractures in the vertebrae are seen on chest or spine X rays. Common situations include back pain with vertebral compression fractures, pain due to a hip fracture following a fall, and fracture of the wrist after falling on outstretched hands. Because of an increased awareness of the occurrence and importance of osteoporosis, many women now seek an assessment of their risk.

Evaluation of Osteoporosis. In general, the physician's evaluation includes a complete physical examination and blood tests to look for possible causes such as thyroid gland abnormalities, diabetes mellitus, various malignant diseases, and liver and kidney disease.

Estimates of fracture risk depend on several clinical factors: racial and genetic background, diet, medications, smoking history, exercise, and body size and weight. However, even when used in combination, these clinical factors cannot adequately predict bone density in an individual person and cannot be recommended as a way to reliably determine the chance of a fracture.

To provide more accurate estimates of the risk of fractures, a special technique called bone densitometry has been developed to measure bone density. This technique uses a low-level X ray source to determine the amount of bone density. The person puts his arm in a box and the bone is scanned in a few moments. Bone density measures can predict the likelihood of fractures up to seven years in advance. The lower the amount of bone density the higher the fracture rate. Bone densities of women under age 60 have been predictive of vertebral fractures, while bone densities of women older than 60 on average have been predictive of hip fractures. Although this predictive capability is impressive, it's still not reliable enough for general application. Bone density screening programs are not recommended at this time.

Treatment and Prevention of Osteoporosis. The treatment for established osteoporosis remains experimental. Sodium fluoride is a recognized treatment, yet its safety and efficacy are still being determined. Fluoride increases bone mineral density, but the resulting bone may be brittle (like porcelain) and fractures may actually be more common during fluoride treatment.

Calcitonin is a hormone that has not yet been shown to reduce fractures, although it is approved for treatment of osteoporosis. It appears to increase bone density up to 8.5 percent over a year. However, this increase in density tends to plateau at about 18 months. Calcitonin is expensive and generally must be used as an injection. However, a nasal spray has been developed and if proved effective may become the preferred mode of administration. Strategies are being developed to try to overcome the plateau effect.

In spite of the progress made in the treatment of osteoporosis, prevention continues to be the main way to address this condition. Men and women should increase their intake of calcium since age-related decreases in calcium absorption occur in both sexes. Good calcium intake early in life can increase the peak of skeletal bone mass. This increased peak can help as bone is slowly lost throughout life. For postmenopausal women, the intake of calcium should be 1,500 milligrams per day, and for elderly men it should be at least 1,000 milligrams per day. Because older men and women have increased requirements for vitamin D, they should take between 600 and 800 international units (IU) of this vitamin. (Two regular multivitamins usually provide 800 IU.) Older people with a history of kidney stones should not take extra calcium or vitamin D.

Weight-bearing exercise should be used as a preventive measure in both men and women throughout life. Exercise three times a week helps maintain bone mass and may reduce the risk of fractures.

Estrogens reduce postmenopausal osteoporosis. There is a 50 percent reduction in the risk of hip and wrist fractures in women who use estrogen.

In addition to providing a substantial benefit of hip fracture prevention, estrogen may also prevent heart attacks. Several studies suggest a 50 to 60 percent reduction of the risk of heart disease, which has led many people to conclude that the benefits far outweigh the risks of estrogens. (See Chapter 25 for more on estrogen-replacement therapy.)

The decision to use estrogens, however, to prevent osteoporosis must be based on an analysis of the benefits versus the risks. If estrogen is used by itself, there is a small increase in the risk of endometrial cancer. The risk of developing endometrial cancer can be avoided by adding progestin, another female hormone, to produce menstrual cycling. The effect of this combination on breast tissue is not known. Using estrogen alone for up to 15 years does not appear to increase the risk of breast cancer; using estrogen and progestin together may increase the risk. Another concern is that adding progestin may change the levels of cholesterol in the blood and reduce some of the potential cardiovascular benefits of estrogen therapy.

It is not clear if a woman is ever too old to begin estrogen replacement therapy (ERT). The rate of bone loss is reduced in women who begin to use estrogen in their eighties, but this may not really reduce their risk of fracture. Some experts have suggested that ERT should begin at menopause and should be stopped at the age of 65. The rationale for this is that it may take approximately 20 years after the menopause for fractures due to osteoporosis to occur. Because of this 20-year interval it is believed that taking estrogen until the age of 65 would delay the onset of hip fractures until the age of 85. However, since this rationale pertains only to the use of estrogen for the prevention of fractures due to osteoporosis, this strategy does not take into account a continued use of estrogen for the potential prevention of cardio-vascular disease.

Osteomalacia

Osteomalacia can be confusing because it may refer to a variety of things, including several symptoms indicating an underlying condition, a specific disease, and a particular, microscopically observed deterioration of bone structure. As a specific disease, osteomalacia is caused by vitamin D deficiency.

Causes of Osteomalacia. The causes of osteomalacia are shown in Table 23. Problems with vitamin D regulation, ultimately, are the common cause of osteomalacia. To understand these causes it is important for us to review how vitamin D is used in the body.

Vitamin D is a naturally occurring constituent of a few foods such as cod liver oil, swordfish, and eggs. It is also made in the skin in the presence of sunlight exposure. A chemically synthesized version of vitamin D is commonly added to milk and other foods. These dietary and skin sources of vitamin D are modified by the liver and in the kidney to more active forms.

Vitamin D has many functions including the regulation of calcium and phosphorus absorption in the intestine, the release of calcium from the bone to regulate calcium levels in the blood, maintaining phosphate balance, and a role in helping bone to mineralize, which is not completely understood. Vitamin D deficiency results in decreased calcium absorption from food, stimulation of parathyroid hormone, decreased phosphorus in the blood, and later on, decreased calcium in the blood.

Table 23. Causes of Osteomalacia

VITAMIN D DEFICIENCY

Anticonvulsant therapy

    These drugs stimulate liver metabolism of vitamin D to inactive metabolites

Chronic severe liver disease

Chronic kidney disease

    Due to impaired formation of active vitamin D by kidneys and to circulating inhibitors of bone mineralization found in kidney failure

Dietary lack, especially in alcoholism

Gut malabsorption

    Vitamin D is a fat-soluble vitamin and fat malabsorption (steatorrhea) leads to vitamin D deficiency

Poor sunlight exposure

Vitamin D-dependent osteomalacia

    Type I inherited deficiency of the enzyme necessary for activating vitamin D; Type II inherited inability of target organs to respond to vitamin D

LOW PHOSPHORUS IN THE BLOOD

Excess ingestion of aluminum hydroxide gels, which decrease phosphate absorption

Hereditary hypophosphatemia

    Inherited phosphate-transport abnormality, with renal phosphate wasting

Tumor osteomalacia

    Some tumors produce a humoral factor that causes renal phosphate wasting

    Other renal disorders

Use of anticonvulsants, chronic severe liver disease, and primary biliary cirrhosis may also be associated with low-turnover osteoporosis.

Source: Adapted from Mundy GR. Osteopenia. Disease of the Mouth. 1987;33:537. Reprinted with permission.

    Any cause of vitamin D deficiency (from poor nutrition to problems in the liver or kidney) disturbs body calcium levels and bone mineralization. There are additional distinct mechanisms that can inhibit bone mineralization and cause osteomalacia. If the level of phosphorus in the blood is persistently low, for example, osteomalacia occurs despite the high levels of active vitamin D. Other causes of osteomalacia appear to exert their effects directly by inhibiting bone mineralization through as yet unknown mechanisms.

Deficiencies of vitamin D, calcium, and phosphorus affect muscles and other biochemical processes as well as bone formation. Vitamin D may be necessary for normal muscles to function. Low calcium levels in the blood can produce numbness or tingling in the hands and feet, muscle cramps, and muscle contractions. Low phosphorus levels in the blood can cause muscle, blood, and heart disorders.

Who Is at Risk for Osteomalacia? Age-related changes in nutrition and body functions place older people at higher risk for vitamin D deficiency. The amount of vitamin D in the diet is generally low because of voluntary avoidance of milk products and foods rich in vitamin D. In addition there is decreased vitamin D absorption by the intestine. Because of these factors vitamin D levels in older people depend more on the amount of sunlight they are exposed to than on the amount they get from food. Therefore, older people who live in northern climates and those who are institutionalized or house-bound are at higher risk for osteomalacia from vitamin D deficiency. Clearly an important contributing role may also be played by the chronic diseases that led to the person being house-bound or institutionalized.

Symptoms and Evaluation of Osteomalacia. Osteomalacia in older adults produces bone pain, especially in the lower spine, ribs, pelvis, and legs; muscle weakness in the thighs and shoulders; and cramps or involuntary muscle contractions if blood calcium is low. Fractures of the hip, spine, ribs, and pelvis also are part of the osteomalacia syndrome. Studies of the bone condition in older people who have had hip fractures suggest that as many as one-quarter have osteomalacia.

Wide-scale screening programs for osteomalacia are currently not being recommended because of the limited knowledge of the extent of osteomalacia and the poor understanding of its relationship to subsequent events such as fractures. However, people who have conditions that are associated with changes in vitamin D or phosphorus as listed in Table 23 should consider an evaluation for osteomalacia. Generally, this can be started by having blood tests for calcium, phosphorus, vitamin D levels, and parathyroid hormone levels. A complete evaluation would include bone X rays.

Treatment and Prevention of Osteomalacia. For all age groups, the standard dose of vitamin D to treat documented vitamin D deficiency is 10,000 International Units (IU). Intermittent larger doses can also be used but are associated with increased risk of developing a dangerously high calcium level in the blood. Two to three grams of calcium is usually taken each day to prevent the low calcium in the blood that may occur as bone is actively being mineralized. For osteomalacia caused by changes in the gastrointestinal tract or liver, or by kidney disease, the treatment must be tailored to the specific cause.

Although the recommended daily allowance for vitamin D for all ages is only 400 IU, the amount needed to maintain bone health in older people is higher. This is due to the previously described changes related to aging. Except for people with a history of kidney stones, the safe alternative is 800 IU per day. This amount can be easily supplemented by taking two multivitamins a day. An alternative method is a single 10,000 IU, high-dose vitamin D supplementation once every six months when the risk of osteomalacia is high and the person's compliance with daily medications is doubtful.

Paget's Disease of Bone

In Paget's disease of bone (named for the 19th-century English surgeon Sir James Paget), the affected bones are larger than normal, are often deformed, and have an increased blood supply. Under the microscope, the bone looks very disorganized, with increased activity of cells. Bone turnover seems to be rapidly accelerated, with increased bone destruction followed by excessive bone growth. Eventually the bone loses its rich blood supply and develops scar tissue in the bone marrow space.

Causes of Paget's Disease of Bone

The exact cause of Paget's disease of bone has not yet been determined. Some evidence suggests a virus as the cause, though so far no virus has been isolated. Other factors such as repeated trauma and a strong family history may play a role in the development of the disease. The prevalence of Paget's disease of bone increases with age and has a peculiar geographic distribution. In the United States, it is seen more commonly in northern rather than southern states, and in Europe it is more commonly seen in England and France than in Sweden and Denmark.

Paget's disease is sometimes obvious if the skull or a superficial bone is involved because the bones appear much larger than normal and are deformed. For most people, Paget's disease is discovered accidentally when tests are done for other reasons. Bone changes revealed in X rays show characteristic features of the disease. Blood tests reflect the increased bone turnover. Bone pain, the most common symptom of Paget's disease, results either from the disease or its complications. The pain is generally worse at night, especially if the person is lying in a warm bed. Severe unrelenting pain that occurs suddenly and is resistant to treatment suggests the development of a malignant tumor and is more likely to affect the bones of the upper arms and the skull.

Evaluation for Paget's Disease

The features and complications of this disorder depend upon which bones are affected. Long bones such as those in the legs tend to bend along the lines of least resistance. For example, the bone in the lower leg, called the tibia or shinbone, bows out to the front or the long bone in the thigh, the femur, may bow out sideways. Other bones commonly affected include the pelvis, skull, and the vertebrae. Nerve compression can occur. In the skull Paget's disease can cause blindness and deafness in some cases (Beethoven's deafness may have been caused by Paget's disease).

Fractures that commonly occur in Paget's disease may happen spontaneously or be caused by trauma. The fractures often have multiple breaks and are difficult to repair. The difficulty in management is due to the increased blood flow and the brittleness of the bone. In addition, even if a support is properly placed around the fracture site, the surrounding bone is weak and may not be able to hold its position.

Additional complications of Paget's disease include an increased level of calcium in the blood caused by the person's reduced mobility and the development of a malignant tumor called osteogenic sarcoma. Osteogenic sarcoma is a rare complication of Paget's disease occurring in less than 1 percent of people with the disease. In rare cases, people with Paget's disease develop high blood pressure, irregular heartbeat, and changes in the heart valves, especially if bone involvement is extensive.

Treatment of Paget's Disease

The treatment of Paget's disease is aimed at relieving pain, avoiding complications, relieving any nerve compressions, and maintaining skeletal function, while minimizing treatment side effects. Specific therapy must be individualized. Since most people do not have any symptoms, they do not require specific treatment. The main reasons for specific treatment include pain that does not respond to mild pain relievers, fractures, and neurologic complications. Some orthopedic surgeons also prefer specific treatment before they operate on an involved bone to reduce its overly rich blood vessel supply.

Traditionally, a hormone called calcitonin that specifically inhibits the cells that normally destroy bone has been used to control the activity of Paget's disease. This hormone is given by nasal spray or by injection. Side effects include nausea and flushing; both tend to disappear over time. The administration of calcitonin usually results in a sharp decline in the biochemical changes in the blood that reflect rapid bone loss and replacement. In most cases, treatment leads to improvement in the bone structure and in the appearance of the bones on X ray.

There are now, however, other medications—diphosphonates and their derivatives—that have largely replaced calcitonin in the treatment and management of Paget's disease. They are easy to take and have relatively few side effects if given in low doses. The remission induced by these compounds appears to be longer lasting than that induced by calcitonin. Diphosphonates are usually taken on an empty stomach since food interferes with their absorption. Some diphosphonates can be given as a single injection and have produced remissions lasting over a year. Because diphosphonates are excreted in the urine, the dose must be reduced in people who have kidney problems.

Bone Fractures

Fractures in the elderly usually result from low-energy injuries and involve bones that have been weakened by osteoporosis or some other disease process. Certain types of fractures happen more frequently among older people. Vertebral compression fractures and hip fractures are relatively rare until the fifth and sixth decades of

Figure 24. Types of Fractures

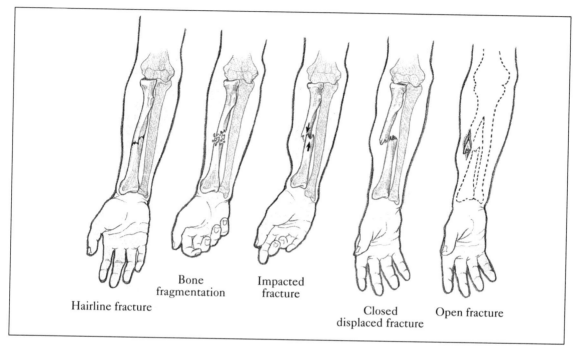

Hairline fracture

Bone fragmentation

Impacted fracture

Closed displaced fracture

Open fracture

life, after which they increase significantly. Other common fractures in old age include those of the wrist, leg, and pelvis.

Causes of Fractures

Most hip, arm, and pelvic fractures in older people are the result of a fall. The older person's ability to ward off the impact of a fall may be reduced by slowed reflexes, decreased muscle strength, and impaired coordination. In fact, most fractures are the result of relatively low-energy trauma caused by a fall on level ground.

Evaluation and Description of Fractures

Fractures are described in terms of their location, the orientation of the break (across, at an angle, or spiral), and the degree of bone fragmentation, called comminution (see Figure 24). If the bone has protruded through the skin it is called an open break, if it is not so exposed, it is a closed break. Another consideration is fracture alignment, referring to the relative position of the broken segments and the orientation of these segments. Finally, the broken ends themselves are identified as overriding, displaced, or impacted (pushed together).

The term "pathologic fracture" refers to any break that occurs in an abnormal bone. The abnormal bone may be weakened by an underlying cancer in the bone, a benign bone tumor, a metabolic disorder, an infection, or osteoarthritis. A person who has a fracture after minimal trauma very likely has had a pathologic fracture. In such cases, the person may have experienced increasing pain in the area of the break before the fracture occurred, pain that is especially noticeable at night and with bearing of body weight. Awareness of any such pain prior to a fracture is important to share with a physician because it can greatly alter the choice of treatment and the likelihood of healing.

Sometimes, a person with a pathologic fracture that has not yet entirely broken through the bone notices pain in the affected area associated with the use of the limb. For example, getting out of a chair can cause thigh pain in a person who has a problem with the large bone in the upper leg (femur). Fixing these partial fractures is often recommended to prevent displacement of the bone sections, provide pain relief, and permit the person to maintain function. Otherwise, if the impending fracture breaks through completely and becomes displaced the treatment becomes considerably more difficult, with increased disability and less chance of an effective bone repair and healing.

Spread of cancer from other places to the bone accounts for the great majority of bone malignancies. The most common spread occurs from breast, lung, prostate, gastrointestinal, kidney, and thyroid cancers. Multiple myeloma and lymphoma can also produce bony abnormalities in older people. (These bone marrow and lymph gland malignancies are covered in Chapter 20.)

How Fractures Heal

The repair process can be divided into three overlapping chronological phases: inflammation, repair, and remodeling. The inflammatory phase usually lasts several days and constitutes the body's initial response to injury. The trauma that breaks the bone also injures surrounding blood vessels, muscles, and other soft tissues. Bones are well supplied with blood and bleeding around the fracture site forms a large clot (hematoma). The bony fragments at the fracture site produce an immediate and intense inflammatory reaction, making the area swollen and tender. The repair stage begins within 24 hours after the injury and reaches peak activity after one to two weeks. During this time, fractures of the bone that are not rigidly stabilized heal by rapid formation around the fracture site of new bone, called external callus. This callus is not visible on the X ray until three to six weeks after the injury. Until enough callus forms to provide stability, collapse and displacement of the fracture can occur. This repair process can take up to several months for a long bone fracture such as in the leg. Fractures at the ends of bones tend to heal faster. During the remodeling phase, the initial callus, which was laid down relatively rapidly, is slowly reabsorbed and replaced by stronger bone. This process may proceed slowly in older people and may account for symptoms of discomfort that last for many months after a fracture.

Principles of Treating Fractures

The outlook for fracture healing in older people differs from that for younger people since there is a greater chance that joints will stiffen as a result of immobilization and there is a higher risk of medical complications with bed rest. The death rate for people during their first year after a hip fracture is 10 to 20 percent higher than for people of the same age and sex who have not had a hip fracture. In addition, 15 to 25 percent of those people who lived at home and were functionally independent before their fracture required nursing home care for more than a year. An additional 25 to 35 percent became dependent on various mechanical aids or help from others.

To avoid these complications, the goals of treatment emphasize a rapid return to the physical activities necessary to maintain independent living. Older people generally place less stress on their musculoskeletal system, so that alignments of bones or prosthetic replacements of joints that would not be suitable for a younger population often work well for this age group.

The injured limb must be properly immobilized to prevent further damage. The movement of sharp fracture ends can cause serious damage to soft tissues, arteries, veins, and nerves. In addition, the skin can be punctured, converting a closed injury into an open one, increasing the likelihood of infection. Immobilization makes it easier to transport the injured person and also relieves pain. Initially, injuries located near or beyond the elbow or knee can often be immobilized with splints. All splints are best fitted by holding the injured part with a gentle, longitudinal traction while someone else applies the splint. A sling can be effective in immobilizing most injuries of the shoulder, upper arm, and elbow. If further restraint is required, the arm can be kept close to the body by adding various wraps. Hip fractures can be treated initially by careful positioning with pillows.

Surgery to stabilize fractures offers compelling benefits for older people, especially when they have hip fractures for which non-surgical treatment would involve prolonged immobility and bed rest. In these circumstances, the risks of surgery are usually outweighed by the likelihood of complications resulting from the bed rest.

Despite these advantages, surgical treatment of most fractures should be postponed until the correction of any acute medical problems has been achieved. Only those fractures that are associated with limb-threatening conditions or open fractures require urgent surgical treatment. There are some situations in which surgery generally should not be performed. For example, the presence of a blood infection prohibits the use of pins or other metal implants. In addition, bones severely affected by osteoporosis or Paget's disease may have poor mechanical properties and the surgeon may be unable to fix the hardware securely to the bone. (Osteoporosis and Paget's disease are discussed elsewhere in this chapter.)

Complications of Fractures

Swelling of injured muscle within a confined space surrounded by a cast or other unyielding constraint can lead to increased pressures that can block the normal circulation. The resulting tissue damage in turn leads to further injury, swelling, and higher pressures. The only solution to this ever-intensifying cycle is to completely remove all of the confining elements around the swollen muscles. This means all casts, splints, and dressings must be loosened immediately if a person complains of increasing pain or numbness in an immobilized limb. Emergency surgery is sometimes necessary to open up the muscle compartment.

The development of large blood clots in the legs and pelvic veins is another complication of fractures. Before the advent of specific treatment to prevent blood clots, deep vein clots developed in about half of people with hip fractures. These clots can be serious because they can dislodge and travel to the lungs causing a "pulmonary embolus," a potentially fatal event. Death caused by such blood clots was once the most frequent fatal complication resulting from lower leg trauma. The major factors that predispose a person to have such blood clots in the legs are advanced age, trauma or surgery involving the legs, a previous history of having one or more blood clots, being immobilized through bed rest, having a malignancy, and being overweight. These blood clots are hard to detect without specialized testing.

The majority of episodes of deep venous blood clots that occur in the hospital are preventable. Thinning of the blood with heparin is necessary for people undergoing hip replacement surgery or who have hip fractures. Treatment to thin the blood before and after surgery has greatly reduced the chance of having deep venous blood clots. Nonetheless, blood clots are still a matter for significant concern when fractures occur in the leg and pelvic areas.

Fractures of the Upper Arm. This injury is most commonly the result of a fall on an outstretched hand. People with this fracture have intense shoulder pain, inability to move the arm, considerable swelling, and discoloration of the lower arm. Fortunately, about 80 percent of these fractures do not have the fractured ends displaced.

Specific Fractures

The treatment and outlook depend upon the number and extent of the fracture fragments. If the alignment and position of the fragments are satisfactory, the arm may be immobilized in a sling. If not, an orthopedic surgeon may be able to realign the fragments by manipulating them without surgery. If a satisfactory alignment cannot be achieved by manipulation, then surgery is necessary to restore the appropriate alignment.

It is very important to begin simple movement exercises as soon as possible, because the most common complication results from the irritated surfaces of the joint capsule in the shoulder sticking together. This can cause severe pain as well as disability due to restricted motion. Physical therapy is often extremely helpful in these situations. It may take several months to regain the ability to perform over-the-head tasks, such as combing the hair.

Wrist Fractures. As with upper arm fractures, wrist fractures are usually the result of a fall on an outstretched hand. The fracture causes pain, tenderness, and swelling of the wrist.

For people with minimally displaced fractures or with low functional demands, the treatment may consist only of a short arm cast or splint. For displaced fractures, the physician may have to manipulate the bone pieces. This can be painful and some form of anesthesia is usually necessary. More severe fractures may require extensive casting.

Because the most frequent complication of a wrist fracture is stiffness of the fingers and shoulder, active motion of the shoulder, elbow, and fingers is usually strongly encouraged. To prevent swelling in the hand, it is important to hold it elevated above the heart. Immobilization of the wrist by a cast is usually maintained for three to eight weeks depending on the nature of the break. The person can expect gradually diminishing pain and weakness in the wrist to last for 6 to 12 months after the injury. Physical therapy and various exercises help to speed the recovery, and most people eventually regain satisfactory, pain-free function.

Hip Fractures. Two common forms of hip fracture involve either the femoral neck or the area between two trochanters (see Figure 25). Femoral neck fractures can be classified as either occult (invisible on ordinary X ray), impacted (wedged together), nondisplaced, or displaced. Elderly people with an occult fracture may have experienced minimal or even no apparent trauma. They typically complain of persistent groin pain with weight bearing, but X rays of the hip reveal no fracture. A bone scan may show the fracture. Weight bearing must be avoided because the crack can extend across the bone, causing complete displacement.

People with impacted and nondisplaced femoral neck fractures can also have groin pain and no deformity on physical examination. These fractures are visible on X rays and are classified according to the disruption of the blood supply to the head of the femur. The classification is very important in determining the treatment and outcome.

Occult, impacted, and nondisplaced femoral neck fractures are usually treated with surgery by using special pins. The stabilization

allows older people to begin movement and weight bearing immediately and prevents displaced fractures. These fractures heal well
because the blood supply to the femoral head is not disrupted.

A displaced fracture severely reduces the blood supply to the
femoral head. While a displaced fracture can heal if it is securely
stabilized, the chance of complications is considerable because of
the poor blood supply. In 15 to 20 percent of people who have suffered a displaced fracture, there is no healing, and severe deformity
of the femoral head occurs in another 15 to 30 percent.

People with displaced fractures have two treatment options—
surgery to stabilize the joint or a hip joint replacement. Surgical
treatment with no prosthetic replacement is usually reserved for
vigorous people who are under the age of 70 and can tolerate a
postoperative treatment of protected, crutch-associated weight
bearing. This treatment preserves the femoral head and, if successful healing occurs, makes for a nearly normal hip. However, if the

Figure 25. Hip Fractures

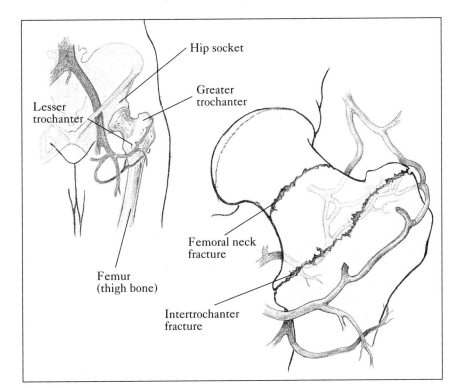

Hip socket

Greater
trochanter

Lesser
trochanter

Femoral neck
fracture

Femur
(thigh bone)

Intertrochanter
fracture

fracture does not mend properly, the joint will become very painful and a second operation will be required.

Partial or complete hip replacement is often recommended as an initial treatment because of the high likelihood of poor healing and deformity of the femoral head. In partial replacement the femoral head fragment is removed and replaced with a prosthesis. A prosthetic hip replacement may be the best choice for those over 70 because it permits immediate full weight bearing and a faster return to independent functioning.

In the group of people who are at highest risk for major complications, such as people from nursing homes who were not able to walk prior to their fracture, nonsurgical therapy may be appropriate. Conservative nonsurgical approach may also be appropriate for people who are confined to bed.

Hip fractures occurring between the two trochanters of the femur, called intertrochanteric fractures, are usually caused by a fall, often on level ground. Bleeding around the site can be significant and can cause shock due to a decrease in blood pressure.

Intertrochanteric hip fractures are treated by surgery unless there is a serious medical reason not to. This is because healing with traction instead of surgery usually requires four to eight weeks and exposes the person to all the hazards of immobilization in bed. Furthermore, healing in traction is often incomplete, as it does not allow for adequate control of the powerful muscles around the hip. The leg can become shortened and be turned slightly to the side, making it difficult to walk. After surgery, on the other hand, most people can begin immediate full weight bearing with a walker for support. Usually 6 to 12 weeks of walker use are required before they are able to switch to a cane and then walk independently.

Compression Fractures in the Vertebrae. In older people, this type of fracture is usually caused by some activity that increases compression stress on the spine such as lifting, bending forward, or missing a step while walking. Usually the person has severe pain that is made worse by sitting or standing, and there is a very specific point of tenderness over the affected part of the spine. There are rarely any neurological problems.

Initially, hospitalization for a short course of bed rest and pain relief may be necessary. As soon as possible, the person should be encouraged to sit up and walk for short periods. It may require a week or longer for independent walking. The person may have significant back pain for 6 to 12 weeks thereafter. As the healing progresses, the pain frequently shifts from the site of the original fracture to a higher or lower location. This is probably due to altered mechanical stresses caused by the deformity.

Back braces, which probably do little to prevent deformity, are only useful in the lower back because adequate support cannot be achieved above this level. Braces sometimes can help to relieve pain and permit a more rapid return to activities. The most effective in providing mechanical support, however, are not necessarily the most comfortable.

Many vertebral body fractures occur without any symptoms in older people, and are only revealed on an X ray. Osteoporosis weakens the vertebral bodies, which are then compressed by excessive stress on the back. This can result in a stooped posture as the fronts of vertebral bones crush in on themselves.

Vertebral body compression fractures always heal since the bone is really just compressed onto itself. The blood supply is not impaired, and neurological problems due to pinching nerves are not common. In addition, these fractures are generally stable because the back components of these vertebrae remain in place. The long-term result is a progressive forward curvature of the spine, due to wedging of these vertebrae, and a loss of height.

Overview

Sensory concerns such as hearing difficulty and vision problems produce a large proportion of the increased impairment we may experience as we age. In fact, the top causes of disability among older people are joint, bone, and muscle problems and sensory impairments. This chapter addresses head, neck, and sensory concerns.

SYMPTOMS
Hearing
Difficulty

Hearing loss is the most common sensory impairment experienced by older people. Approximately 30 percent of people over the age of 65 report problems with their hearing. This impairment becomes increasingly common with advanced age, rising to about 50 percent in 85-year-old people. Among people in nursing homes, the prevalence of hearing impairment approaches 60 percent. In all older age groups, impaired hearing and deafness are more common in men than in women; almost 20 percent of very old men have significant

Figure 26. The Ear

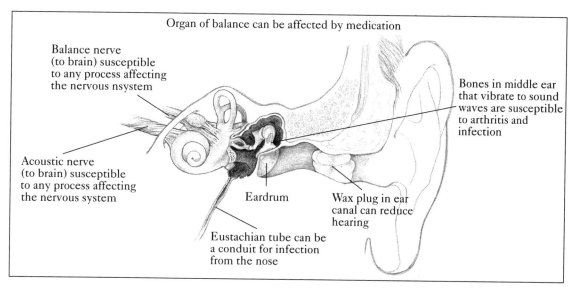

Organ of balance can be affected by medication

Balance nerve (to brain) susceptible to any process affecting the nervous nsystem

Bones in middle ear that vibrate to sound waves are susceptible to arthritis and infection

Acoustic nerve (to brain) susceptible to any process affecting the nervous system

Eardrum

Wax plug in ear canal can reduce hearing

Eustachian tube can be a conduit for infection from the nose

hearing loss in both ears. Approximately two million elderly people use hearing aids, but about 20 percent of these people report that they still have difficulty hearing. People with Alzheimer's disease have a higher rate of hearing loss than other people of the same age. Hearing loss is also associated with poorer cognitive function in people without dementia.

How Normal Hearing Works

Normal hearing depends upon the functioning of three systems: the ear, the central auditory system in the brain that controls hearing, and processes in the brain that are not strictly limited to auditory signals (see Figure 26). The ear modifies the sense of sound, while the brain's activities help us perceive and interpret sound.

Sound is quantified by frequency (pitch) measured in cycles per second, and by intensity (loudness) measured in decibels (see Figure 27). In young people, the frequency range of normal hearing runs from 30 cycles per second to about 20,000 cycles per second. In older people, the range is from 250 to 8,000 cycles per second. Normal speech occurs within a frequency range of 500 to 2,000 cycles per second. The intensity at which a sound must be generated to be heard by a person is termed that person's threshold; the higher the threshold the poorer the hearing.

Figure 27. Frequency Spectrum of Familiar Sounds

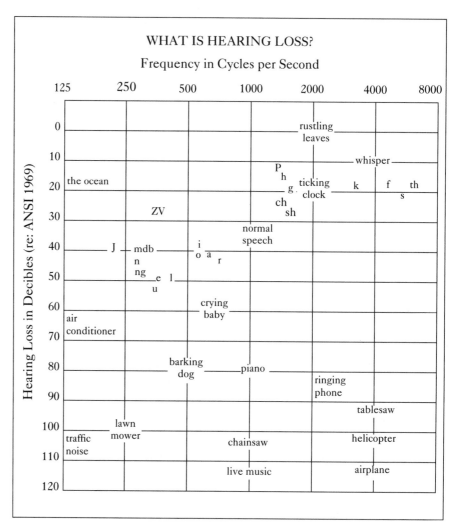

Common Causes of Hearing Loss

While hearing impairment is not a universal aspect of aging, it is exceptionally common. Hearing loss in elderly people usually fits a characteristic pattern that is called presbycusis. Presbycusis is a gradual, progressive, high-frequency hearing loss that affects both ears equally.

Even if the hearing loss is very mild, a person may still have difficulty understanding speech. Studies of otherwise normal older people indicate that up to half of them may have difficulty understanding speech on formal testing. A problem within the brain in processing sounds is believed to be responsible. Changes in memory and overall slowing of mental processes may also affect speech understanding and hearing.

Some specific changes in the ear and brain are associated with hearing loss, including atrophy of the sensory part of the ear, loss of sensory cells, and loss of nerves in the central nervous system. The influence of environmental factors such as excess noise has not been clearly defined.

Other Causes of Hearing Loss

In addition to presbycusis, other ear and hearing disorders are classified in three general categories: (1) conductive hearing loss disorders that affect the normal transmission of sound waves from the eardrum to the sensory apparatus; (2) sensory neural hearing loss disorders that are caused by problems of the auditory nerves; and (3) central hearing loss disorders that are due to disturbances in the brain. When hearing loss is due to more than one of these conditions, it is called a mixed hearing loss. Earwax can be a major cause of hearing loss, reducing sound intensity as much as 35 percent. Earwax clogging the ear canal is one important and easily correctable cause of conductive hearing loss found in about a third of older people.

Most causes of conductive hearing loss are not very common in older people. These include severe ear infections, arthritis affecting the bones of the ear, and trauma. However, Paget's disease of bone, which may affect the ear, is a cause of conductive hearing loss that is of particular importance to older people.

Sensory hearing loss may be due to Ménière's disease or medications, especially antibiotics and diuretics. Table 24 shows a partial list of drugs that can produce hearing impairment. Sensory hearing

Table 24. Drugs That Can Cause Hearing Loss

Antibiotics	Cancer chemotherapy
Erythromycin	NSAIDs
Vancomycin	Diuretics
Others	Drugs used to treat malaria

loss can also be caused by brain tumors, hemorrhage into the brain, and other diseases. Causes of central hearing loss are extremely rare and involve damage of both hemispheres of the brain.

Evaluation of Hearing Loss

The evaluation of hearing loss begins with telling the physician about any difficulties related to hearing. Some individuals may not readily want to volunteer this information or may attribute the difficulty to aging. The person's ears are inspected for earwax, which should be completely removed by the physician before any further testing is performed.

Pure tone audiometry has emerged as the basic test of hearing. The test can define the extent of hearing impairment and determine the location of the problem. It can also suggest some causes of the hearing difficulty.

Although the magnitude and pattern of hearing loss can be determined by use of pure tone audiometry, the value of these findings is limited because hearing in social situations rarely depends upon pure tone hearing.

Hearing Aids

Many older people use hearing aids to amplify sound. Some people and their physicians, however, have been led to believe that sensory hearing loss will not benefit from amplification—this is not true. In fact, well-selected hearing aids can improve the efficiency of speech perception even for people with severe sensory neural hearing loss.

In general, hearing aids should be worn in both ears to preserve the directional clues that help to localize sound. If only one hearing aid is used, however, the condition of the poorer ear will determine which ear is amplified. If the poor ear has internally generated distortion, amplification is likely to make matters worse. Because of this, the person should be tested with the hearing aid applied to the good ear, then the poor ear, and then both ears.

The most popular hearing aids are the behind-the-ear and in-the-ear models. Behind-the-ear hearing aids have the advantage of being durable, easily repaired, and more easily adjusted. Although the in-the-ear models may be easier to insert in the ear, they may be more difficult to adjust, and they may produce more acoustic feedback. Hearing aids that fit in the ear canal have the advantage to some of being the least visible hearing aids. They also improve hearing at higher frequencies due to better sound transmission.

Regardless of which type of hearing aid is selected, a person should purchase it from a comprehensive hearing aid center on a 30-day trial basis. These centers provide assessment, service, and rehabilitation. Immediately following the purchase of the hearing aid, the person should begin the aural rehabilitation program. This includes counseling regarding the benefits and limitations of hearing aids and suggestions for communicating with others. Some suggestions for improving communication with hearing impaired people are provided in Table 25.

A common problem limiting the effectiveness of hearing aids is their lack of use. Less than one-third of people over age 70 with hearing difficulty use the hearing aid for more than eight hours a day. Approximately one-third use hearing aids only for a few hours per week. Reasons people give for not using hearing aids include diminished dexterity, noise (such as the amplification of background noise), and the belief that the aid is not needed. Another problem that limits the use of hearing aids is the cost, which is usually around $500 per hearing aid.

The hearing mechanism can also be simulated electronically by means of an implanted electrode in the middle ear that stimulates the nerves directly. Unfortunately, the hearing provided by these implants is only rudimentary and their use is restricted to those who are totally deaf, which is rare among elderly people.

In addition to hearing aids, other helpful assistive listening devices (ALDs) are available. All of these devices rely on a microphone that is moved close to the sound source; the sound is usually clearer with less background noise. Systems differ, however, as to the method of transmitting the sound from the signal source to the ear. Infrared systems, which use nonvisible light waves as the carrier signal, are available as individual systems and cost several thousand dollars. These are principally helpful for home use to amplify home entertainment systems. Infrared technology has also been used for sound systems in public buildings, auditoriums, and churches. More costly than infrared systems, FM broadcasting systems are similar to infrared systems except that they use radio frequencies as the carrier signal.

Table 25. Suggestions for Improving Communication with a Hearing-Impaired Elderly Person

- Reduce or eliminate background noise. Close doors and turn off TV or running water.

- Face listener. Keep your face at level of listener's eyes. Maintain eye contact.

- Allow adequate light to fall on your face.

- Give listener a clear view of your face. Keep hands or other objects down. Avoid chewing gum. Beards or mustaches should be trimmed so as not to interfere with speech reading.

- Use facial expressions and gestures to convey meaning.

- Avoid writing or walking around the room while talking.

- Gain person's attention before beginning to speak.

- Speak in normal tone of voice or slightly louder. Shouting does not help because hearing loss is not simply reduction in loudness of sound.

- Speak clearly, a little more slowly, and in short sentences, using simple words.

- Have the person repeat the message to be sure it is understood. (Some people do not admit to a handicap.)

- Repeat or rephrase in a different way.

- If the person can read, write down key words.

- If the individual has a hearing aid, learn how to help with it.

- Learn how to use assistive listening devices.

- Arrange for the individual to have a vision exam.

Source: Adapted from Voeks SK, Gallagher CM, Langer EH, et al. Hearing loss in the nursing home: an institutional issue. *Journal of the American Geriatrics Society.*1990;38:145. Reprinted with permission.

The telephone company offers several assistive devices for the deaf or hearing impaired. These are usually provided at no additional charge if a physician has certified that the person is hearing impaired. These devices include amplifiers, louder bells, and light signals that flash on and off when the phone rings. Telecommunication Device for the Deaf (TDD) service, which links a typewriter source and a destination over the telephone lines, is also available.

Nonauditory communication aids, such as closed-captioning television and text messages, and interactive services on the computer are also available to help hearing-impaired people.

Vision Problems

Visual impairment increases with advancing age. Approximately 15 percent of people over the age of 65 report having vision impairment, and this figure rises to nearly 30 percent of those 85 years old and older. More than 90 percent of older people require eyeglasses, and over 20 percent of those over 85 report that even with the aid of glasses they have a great deal of difficulty seeing. Age-related changes in the lens of the eye causes a scattering of light over the retina, which decreases the older person's resistance to glare (see Chapter 2). This can constitute a significant threat to safe driving at night. In addition, there is an almost universal age-associated change in near vision that makes the eye lens more rigid, less flexible, and thus less able to focus at a close range.

The health consequences of impaired vision can be significant. For example, five-year survival rates decline with progressively worse vision. Hip fractures may be more common in people with impaired vision: The authors of one survey estimated that 18 percent of hip fractures occurred because impaired vision led to tripping, stumbling, missing a step, and falling.

Causes of Visual Impairment

There are four major eye diseases that cause visual impairment in older adults: cataracts, macular degeneration, glaucoma, and diabetic eye disease. The prevalence of cataracts and macular degeneration increases with age. This is less the case with diabetic eye disease and glaucoma. Approximately 13 percent of people between the ages of 65 and 74 have cataracts; this figure rises to over 40 percent in people 75 years and older. For people living in nursing homes, the incidence of cataracts is estimated to be between 60 and 80 percent. Age-related macular degeneration (ARMD) also rises with advancing age, from 6.4 percent in people between the ages of 65 and 74 to almost 20 percent in those over the age of 75. The incidence in nursing homes is estimated to be between 30 and 40 percent. Open-angle glaucoma and diabetic eye disease rates also increase with age, but the prevalence of either disease does not exceed 3.5 percent even in the oldest age group. However, the prevalence of open-angle glaucoma in nursing homes may be considerably higher; it is estimated at approximately 10 percent. There is some evidence that sunlight causes damage in the eyes that relates to the formation of cataracts. In particular, an association between ultraviolet B light and cataracts has been demonstrated in one study.

Cataracts. Cataracts are defined as a clouding or opacity in the lens of the eye (see Figure 28). A variety of changes in the lens have been noted with aging, and some of these are believed to be important in the development of cataracts. For example, the aging lens develops a yellow-brown pigmentation caused by protein in the lens that increases with age.

Symptoms of cataracts differ in composition and location, but regardless of the type of cataract involved people with cataracts have a painless, progressive loss of vision that may involve either one or both eyes. Early on, the location of the cataract may influence the nature of the vision loss. For example, the ability to see things far away particularly at night and in bright daylight is most severely compromised by one type of cataract while near vision may be affected by another. Months to years later when the cataract is fully developed, the entire range of vision has been impaired. Once the presence of a cataract has been established, people whose vision is poorer than expected on the basis of the cataract alone should have further testing to assess whether there are additional vision problems.

Treatment of Cataracts. As with any vision disorder, the impact of the vision loss upon daily activities must guide the treatment. If the severity of the vision loss does not affect a person's ability to function, nonsurgical management is certainly appropriate, especially when the person does not wish to have surgery, or when other medical or eye problems make surgery too dangerous. Under these circumstances, eyeglasses, contact lenses, and aids for low vision should be used. Specific measures to prevent the progression of cataracts include controlling the blood sugar of people who have diabetes mellitus and protecting the eyes against ultraviolet light with sunglasses.

Cataract surgery with lens implants improves vision as well as a person's subjective and objective capacity to function. Ophthalmologists are generally very accurate in their predictions of the amount of visual improvement following surgery. Mental function and performance of daily activities also seem to improve.

The surgical removal of a cataract is accomplished either by removing the entire lens with its enveloping capsule, or by extracapsular extraction, which leaves the transparent back of the lens in place. About 90 percent of cataract extractions are done by this extracapsular method. This method requires a smaller incision and

Figure 28. Common Visual Impairments in Old Age

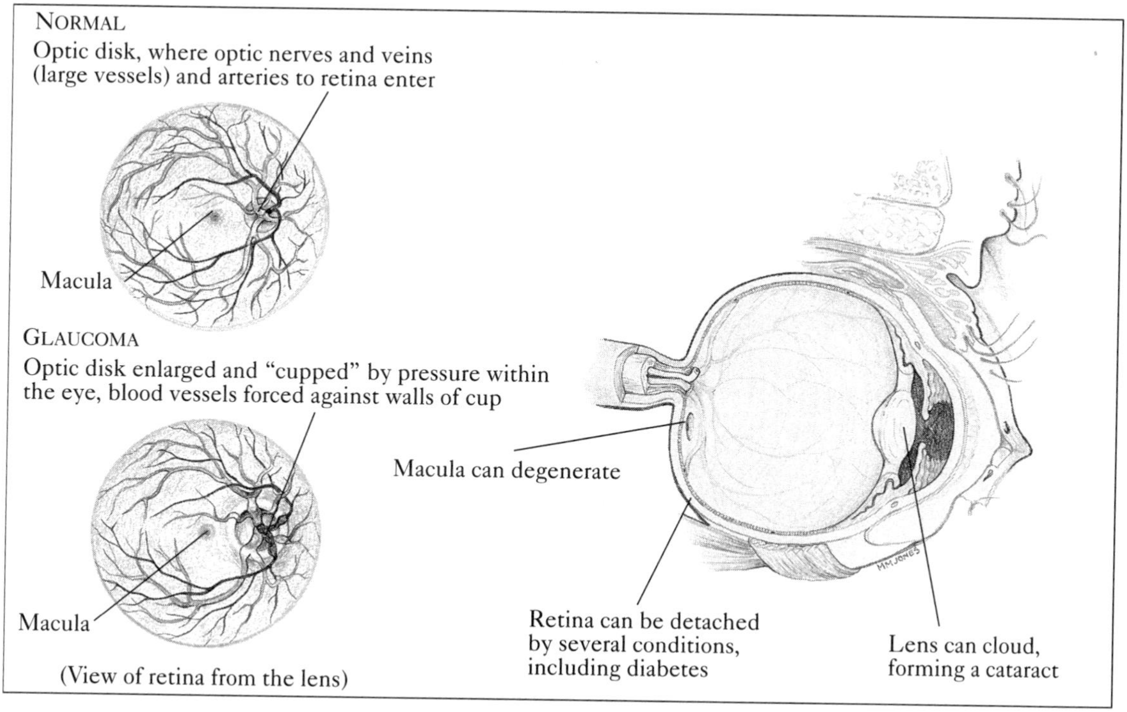

NORMAL
Optic disk, where optic nerves and veins (large vessels) and arteries to retina enter

Macula

GLAUCOMA
Optic disk enlarged and "cupped" by pressure within the eye, blood vessels forced against walls of cup

Macula can degenerate

Macula

(View of retina from the lens)

Retina can be detached by several conditions, including diabetes

Lens can cloud, forming a cataract

leaves the posterior capsule in place, providing a stabilizing membrane to hold a lens implant and to maintain the natural compartments of the eye.

A technique that uses sound waves to pulverize the lens and vacuum it out of the eye using special instruments has been devised. The incision for this appears to be even smaller than for usual extracapsular cataract extractions. This technique, however, appears to be less valuable for those people who have very hard cataracts.

Once the cataract has been removed, the magnifying power of the lenses must be replaced by one of three options: eyeglasses, contact lenses, or lens implants. Although eyeglasses are safe and inexpensive, they are usually less than optimal and people who have had only one eye operated on frequently experience double vision with the glasses. Other common deficiencies of cataract glasses are visual distortions, spatial dislocation, and reduced fields of vision. Contact lenses help correct these optical problems but they may be difficult for very old people to manage, especially because of the manual dexterity that they require. They may also cause corneal ulcers. In contrast, lens implants provide the best result on vision and do not require special care.

Lens implants can be placed in front of the iris, in the iris plane, or behind the iris (see Figure 28). By far the most common lens implant (used in more than 90 percent of replacements) is that which is placed in the back chamber behind the iris. This capitalizes on the presence of the natural lens capsule to help support the implant. The appropriate power of the lens implant can be determined by special testing before surgery. Most people can have their cataracts removed and the lens implanted as a single procedure done on an outpatient basis. Delayed clouding of the posterior capsule may develop in as many as 50 percent of people over a three-year period after this type of surgery. Fortunately, this complication can be treated nonsurgically using a special laser technique. This treatment results in improved vision in up to 90 percent of affected individuals.

Macular Degeneration. Although the exact cause of macular degeneration is not entirely clear, it is the leading cause of permanent central vision loss in older people. Changes in the pigmented tissues of the retina, or retinal pigmented epithelium (RPE), are related to the development of macular degeneration. This thin layer of cells is vitally important in the metabolic chemistry of vitamin A, in maintaining the blood vessels in the retinal area, in transporting various substances in and out of the eye's light receptor (photoreceptor) cells, and in removing depleted photoreceptors.

An initial deterioration of the RPE or a disturbance between the RPE and the photoreceptor cells may be the original event leading to macular degeneration. The result of this is the accumulation of material within the RPE and the formation of deposits between the base membrane of the RPE and the remaining membranes. The medical name for these deposits is drusen (from the German, meaning "strong nodule"). Drusen usually appear as hard pinhead-size areas in the retina that are visible to the physician looking into the eye with an ophthalmoscope. Other eye changes in macular degeneration include atrophy of the photoreceptors and the proliferation of new blood vessels. These new vessels may leak or bleed, leading to hemorrhage and possible detachment of the RPE. Blood stimulates the formation of scar tissue.

Ophthalmologists often classify macular degeneration into dry or wet macular degeneration. The dry form accounts for approximately 80 to 90 percent of macular degeneration and causes loss of central vision. A person with the dry form will see a dark fuzzy spot in the middle of the visual field.

Generally the vision of only 10 percent of people with dry macular degeneration is impaired to the extent of legal blindness, which is corrected vision of 20/200 or worse in the best eye—20/200 vision means that a person can only see at 20 feet what a normal person can see 200 feet away. Twenty feet is the distance at which the eye relaxes from the work of near vision. It is important to note that people with age-related macular degeneration still retain good peripheral vision despite meeting the criteria for legal blindness.

No specific medical treatment for dry macular degeneration has gained widespread clinical acceptance, but oral zinc supplementation may be effective in slowing the progression of visual loss. Progressive loss of vision seems less common and less severe in people who are given zinc. An Amsler grid (essentially a piece of graph paper) may help in monitoring people with early macular degeneration. A person can use it on a daily basis to check for changes in vision that may indicate fluid accumulation in the back of the eye and possible retinal detachment. These abnormalities distort the appearance of the grid, making some of the lines seem wavy or curved. Other indications that a problem has developed in a person who has macular degeneration include sudden or recent loss of central vision, blurred vision, visual distortion, or a new blind spot. Medical management of dry macular degeneration also makes use of aids for low vision, which are described below.

Wet macular degeneration is much more likely to cause very severe visual loss. This condition is present in 80 to 90 percent of eyes with 20/200 vision or worse. Wet macular degeneration is characterized by the formation of new blood vessels with consequent separation of the RPE from the retina. For people under the age of 55 with a pure detachment of the RPE, the prognosis is excellent, but older people have a much higher risk of complications and visual loss. Generally, simple RPE detachment is usually managed without surgery or lasers in elderly people. Treatment with lasers is indicated in people with macular degeneration and new blood vessel growth. This use of laser is best regarded as postponing rather than preventing severe visual loss in people with this problem. In only a minority of people with wet macular degeneration is this problem confined to the avascular zone, and laser treatments are not of value within the zone. The complications of laser treatment include decreased vision and laser injury to areas adjacent to and beyond the intended area of treatment.

Glaucoma. In glaucoma, vision loss is due to increased fluid pressure within the eye that damages the optic nerve. This affects approximately 3 percent of people over the age of 65. To the examining physician, glaucoma is detectable as increased pressure within the eye, atrophy and cupping of the optic nerve, and defects in the visual field. Approximately 95 percent of people with glaucoma have open-angle glaucoma (OAG). Virtually all of the rest have angle-closure glaucoma.

Causes and Symptoms of Glaucoma. In OAG, the aqueous humor (the fluid that circulates in the chamber between the cornea and the lens) that is formed in the eye travels to the front of the eye and gets reabsorbed. In angle-closure glaucoma, the chamber angle is closed by a bowing of the iris. As the pupil dilates, the iris blocks the flow of aqueous humor out of the eye, which causes the pressure in the eye to rise rapidly and precipitates halos, blurred vision, and eye pain, and is an emergency. Angle-closure glaucoma needs to be treated immediately with special eyedrops to constrict the pupil.

Treatment of open-angle glaucoma is not usually started simply on the basis of finding a high pressure within the eye, except for when this pressure is extremely high. More commonly, treatment is started only if there is evidence of glaucoma damage to the eye, such as changes in the optic disk or in the optic nerve fibers. Drops that constrict the pupil stimulate the muscles of the eye and open the pores that reabsorb the fluid. Adrenaline eyedrops decrease the pressure within the eye by decreasing the production of aqueous humor and by increasing its removal. Other medications may be prescribed by an ophthalmologist. These other medications, including beta-blockers and carbonic anhydrase inhibitors, must be used carefully in older people because they can produce confusion, drowsiness, poor appetite, numbness in the hands and feet, and can precipitate kidney stones.

When medical therapy fails to provide adequate control of the pressure, surgery is necessary. Laser treatment can help the flow of aqueous humor and lower the pressure within the eye.

Diabetic Eye Disease. Diabetic eye disease is called diabetic retinopathy, and appears to be more closely related to the length of time the person has had diabetes mellitus than to the age of the person. Nonetheless, approximately 3 percent of people over the age of 85 have this condition. (Diabetes mellitus is discussed on page 436.) The disorder is usually classified as either background retinopathy or proliferative retinopathy. Background retinopathy includes hemorrhages, small blood vessel defects called microaneurysms, and the accumulation of fluid around the macula. Proliferative retinopathy is characterized by new blood vessel formation, bleeding within the eye, and retinal detachment. There is less risk of proliferative retinopathy in older people, but the large number of elderly people who have diabetes mellitus justifies its importance.

Whether or not tight control of diabetes can prevent diabetic retinopathy remains an unsettled question. Regular eye checkups are a valuable part of care for every person with diabetes.

Other Causes of Blindness. Although much less common, other causes of blindness can occur in older people, such as reduced blood flow to the optic nerve; inflammation involving the arteries of the head; inflammation to the optic nerve; and masses in the brain. Inflammation around the arteries that run along the temples (temporal arteries) is a rare but serious disorder because this inflammation can lead to irreversible blindness.

Other Disorders of the Eye. While they are not directly related to vision loss, several other disorders commonly occur in older people. With aging, increased relaxation of the skin around the eyelids and decreased muscle tone can lead to an in-turning of the eyelid margin toward the cornea (entropion) with subsequent irritation by the eyelashes. Another condition (ectropion) is when the eyelid sags and causes a loss of tears, drying out the tissue at the base of the eye. Both of these conditions can be corrected with simple surgical therapies. A number of underlying diseases, especially those related to rheumatoid arthritis can affect the tear system leading to dry eyes. Replacement of the fluid with artificial tears is the most common treatment for these conditions, but some people become sensitive to the preservatives used in the artificial tears and experience further irritation because of them.

Aids for Low Vision. Providing adequate lighting is one of the keys to improving vision in older people with impaired sight. Precautions must be taken to avoid glare. Because of this, filters, visors, and sunglasses may be valuable. Reading glasses with magnifying lenses can add some lens power and are the most commonly prescribed low-vision aids for older people. Once the simple magnifying glasses move beyond low power, the preservation of binocular vision becomes very difficult. Magnifying glasses usually allow broad fields of vision, but require that objects be held relatively close to the eye. Handheld magnifying glasses, which can be used as either a major or supplemental low-vision aid, can be helpful for simple tasks conducted at about arm's length. Stand magnifiers require an additional reading lens to focus the image, but have the advantage of eliminating the problem of hand unsteadiness. For longer working distances, near vision and distance telescopes provide magnification, but they tend to distort images and create a tunnel vision effect. Video and computer magnifiers may be valuable, but their use is limited by their high cost and lack of portability. Nonvision aids such as talking books may eliminate some of the handicaps that are caused by visual loss.

Dry Mouth

Three major pairs of salivary glands and hundreds of minor salivary glands secrete saliva into the mouth. In general, saliva serves as a primary defense for all oral tissues. It lubricates the soft tissues, helps in remineralizing the teeth, and also helps to control bacterial and fungal populations in the mouth. Because of this, dry mouth caused by lack of salivary secretion can have severe consequences.

Causes of Dry Mouth

In older people, a dry mouth with reduced saliva may be caused by a variety of diseases and treatments. For example, dryness of the mouth is a side effect of over 400 prescription medications. Many antidepressant, antihypertensive, anti-inflammatory, and diuretic medications commonly used by elderly people can reduce salivary gland performance. People taking these medications frequently develop oral dryness and have a very high rate of cavities.

Sjögren's syndrome (named for the Swedish physician who first described it) is the single most common disease affecting salivary glands. This is an illness that affects the immune system of about a million Americans, the majority of whom are postmenopausal women. The condition diminishes salivary gland function, causing a dry mouth and difficulty in swallowing dry foods such as bread. The person may notice that lipstick sticks to the teeth.

The management of dry mouth requires a careful examination by a physician or dentist to check the three major pairs of salivary glands and to look for Sjögren's syndrome.

If the cause of the dry mouth is due to medication, it is important to reduce the medication levels or to replace them with alternative preparations. Sometimes special medications can be used to stimulate saliva production gently if some functioning salivary glands remain. However, no satisfactory salivary substitutes are available for people when the glands cease to function. Artificial saliva can be useful in controlling dental disease, but it has minimal effects on problems with the soft tissue in the mouth. All people with dry mouth should receive comprehensive and frequent preventive dental care, including regular fluoride treatments.

Difficulty Chewing

Among older people, the most common difficult mouth movement is chewing. Older people with an intact set of teeth even show a modest increase in the time they take to chew a mouthful of food before swallowing. In those with poor dentition or those wearing dentures, the time needed is even longer.

Causes of Difficulty Chewing. The causes of difficulty chewing in an older person are jaw pain, limited ability to open the jaw, or a shift in the jawbone as the mouth opens. These problems sometimes result from difficulties in the joint at the base of the jaw (under the ear) and can either be muscular or dental in origin. A form of blood vessel inflammation called temporal arteritis can cause chewing difficulty by reducing blood flow to the masseter, the muscle that allows chewing. A thorough medical and dental evaluation usually uncovers the cause and leads to appropriate treatment.

Oral and Dental Problems

The mouth serves two essential functions: the production of speech and the initial preparation of food for proper digestion. Together these functions require intact teeth, healthy lining of the tissues (mucosa), good sensation, and proper salivary gland function (see Figure 29). If disease affects any of these components, the consequences can be serious. There is no evidence that oral health and function decrease with age. Older people experience more medical problems in general, and it is likely that illness and medications contribute to oral problems. However, in many older people, oral tissues remain healthy.

Dental Disease

Dental disease refers to disease affecting tooth surfaces. It is classified according to which tooth surface has been affected by decay. The most common form of dental disease are the cavities in children and young adults on the chewing surface, or crown, of the

Figure 29. Healthy Jaws and Oral and Dental Problems

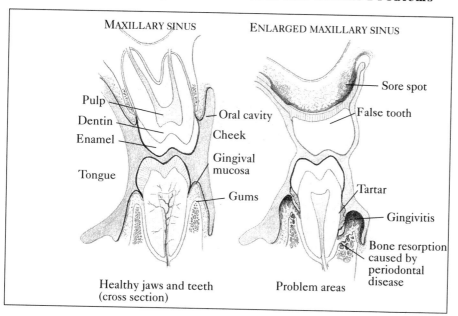

Healthy jaws and teeth (cross section)

Problem areas

tooth. Cavities along the root surface are more prevalent among older people and occur when gums recede to expose the root. Older adults and younger adults have about the same amount of cavities.

Oral hygiene is the major determinant of cavity disease. Adults with untreated cavities have more amounts of plaque, tartar, and inflammation of the gums (gingivitis) than adults without cavities. Because of this, good oral hygiene—care of the teeth and gums—is important for all people regardless of their age to reduce the risk of dental decay. Fluoride treatment is usually given to prevent cavities in children and in certain high-risk groups of adults, such as those who have had radiation treatment to the head or neck. People of all ages who have high amounts of fluoride in their water have significantly fewer cavities compared with lifelong residents of nonfluoridated communities. Fluoride is helpful in older adults, even when fluoride exposure does not begin until late adulthood. Because of this, fluoride treatment to prevent dental cavities should be seriously considered for people of advanced age, especially those with diminished salivary gland function.

Preventing Cavities

Periodontal Disease

The periodontium consists of the tissues that support the teeth; these tissues are divided into the gums and the attachment apparatus, that is, the structures that hold the teeth in place below the gums. Gingivitis refers to inflammation of the gums primarily caused by infection. Antibiotics can help the condition, but they may have to be used for several weeks.

Inflammation and loss of the attachment apparatus is called periodontal disease. A variety of oral bacteria have been linked to this inflammation. Eventually the process results in bone loss in the jaw and loss of teeth. It appears that this process occurs over time as a series of specific attacks, rather than as a slowly eroding process.

Osteoporosis may have oral complications. Some experts suggest that postmenopausal women are at increased risk for developing loss of bone in the structures that support the teeth. (Osteoporosis is discussed in Chapter 17.)

Disorders of the Oral Tissue

Age-related changes in the skin can produce similar changes in the lining of the mouth. Most often, oral changes in older people correspond to the state of their dental hygiene; the condition of dentures; the consumption of drugs, alcohol, and tobacco; and the secretion of saliva. Medical conditions can also affect the lining, allowing yeast infections in the mouth to become established. Older people taking antibiotics on a long-term basis can also develop yeast infections. People who wear dentures may experience irritation due to yeast on the upper part of the mouth beneath the dentures. Approximately 50 percent of these people also have reddish cracks at the corners of their mouth, again due to yeast. Most of these yeast infections respond well to oral medication or ointments.

Tobacco and alcohol use contributes to the development of premalignant and malignant disorders of the mouth. These disorders are not common but are more likely to occur in older people. Oral cancers account for about 5 percent of all malignancies. Approximately 95 percent of all oral cancers occur in people over 40 with the highest incidence in people in their seventies. While oral cancers can arise in any soft tissue, the back of the tongue on either side and the floor of the mouth are the most susceptible areas, presumably because secretions tend to pool in these areas.

The mouth contains many sensory systems that are essential for normal functioning and quality of life. For example, taste is critical to food enjoyment and for distinguishing spoiled from acceptable food. Other sensations help prepare for swallowing. Many conditions and medications can alter gustatory function. Poor oral hygiene and severe dental disease are common causes that respond to appropriate dental care.

Sensory Disorders

The normal function of the thyroid gland is to manufacture and secrete thyroid hormones, which directly influence a wide variety of body processes. Thyroid disease is twice as common in older people as in younger people. About 4 percent of people over age 65 have either hyperthyroidism (overactive thyroid that produces too much thyroid hormone) or hypothyroidism (underactive thyroid that does not produce enough thyroid hormone). Up to 9 percent of people in the hospital in this age group have significant thyroid disease. In addition, "subclinical hypothyroidism," where the levels of thyroid hormones in the blood are normal but where the signals from the pituitary gland suggest decreased thyroid activity, occurs in about 10 percent of older people.

CONDITIONS
Thyroid Disease

    Thyroid disease in elderly people differs from that found in younger age groups. The illness can produce nonspecific, atypical symptoms, often confused with other illnesses and frequently attributed to old age. Older people often have multiple concurrent diseases, and thyroid disease may mask or mimic any one of them, making it difficult to recognize that thyroid disease is present and probably exacerbating the situation. Conversely, coarse hair, dry skin, and constipation, which are important clues to hypothyroidism in younger people, are common complaints in older people with normal thyroid function. Furthermore, when hyperthyroidism develops in older people, the fine hair, moist skin, and diarrhea that are seen in younger people may not be present. Also, some of the drugs used by older people for blood pressure control can hide the presence of hyperthyroidism.

Hyperthyroidism means that there is too much thyroid hormone in the blood. While the chance of having an enlarged thyroid with one

Hyperthyroidism

or many nodules increases with age, the more common cause of hyperthyroidism in elderly people is Graves' disease. Graves' disease (named after the 19th-century Irish physician Robert James Graves) is an immune problem caused by an antibody with the remarkable property that it stimulates the thyroid cells.

Symptoms of Hyperthyroidism. People with this condition may have loss of weight, an irregular heart rate, congestive heart failure, and an increased chance of heart attacks. However, they may also have apathy, depression, confusion, loss of energy, and gastrointestinal problems such as constipation, loss of appetite, or a general loss in vitality. As mentioned earlier, the signs that physicians would ordinarily rely on to diagnose hyperthyroidism may be less evident or even absent in elderly people.

Evaluation of Hyperthyroidism. The physician can diagnose hyperthyroidism with specific blood tests that show elevated levels of thyroid hormone. Sometimes an older person with a goiter (a large, swollen thyroid gland) develops temporary hyperthyroidism if given an excessive dose of iodine. This typically occurs after the person has had X ray procedures requiring iodine-containing dye.

Treatment of Hyperthyroidism. In treating hyperthyroidism, the options include antithyroid medicines, surgery, and radioactive iodine ablation (destruction)—the radioactive approach is the simplest, least expensive. Older people generally have normal levels of thyroid hormone 6 to 12 weeks after treatment with radioactive iodine. Four out of five people given this treatment will eventually develop hypothyroidism; consequently, anyone treated with this approach needs to be carefully monitored. In addition, the body's ability to chemically break down various medications may decline after this therapy, and it is important to review and possibly adjust the doses of any such medications. Surgery has a limited role in treating hyperthyroidism. The prolonged use of antithyroid medications usually does not produce a remission in Graves' disease. Permanent remission does not occur if the hyperthyroidism is due to a sudden overgrowth or swelling of part of the thyroid.

Hypothyroidism means that the thyroid gland is not secreting enough thyroid hormone and that blood levels of thyroid hormones are low. In older people, it is most often due to an immune form of thyroid destruction (called Hashimoto's disease after the Japanese surgeon who first described it), or because of earlier treatment for hyperthyroidism (described above).

Hypothyroidism

Symptoms of Hypothyroidism. While most of the signs of this disorder are not very specific in older people (fatigue, constipation, feeling cold, and so on), a puffy face, especially around the eyes, and delayed tendon reflexes (measured by a physician during a neurologic examination) help point to the diagnosis.

A diagnosis of hypothyroidism can easily be confirmed when blood tests show low levels of thyroid hormone associated with an elevated serum thyroid stimulating hormone (TSH). This elevated TSH is the pituitary gland's attempt to signal the thyroid gland to produce more thyroid hormone.

Treatment of Hypothyroidism. Since thyroid hormone requirements decrease with age, older people who need replacement are started on very low doses of thyroid hormone. Particular caution must be observed when starting treatment in people with underlying heart disease. Usually the blood is checked for the level of thyroid hormone approximately six to eight weeks after treatment is begun. Once the hypothyroidism has been corrected, the chemical breakdown of other medications the person is taking will change, which may require adjustment of their dosage. Older people who have had long-term treatment with dried thyroid extracts called desiccated thyroid preparations should consider a change of treatment using more recently developed synthetic thyroid hormone. The older desiccated thyroid preparations have a very short shelf life and do not maintain a steady level in the blood.

CHAPTER 19

HEART AND CIRCULATION CONDITIONS

Overview   The heart is a muscle pump that sends blood throughout the body. The heart has two main chambers: one that pumps blood through the lungs to receive oxygen and one that sends blood through the arteries. Valves in the heart keep the blood flowing in the proper direction. Coronary arteries supply energy and nutrients to the heart. If this supply of blood is reduced or stopped, chest pain or a heart attack can occur.

Age-related changes in cardiovascular function probably occur but are hard to document because heart disease is so common. Most declines in cardiac function are due to diseases. Physical activity, nutrition, cigarette smoking, and socioeconomic status and other lifestyle factors contribute to the presence of heart disease in elderly people.

Pain in the chest implies something ominous like a heart attack for most older people. Although chest pain may be preceded by a series of events that went unreported, most people will complain of chest pain out of concerns for underlying heart trouble.

SYMPTOMS
Chest Pain

Chest pain can be produced by a number of conditions; sometimes a specific cause cannot be pinpointed. Chest pain can be divided into heart-related (cardiac) and nonheart-related causes. Pain from the heart is usually felt under the breastbone, but it can be felt anywhere in the chest, upper abdomen, in the jaw, or down the inner part of the arm. The discomfort ranges from minimal to severe and often provokes a feeling of squeezing, pressure, or burning in the chest (as if someone were standing on the chest). Cardiac pain that occurs during an activity usually causes the person to immediately stop until the pain subsides. If the pain is related to activity and immediately goes away when the person rests, it is called angina (from the Latin, meaning a choking or suffocating pain). Angina means that the heart muscle is not receiving enough blood, usually due to narrowing in the arteries that supply the heart (coronary arteries). The pain of a heart attack is similar to angina but usually lasts longer and is more severe. It is sometimes described as "crushing" or "viselike" and usually produces considerable shortness of breath.

Causes of Chest Pain

Nonheart-related chest pain can come from any of the numerous structures in the neck, chest, or upper abdomen. Pain in the chest wall (ribs, muscles, cartilage, and ligaments) can sometimes be produced or worsened by pressing on the site of the discomfort. Shingles (herpes zoster) is a skin disorder that can cause chest pain. Usually a rash is present. (Shingles is discussed on page 230).

Any new chest pain warrants a complete medical evaluation. Chest pain and sweating, dizziness, fainting, shortness of breath, or an irregular pulse require urgent medical attention. The physician will want to determine whether the chest pain is due to a heart attack. A

Evaluation of Chest Pain

complete internal examination and electrocardiogram are essential parts of this evaluation.

Treatment of Chest Pain

The treatment of chest pain depends upon its underlying cause. However, the outlook is good even if the pain is due to a heart attack. The most important consideration is prompt medical attention.

Swollen Ankles

Ankle swelling results from fluid accumulation. It usually affects both ankles and occurs there because of the effects of gravity.

Causes of Swollen Ankles

Ankle swelling is caused by increased pressure in the veins or a low albumin in the blood. Increased venous pressure in the legs often results from problems in the leg vein valves that slow down the blood return to the heart. Blood tends to settle in the lower legs, and the pressure increases to the point that fluid leaks out and causes the ankle to swell. Heart failure, serious lung disease, and liver and kidney diseases can also produce leg swelling. Ankle swelling and chest pain, shortness of breath, or any ankle or leg pain need prompt medical evaluation.

Evaluation of Swollen Ankles

A physician's evaluation includes a complete examination of the heart and lungs to look for signs of heart failure and conditions that produce venous obstruction or a low albumin.

Treatment of Swollen Ankles

Mild swelling of the ankles with no other symptoms frequently does not require treatment. Elevating the legs can help the swelling by allowing blood to drain back toward the heart. Avoiding constricting garments and prolonged standing or sitting can reduce fluid accumulation. Support hose can be helpful. Sometimes a physician will prescribe medication to help reduce the amount of body fluid accumulation.

CONDITIONS High Blood Pressure

In industrialized societies, blood pressure progressively increases with aging; nearly half of people older than age 65 have mild elevated blood pressure.

The risk of cardiovascular complications such as heart attacks and strokes increases as blood pressure rises, and there is no particular value that can be specified as too high. Definitions of blood pressure based on recommendations from the National Heart, Lung and Blood Institute will be used in this section. Blood pressure measurements are composed of two factors: the pressure when the heart muscle is contracting and pushing blood out, or the systolic pressure, and the pressure when the heart muscle is relaxing and letting blood into the heart, or diastolic pressure. Normal systolic pressure is about 120 to 130 mm Hg; normal diastolic pressure is around 70 to 80 mm Hg.

Blood pressure is measured in terms of millimeters of mercury (mm Hg). Millimeters of mercury are used to measure atmospheric pressure and define the unit of pressure needed to support a one millimeter column of mercury. These technical units of measurement are called "torr," for the Italian scientist Evangelista Torricelli.

According to the National Heart, Lung and Blood Institute systolic pressure equal to or greater than 160 mm Hg and diastolic pressures at 90 mm Hg or below present a condition called isolated systolic hypertension. When diastolic pressure rises above 90 mm Hg, the condition is called systolic–diastolic hypertension.

Most people's average systolic blood pressure increases throughout their life, while the average diastolic blood pressure rises until about the age of 55 to 60 when it tends to level off. This age-related increase in blood pressure is not, however, a universal phenomenon. For example, the populations of nonindustrialized societies and people living their lives in mental institutions do not show a rise in average blood pressure with age.

The Epidemiology of High Blood Pressure

For older people, the systolic blood pressure is more predictive of future cardiovascular problems than is the diastolic blood pressure. However, both systolic and diastolic blood pressure are independently useful in predicting blood vessel problems. Approximately 40 percent of strokes in elderly men and 70 percent of strokes in elderly women are directly related to high blood pressure.

Aside from age itself, an increased level of systolic blood pressure is the single greatest risk for cardiovascular disease in people over 65. In addition, increased blood pressure contributes to other cardiovascular risk factors, increasing the overall risk of heart diseases.

What Produces High Blood Pressure?

High blood pressure in elderly people is caused by increased resistance in the blood vessels of the body. This increased resistance results from an age-related decline in elastic tissue in the blood vessels and an increase in stiffness in the aorta and large blood vessel walls. The blood vessels also lose their ability to dilate, which increases the resistance in the small blood vessels. In addition, as people age, their blood vessels often become clogged with fatty tissue, a condition called atherosclerosis. Changes in the hormonal regulation of salt and water in the aging body may also play a role in the development of high blood pressure in the older person.

Treatment of High Blood Pressure

The goal of treatment in high blood pressure is to bring the pressure into a range where cardiovascular risks are lowered and drug side effects are minimized. Generally this means a systolic blood pressure of around 140 mm Hg and a diastolic blood pressure around 90 mm Hg. Nondrug therapy for high blood pressure may avoid the need for medications. This approach appears to be effective for some people with mild or borderline high blood pressure. Methods used include weight loss if overweight, sodium (salt) restriction, moderate and regular exercise, and a reduction of alcohol intake. The value of these measures has been inconsistent. It appears, however, that weight loss, provided it can be maintained, is effective in people who are overweight.

If nondrug treatment fails, the alternative is medications. Moderate doses of diuretics are as good as other drugs in lowering blood pressure. Since diuretics are effective, inexpensive, and only need to be taken once a day, they are usually the first treatment for most older people with high blood pressure. Diuretics are not a good choice if a person has increased heart muscle mass or signs of heart stress or strain on the electrocardiogram. People with poorly controlled diabetes should also avoid certain types of diuretic medicines. Diuretics increase urine production, and people who have urinary difficulties can experience incontinence. Moreover, in some men diuretics can cause impotence. Many other medications for high blood pressure are available.

The cost of antihypertensive medication over a long time can be substantial if several drugs are used. In effect, there can be a 20- to 30-fold difference in cost between the less expensive diuretics and the latest patented medications. The quality and effectiveness of antihypertensive drugs is not necessarily related to their cost. Once a person's blood pressure has been consistently controlled on a certain medication for over six months, dosage should be slowly tapered down. In some cases drug treatment can be replaced entirely by nondrug intervention.

A number of studies on assorted age groups indicate that high blood pressure is treatable. The problem in treating people with mild to moderate hypertension is that the benefits of treatment for each person are fairly low. For example, at least 300 people with mild to moderate high blood pressure need to be treated to prevent one of them from having a heart attack or a stroke (some studies suggest that over 800 people need to be treated to prevent one stroke or heart attack). This means that many people must be treated to benefit only a few. However, the benefits seem more obvious for people with severe high blood pressure.

How Beneficial Is the Treatment of High Blood Pressure?

It is worth noting that the goal should be modest when lowering blood pressure. There may be a J-shaped relationship between the treated level of diastolic blood pressure and the likelihood of heart attack or death. This means that people whose diastolic blood pressure lowers most dramatically may have higher rates of death or heart attacks than people whose blood pressure is more modestly lowered. Therefore, modest lowering of the diastolic blood pressure to about 85 to 90 mm Hg and lowering of systolic blood pressure to around 150 mm Hg appear to be the most appropriate targets for most elderly people.

Because of the concerns about the side effects of drug treatment for high blood pressure, some experts have advised restraint or even no treatment at all for high blood pressure in elderly people because they are particularly susceptible to many of the side effects. For example, they are more likely than younger people to develop a low sodium or a low potassium in the blood with the usual doses of diuretics. They are also more likely to develop depression and confusion when they are treated with antihypertensive medications that affect the central nervous system. The body reflexes that control posture and balance become less sensitive with age, which

The Dangers of High Blood Pressure Treatment

makes older people more susceptible to falls and fractures if they are given high blood pressure medicines.

Some people have argued that older people with hypertension actually need the higher blood pressure to provide blood adequately to vital organs such as the brain or kidney. Despite this theoretical concern, judicious use of high blood pressure medications in older people does not adversely affect either the kidney or the brain. Long-standing high blood pressure should be lowered cautiously and slowly. A gradual, controlled reduction of high blood pressure will reset the blood flow in the brain to a more normal pattern without undue stress.

Coronary Artery Disease

Coronary artery disease is the progressive narrowing of the arteries supplying blood to the heart (see Figure 30). Although coronary artery disease remains the most common cause of death in people over the age of 65, the rate of coronary deaths has decreased by 28 percent for those older than 80 over the past 30 years and by more than 44 percent for those ages 65 to 70. During the same period, deaths due to stroke also decreased by 40 percent in older people. These findings suggest that even in the older age group the specter of cardiac disease does not loom as ominously as it used to: Lifestyle changes and possibly medical therapies have had an impact on the progression of vascular disease.

Risk Factors for Coronary Artery Disease

Smoking significantly increases the risk of cardiovascular deaths in older people. The mortality due to coronary artery disease increases with the number of cigarettes smoked. Smoking also accelerates the development of blood vessel disease. For all of these and for other health reasons, people who smoke should seriously consider giving it up immediately.

High blood pressure is a risk factor for coronary artery disease. One large study showed a decrease in heart-related deaths as a result of treatment for high blood pressure. There was a decrease in deaths from heart attacks, but not a decrease in the number of heart attacks per se.

The levels of different fatty substances in the body are predictive of heart disease. For instance, levels of high-density lipoprotein (HDL, which is considered healthy) and low-density lipoprotein

(LDL, which is considered unhealthy) are related to the likelihood of having heart attacks. The total level of a person's cholesterol (yet another fatty substance) may be an independent risk factor for heart disease. There is not, however, a scientifically established exact level that can be considered the line between acceptable and too high cholesterol levels. Furthermore, maintaining a low cholesterol level may be at odds with a healthy diet. A diet that is restricted to 300 milligrams of cholesterol or less, for instance, may be deficient in calcium; people on such a diet would probably need to take calcium supplements to prevent loss of calcium in the bones. Drug treatment for elevated cholesterol in older people who have no

Figure 30. Coronary Artery Disease and Heart Attack

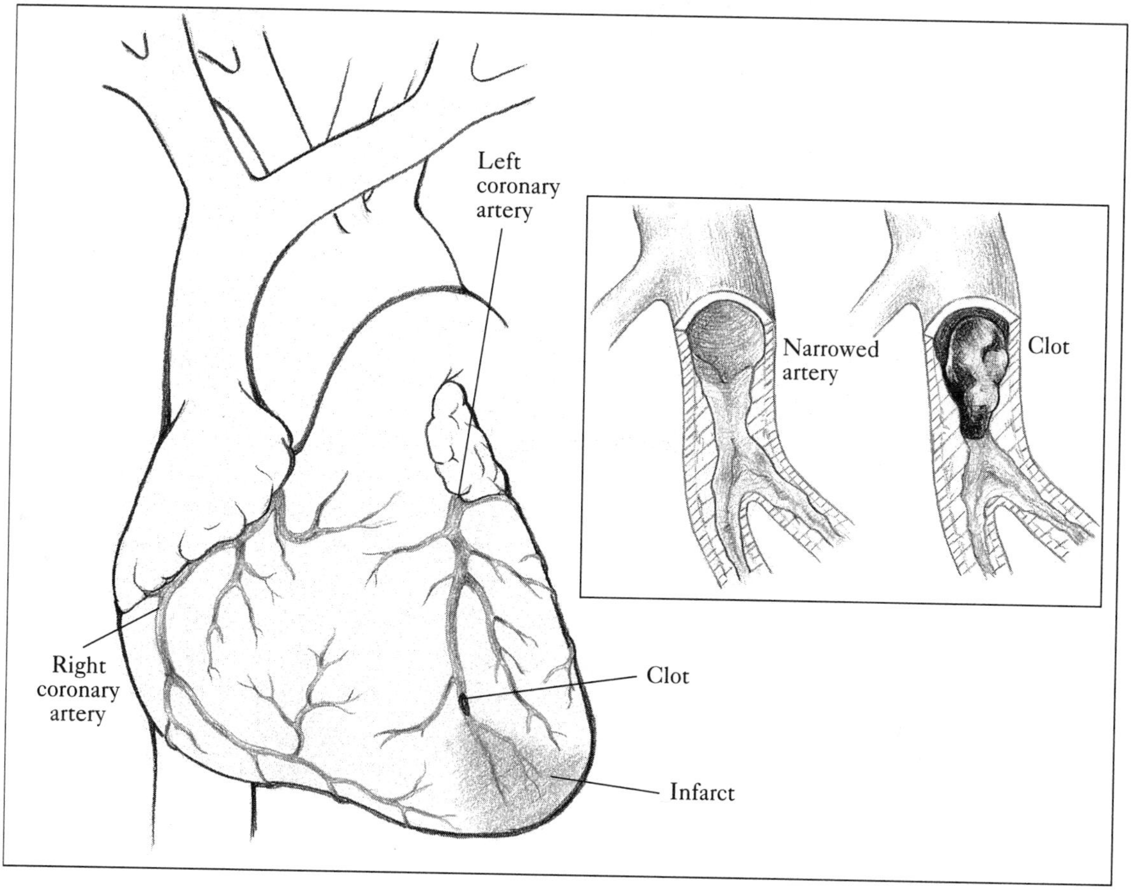

history of heart disease is very controversial. Low-cholesterol diets are usually inappropriate for disabled older people.

Older women with heart disease should discuss the question of estrogen replacement with a physician. Estrogen levels fall after menopause, causing HDL levels to decrease and LDL levels to increase in the blood. These changes can be reversed by estrogen replacement therapy; however, when estrogens are combined with progestins some of the beneficial effects are reduced. It does appear, however, that estrogen replacement therapy lowers the rate of subsequent cardiovascular events such as heart attacks.

Symptoms of Coronary Artery Disease

As people age, symptoms of heart disease can change. For example, the chest pain on exertion, called angina pectoris, may not be as intense; an older person may only experience significant shortness of breath on exertion. Nonetheless, chest pain remains the major symptom of a heart attack in people over the age of 65. Loss of consciousness, severe shortness of breath, nausea and vomiting, and changes in mental function become more common presenting symptoms of a heart attack. In people over the age of 80, shortness of breath is increasingly more common as an initial symptom of a heart attack. In disabled older people, changes in mental function may be the initial symptom. Despite these differences in initial symptoms, the physical examination and laboratory tests that physicians perform are the same for older people as they are for younger age groups.

Evaluation of Coronary Artery Disease

Various medical tests used to evaluate heart disease, such as the exercise electrocardiogram, are just as accurate in older people as they are in younger people. The accuracy of coronary angiography (cardiac catheterization) for detecting coronary heart disease in older people is also reliable. However, the decision to use these tests should be based on individual circumstances. Older people should drink plenty of fluids before and after the procedure to avoid kidney damage caused by the X ray dye given during the catheterization.

During their stay in the hospital, the major difference between older people with a heart attack compared to their younger counterparts is a marked increase in mortality. For people in their fifties, the mortality rate for an acute heart attack is between 5 and 10 percent. In people past the age of 75 it is about 30 percent. In addition, the complication of congestive heart failure develops in about 60 percent of older people after a heart attack.

The medical treatment of heart disease is similar in both younger and older people. It is important to rest after eating, avoid vigorous activities in excessively cold weather, and avoid significant emotional stress. A regular exercise regimen and a good diet are also useful.

Treatment of Coronary Artery Disease

The use of nitroglycerin is helpful for chest pain or pressure. It causes the blood vessels feeding the heart to dilate, reducing the work of the heart, which in turn helps relieve the pain. It also helps make breathing a little easier. Because fainting is a possible side effect of placing a nitroglycerin pill under the tongue, it is wise to take any nitroglycerin dose when seated. Nitroglycerin can also be given as a cream, in a patch worn like a bandage, or as an aerosol spray as directed by a physician.

Chest pain on exertion (angina) is sometimes helped by medications called beta-blockers. These drugs can have a sedating effect and cause decreased mental function. Calcium channel–blocking drugs can also be helpful in controlling exertional chest pain and high blood pressure. These medications can cause constipation and difficulty urinating and may cause the blood pressure to drop when a person is standing. Calcium channel blockers can also cause the feet and ankles to swell uncomfortably.

Treatment with drugs (called thrombolytic agents or clot busters) appears to present a major breakthrough in the treatment of acute heart attacks in older people. Because these drugs can cause significant bleeding complications, they should be used only after careful consideration of a patient's past history of bleeding disorders. Other medications, such as beta-blockers, may reduce by one-third the rate for having an additional heart attack.

The heart valves keep the blood circulating in the appropriate direction (see Figure 31). Diseases of the heart valves due to wear and tear are more common in older people than problems due to rheumatic fever or congenital valve conditions.

Diseases of the Heart Valves

People with significant heart valve disease may be advised, with particular instruction, to use antibiotics prior to various procedures, such as dental care. The antibiotics will reduce the chance that bacteria released into the blood through such procedures will infest the damaged valve, thereby causing the very serious condition known as endocarditis.

Aortic Valve Narrowing

Narrowing of the aortic valve, called aortic stenosis, often results from wear and tear on a previously normal valve for people over age 70. Injurious changes on the valve are composed of scar tissue, calcium, and fat deposits. Scar tissue and calcium on the valve keeps it from opening normally, leading to obstruction of blood flow. People with diabetes mellitus have an increased risk of developing this form of aortic stenosis. In addition, nearly one-half of people with this disorder also have coronary artery disease.

Symptoms of Aortic Valve Narrowing. People with aortic stenosis often complain of exertional chest pain, shortness of breath, and loss of consciousness (fainting). Older people who are not very active may show weight loss, fluid buildup in the lungs, and kidney or liver failure. These symptoms may also be caused by a change in the normally regular heart rhythm (in addition to heart valve disease) leading to congestive heart failure.

Treatment of Aortic Valve Narrowing. If left untreated after the onset of symptoms, aortic stenosis leads to death within a year for 30 to 50 percent of older people. The older person without any symptoms does not require surgery unless there is very poor function on the left side of the heart, often determined by an echocardiogram. Valve repair is needed, however, when symptoms such as chest pain, congestive heart failure, or fainting occur.

In the healthy older adult, the surgical procedure should be an aortic valve replacement, which, for people between the ages of 65 and 75, has a mortality rate of less than 5 percent. In people older than 80, a 10 percent mortality rate due to this operation is a realistic estimate. Replacement with specially treated valves from pig hearts is preferable to replacement with mechanical valves because they do not require as much blood-thinning medication afterward.

Other procedures are available for people who cannot undergo heart surgery. One of these procedures is called balloon valvuloplasty. This enlarges the valve opening by passing a deflated balloon across the valve and then inflating it. The procedure carries a 2 to 3 percent mortality rate as well as a significant chance of stroke and other complications. In addition, the valve recloses in about half of the people within six months and in 70 percent within one year. The procedure may be helpful in the preoperative management of older people with aortic valve disease who are getting ready for nonheart surgeries such as the repair of a broken hip.

The medical (i.e., nonsurgical) treatment of aortic stenosis consists of close observation and taking diuretics if heart failure is present. It is important to monitor any other medications a person may be taking for their effect on the heart in order to avoid heart failure or significant drops in blood pressure.

Aortic Valve Leaking

When an aortic valve leaks, the condition is called aortic valve insufficiency. In older people this may be due to rheumatic heart disease, but if it is, disease of the mitral valve (the valve controlling blood flow between the left atrium and left ventricle of the heart) must also be present (see Figure 31). Sometimes, the leaflets of the valves in people with high blood pressure and kidney disease develop holes that ultimately lead to leakage. Normal wear and tear on the aortic valve, however, is very rarely the cause of any major leakage.

Symptoms of Aortic Valve Leaking. People with aortic valve insufficiency usually tolerate it quite well. In some people, shortness of breath while lying flat, chest discomfort, and shortness of breath while at rest may be the early clues to this problem. Congestive heart failure is usually the prominent symptom of a leaky aortic valve. Physicians can identify the condition through careful listening to the heart.

Treatment of Aortic Valve Leaking. In older people, surgical replacement of the aortic valve is associated with a mortality rate of under 5 percent compared with 1 to 2 percent mortality for younger people undergoing the same surgery. These rates are doubled if other procedures, such as coronary artery bypass grafts, are performed during the same operation. The outlook for elderly people is excellent after a successful valve replacement and comparable to that for younger people who have had successful valve replacement.

Figure 31. Heart Valve Conditions

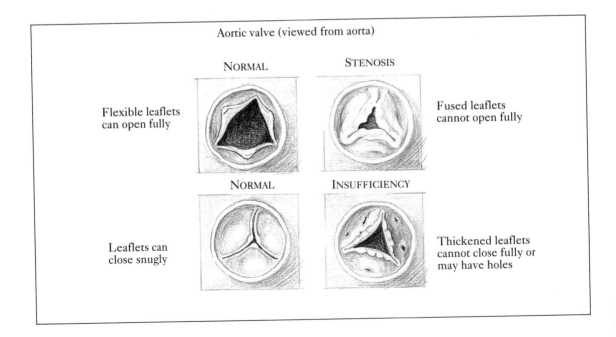

Pulmonary valve

LA

Mitral valve

Aortic valve

RA

LV

RV

Tricuspid valve

A papillary muscle with chordae tendonae attached to valve leaflet

1. Right atrium (RA) receives blood from upper and lower body and pushes it through the tricuspid valve into the right ventricle (RV)

2. Right ventricle (RV) forces blood through the pulmonary valve toward the lungs for oxygenation

3. Oxygenated blood is returned from the lungs into the left atrium (LA), which pushes it through the mitral valve into the left ventricle (LV)

4. The left ventricle (LV) forces the oxygen-rich blood through the aortic valve into the aorta for circulation throughout the body

Aortic valve (viewed from aorta)

NORMAL

STENOSIS

Flexible leaflets can open fully

Fused leaflets cannot open fully

NORMAL

INSUFFICIENCY

Leaflets can close snugly

Thickened leaflets cannot close fully or may have holes

The presence of coronary disease, however, worsens the postoperative outlook.

Narrowing of the mitral valve, called mitral stenosis, sometimes occurs in older people.

Mitral Valve Narrowing

Symptoms of Mitral Valve Narrowing. Often the person will feel tired and have congestive heart failure that gets worse because of a change in the heart rhythm. Blood clots can sometimes form in the heart and may lead to a stroke or other vascular trouble. Mitral stenosis can be determined through physical examination by a physician. Older people with mitral stenosis who have evidence of congestive heart failure or an irregular heart rhythm (or both) should be treated with anticoagulants (blood thinners) to reduce the likelihood of blood clots.

Treatment of Mitral Valve Narrowing. As with aortic valve replacement, mitral valve replacement is associated with a higher mortality in older people than in younger people. In people ages 65 to 75 the mortality rate may be as high as 5 percent; it exceeds 10 percent in people over age 80. The outlook for such surgery, however, is significantly worse if there is coronary artery disease present. With careful medical management, however, a reasonably comfortable lifestyle may be possible.

A leaking mitral valve, called mitral insufficiency, is fairly common in older people. This may be related to dysfunction of the heart muscles that control the valve, dilation of the heart, degeneration of the supporting tissues around the valve, or rupture of the delicate structures, called chordae tendineae, that help the valve stay in place. Sometimes the area around the valve has become calcified.

Mitral Valve Leaking

Symptoms of Mitral Valve Leaking. People with mitral valve leakage may have symptoms of congestive heart failure or irregular heart rhythms or both. Again, diagnosis is made through examination by a physician, who may want to include an echocardiogram as part of the examination to check the size of the heart muscle.

Table 26. The Causes of Heart Failure in Older People

INEFFECTIVE PUMPING	HIGH RESISTANCE TO BLOOD FLOW
Damaged heart muscle	High blood pressure
Drugs	Valve narrowing
TOO MUCH FLUID TO PUMP	PROBLEMS FILLING THE HEART
Increased blood volume	Ineffective heart relaxation
Increased body needs	Heart muscle enlargement
Leaking valves	

Treatment of Mitral Valve Leaking. Replacement of the mitral valve is necessary for people suffering such symptoms as profound fatigue, severe shortness of breath, difficulty breathing when lying flat, and severe edema or swelling of body tissue due to fluid retention. Severe mitral valve disease can also lead to weight loss. Because the mortality rate associated with surgical treatment of mitral valve disease is related to the presence of coronary artery disease, medical management of a patient with both diseases before and after surgery requires particularly careful attention. In people whose mitral disease is not related to coronary artery disease, surgical replacement of the mitral valve is a less risky procedure. People who have an irregular heart rhythm as well as mitral insufficiency are often given blood thinners (anticoagulants).

Congestive Heart Failure

Congestive heart failure occurs when the heart cannot meet the body's demand for blood. Heart failure commonly occurs in older people. The main causes of heart failure are shown in Table 26. The symptoms of congestive heart failure are not very specific, such as shortness of breath, swelling of the ankles, fatigue, weakness, or confusion. Unusual or atypical symptoms can be seen, especially in extreme old age.

Types of Congestive Heart Failure

It is very important to distinguish between two types of congestive heart failure, systolic (when the heart beats) and diastolic (when the heart rests), because the treatment for each type may differ. (The characteristics of each type are shown in Table 27.) People with diastolic heart failure often have a history of high blood pressure; the walls of the heart are thickened, making it difficult for the heart to relax and fill with blood. In contrast, systolic heart failure commonly occurs after a person suffers a heart attack. People with systolic heart failure may have weight loss and low blood pressure. These people often have a history of coronary artery disease and multiple heart attacks. The heart is usually enlarged and its walls are thin. The heartbeats are often weak, thereby limiting the amount of blood flow out of the heart. Sometimes individuals will have elements of both diastolic and systolic heart failure.

Evaluation of Congestive Heart Failure

The physician's evaluation usually includes an interview, physical examination, electrocardiogram, echocardiogram, and a chest X ray. Other tests are ordered if it is the first episode of congestive heart failure.

Treatment of Congestive Heart Failure

Diuretics are medications that increase the amount of urine produced and therefore loss of fluid from the body. They are usually the first line of treatment in both systolic and diastolic forms of heart failure. People with significant heart failure may not absorb oral tablets fast enough into the bloodstream. Intravenous therapy may be required to get the medicine into the bloodstream more quickly.

Table 27. Clinical Characteristics of Systolic Versus Diastolic Congestive Heart Failure

	SYSTOLIC	DIASTOLIC
History	Previous heart attack	Hypertension
Physical examination	No elevated blood pressure Mitral valve leakage	
Echocardiography	Dilated chambers with thin walls Poor heart contractions	Chambers with thick walls Vigorous heart contractions
Treatment	Diuretics, ACE inhibitors, digitalis	Diuretics, calcium channel blockers
ACE, angiotensin-converting enzyme.		

Digitalis is an important medication for treating systolic dysfunction. Long-term therapy with digitalis improves heart function. A third type of medication often considered for treating systolic heart failure is called ACE (angiotensin-converting enzyme) inhibitors.

People started on any of these three medications need to have their blood pressures checked regularly and their kidney function carefully monitored. In older people, ACE inhibitors may produce a low blood pressure on standing and sometimes the loss of taste. A troubling cough has also been associated with their use.

Anticoagulants (blood thinners) are sometimes used in people with very poor heart muscle contractions. However, anticoagulants are not indicated for frail older people who are at risk for falls and injury because of the greater chance they will have a serious bleeding complication.

Diastolic dysfunction is present in 30 to 40 percent of older people who experience congestive heart failure. Initially these people are best treated with diuretics. People in this group may not be suited to treatment with digitalis or nitroglycerin. Digitalis is not necessary because the problem is not one of decreased contraction of the heart. Nitroglycerin preparations may cause fainting due to a sudden drop in the blood reaching the heart. ACE inhibitors and calcium channel blockers may decrease the size of the thickened heart muscle.

Abdominal Aortic Aneurysm

Abdominal aortic aneurysm is the widening or ballooning of the major blood vessel leading from the heart. About 2 percent of people over age 65 have aneurysm in the abdominal aorta. People with high blood pressure and atherosclerosis are at greatest risk for aortic aneurysm.

Symptoms and Evaluation of Abdominal Aortic Aneurysms

Such aneurysms are often not noticed but can be detected through physical examination by a physician. Aneurysms are sometimes discovered during an abdominal X ray performed for another reason or during surgery. If an aneurysm balloons to the point of rupture, it causes pain in the groin, lower back, or lower abdomen, along with symptoms of shock. An aneurysm that is smaller than 4.5 centimeters (about 1¾ inches) should be watched carefully. When an aneurysm is found to be more than that in diameter or if it increases in size every year by more than half a centimeter, it may be close to rupture. Fifty percent of people who have a ruptured aneurysm die, and those who survive are usually left with considerable disability. Because of this, a person usually elects to have the vessel repaired surgically. Aneurysms that are larger than 6 centimeters (about 2 inches) generally should be repaired in most older people. In people over 80, a more conservative approach may be useful, depending upon other medical conditions. The death rate from abdominal aortic aneurysm repair is between 5 and 15 percent, the greatest risk being due to heart disease.

Disease in the blood vessels of the limbs—particularly the legs and feet (peripheral vascular disease)—occurs in 2 percent of men and 1 percent of women who are older than 65. Peripheral vascular disease encompasses conditions that affect both arteries and veins. Poor circulation is due to peripheral arterial disease.

Poor Circulation

Peripheral arterial disease occurs with cigarette smoking, diabetes mellitus, and high levels of cholesterol and fat in the blood. Decreased physical activity can also cause poor circulation.

Causes of Poor Circulation

People with poor circulation often complain of calf, leg, or buttock pain when they exert themselves. Some elderly people have severe reduction in blood flow and even subsequent tissue death without feeling pain. The absence of pain may be because simultaneous or associated problems in the nervous system blunt the sensations. Signs of poor circulation such as changes in skin color or texture tend to occur in the extremities or the feet, and may not be seen by elderly people who have poor vision. The sudden onset of leg pain can indicate a blood clot (thrombosis) in a diseased vessel or a piece of such a clot or other undissolved material in a blood vessel (called an embolus) that has migrated downstream from a large vessel to a small vessel where it causes obstruction. The source of the embolus is often the heart or the aorta.

Symptoms of Poor Circulation

A person being treated for poor circulation should stop smoking immediately, keep to a diet designed to lower fat and cholesterol in the blood, and, if possible, begin a regular walking program. A

Treatment of Poor Circulation

Figure 32. Varicose Veins

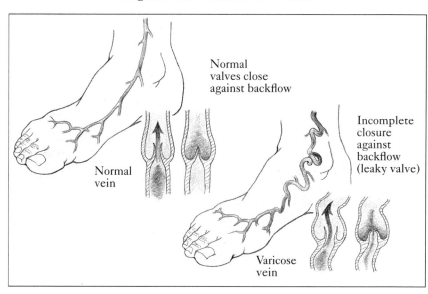

Normal
valves close
against backflow

Incomplete
closure
against
backflow
(leaky valve)

Normal
vein

Varicose
vein

medication called pentoxifylline can help in severe cases of peripheral arterial disease, but its effectiveness for older people has not been specifically tested.

Surgical procedures to improve the blood flow are controversial. Age does not seem to reduce success rates of surgery performed for the relief of symptoms or for the salvage of tissue.

Varicose Veins and Other Venous Disorders

Varicose veins result from leaky valves in the veins in the legs (see Figure 32). This disorder is usually caused by degeneration of the valves for which a person has a hereditary predisposition. Sometimes it is secondary to problems deep in the veins.

Symptoms of Varicose Veins

Aching in the legs that becomes worse when a person is standing is the chief symptom of varicose veins. Most older people with varicose veins will find that wearing elastic support stockings provides relief.

Treatment of Varicose Veins

Although treatment by injection of substances that burn and scar the veins is becoming more common, its purpose is primarily cosmetic, and the condition usually comes back. More invasive surgery such as stripping or tying off these veins should be avoided in older people, because the risk from anesthesia is not worth the essentially cosmetic results. In rare situations, ulcers or repeated bleeding from varicose veins or repeated blood clots may require surgical intervention.

Venous Insufficiency

Chronic problems of the deep venous circulation in the legs is usually the result of a previous blood clot in the deep veins called a deep venous thrombosis. Since this original clotting can occur without any symptoms, some people who develop chronic deep venous insufficiency have no history of deep vein thrombosis.

Symptoms of Venous Insufficiency. Individuals with this condition usually have swelling of the legs that becomes worse at the end of the day. This can evolve to a browning discoloration of the skin and can cause an ulcer above the ankle on the inside of the leg. The pain associated with this condition ranges from mild to severe.

Treatment of Venous Insufficiency. In addition to wearing elastic support stockings, which help prevent the progression of the disorder, the legs should be elevated intermittently throughout the day and long periods of standing avoided. Walking, however, should not be limited. If an ulcer occurs, antibiotic therapy and soaking the ulcer in warm solutions are recommended. Surgery is generally not indicated for deep venous insufficiency.

CHAPTER 20

BLOOD DISORDERS

Overview Blood is the fluid that circulates through the arteries, capillaries, and veins, delivering oxygen and nutrients to body cells. Blood rich in oxygen has a bright red color, but after providing oxygen to body tissues, it is dark purple. The liquid portion of blood is called plasma, and the cellular portion is made of red cells, white cells, and platelets. Red blood cells hold hemoglobin, which carries oxygen to body tissues. White blood cells actively participate in the immune system to provide defense from bacteria, viruses, and other environmental hazards. Platelets assist in blood clotting. In general, the blood and its components change very little with aging, but diseases that produce abnormalities in the blood are commonly seen in older people.

Anemia Anemia is defined as a low level of hemoglobin in the blood—hemoglobin is the essential oxygen-carrying component of red blood cells. For practical purposes, physicians consider the lower limit of normal hemoglobin in both elderly men and women to be

Table 28. Causes of Anemia in Elderly People

DECREASED RED BLOOD CELL PRODUCTION	INEFFECTIVE RED BLOOD CELL PRODUCTION
Blood loss	Folic acid deficiency
Bone marrow dysfunction	Heredity disorders
Chronic diseases and inflammation	Vitamin B_{12} deficiency
Hormone disorders	INCREASED RED BLOOD CELL DESTRUCTION
Iron deficiency	Drugs
Kidney disease	Heredity disorders
Malnutrition	Immune disease
	Mechanical heart valve
	Tumor

12 grams per deciliter of blood. This is roughly equivalent to a hematocrit of 36 percent (the hematocrit is the percentage of the blood volume composed of red blood cells). In healthy people, anemia is not a consequence of advancing age. However, it is a common finding in older people and an attempt should be made to discover the reason for its occurrence.

The causes of anemia are summarized in Table 28.

Causes of Anemia

Anemias Caused by Decreased Red Cell Production. The majority of anemias found in older people are caused by decreased production of red cells due to (1) chronic inflammation, (2) malnutrition, and (3) blood loss. These anemias are usually characterized by an iron deficiency in the bone marrow, which in turn limits the production of red blood cells. While this iron deficiency can be caused by a lack of iron in the body, chronic anemia can be associated with normal or even high iron stores. Special blood tests can determine the size of the iron stores and whether the iron is binding appropriately to various proteins. The problem appears to involve the body's difficulty in recycling the iron released when older red blood cells are destroyed. This problem is different from anemia due to bleeding in the gastrointestinal tract, which reduces the body's iron stores.

In both men and women, a progressive increase of iron stores occurs with advancing age. Therefore, nutritional iron deficiency is very rare in elderly people despite the prominence of other nutritional problems. When unexplained iron deficiency does occur, it is almost exclusively due to blood loss from the gastrointestinal tract often due to ulcers, polyps, irritation of the lining of the gastrointestinal tract, or cancer.

Inflammation associated with chronic disease is another important cause of anemia among older people. Such inflammation can result from bacterial infection, tissue damage, various forms of arthritis, and benign or malignant tumors. Treatment of this form of anemia consists of addressing the underlying cause of the inflammation. This anemia is almost never severe enough to require transfusion; iron therapy is usually not effective because absorption of iron is very limited in the presence of inflammation.

Malnutrition in elderly people can cause an anemia with normal-appearing blood cells. This type of anemia is usually seen in hospitalized individuals, and is usually accompanied by a history of weight loss; laboratory studies may indicate a reduced level of albumin in the blood. Correction of the nutrient deficiency and its underlying cause can significantly improve the hemoglobin level, thereby eliminating the anemia.

Bone marrow failure due to a problem with the marrow cells that produce red blood cells also occurs in older people. The disorder is usually associated with reductions of all the blood elements (red blood cells, white blood cells, and platelets). Common causes include drugs, immune diseases, intrinsic problems in the bone marrow, and replacement of the bone marrow by malignant cells or fibrous tissue.

Anemias Caused by Ineffective Red Cell Production. These anemias indicate that although there may be a sufficient level of red blood cells, there is a problem with their maturation. Red blood cells with maturation problems are unable to leave the bone marrow and enter into circulation. The red blood cells in the circulation can be large, small, and normal, and anemias of this type can be classified according to the size of the red blood cell. Anemias with small and normal-sized cells are usually due to heredity diseases or rare disorders.

Anemias with very large blood cells in older people are almost always due to deficiencies in either vitamin B_{12} or folic acid (another vitamin). When anemia is caused by such deficiencies, the bone marrow generally contains mature-looking cells with immature-looking nuclei (the nucleus is the site of the maturation problem).

Vitamin B_{12} deficiency (also called pernicious anemia) increases significantly with advancing age, and occurs when the body cannot absorb adequate vitamin B_{12}. This condition develops more frequently in women over the age of 60 and produces many different symptoms. A person may be weak; have a lemon yellow skin color; and experience changes in the nervous system, including a clumsy gait or numbness and tingling in the arms and legs. There may be behavioral abnormalities and confusion in severe cases. A low level of vitamin B_{12} in the blood confirms the diagnosis. Regardless of the underlying cause of B_{12} deficiency, treatment consists of periodic (usually monthly) injections of vitamin B_{12}.

Older people can have low levels of vitamin B_{12} but no evidence of anemia. They can also have dementing illness and other neurological problems that are caused by vitamin B_{12} deficiency, but have no evidence of anemia or other abnormalities in the blood. Therefore, physicians often check the blood for the level of vitamin B_{12} even if anemia is not present.

A deficiency of folic acid severe enough to cause anemia in older people is most frequently seen with malnutrition and excessive alcohol consumption. Alcohol and other drugs can interfere with the body's absorption of folic acid. When the need for folic acid is increased, such as when there is an inflammation, cancer, or red cell destruction, there is a risk of developing folic acid deficiency. A diagnosis of folic acid deficiency is confirmed by finding significantly reduced quantities of folic acid in the blood. If folic acid deficiency is discovered, it is very important to also check for vitamin B_{12} deficiency because treatment with folic acid will correct the anemia but not the changes in the nervous system if both deficiencies are present.

Anemias Caused by Increased Destruction of Red Blood Cells.
These are called hemolytic anemias. The causes of anemia due to increased red blood cell destruction in older people differ from

those in younger patients. Destruction of red blood cells by the body's immune system is common in the elderly whereas it is rare in younger people. In older people, this anemia is likely to be associated with a lymph gland malignancy such as non-Hodgkin's lymphoma or a lymphocyte disease such as chronic lymphocytic leukemia (see pages 333–334 for a more complete discussion of these diseases). Immune system diseases and medications are also causes. A physician may prescribe corticosteroids or surgical removal of the spleen. Most older people with congenital disorders have had these conditions diagnosed at a younger age.

Symptoms of Anemia

The symptoms of anemia are fatigue, weakness, shortness of breath, dizziness, and pallor. Apathy, confusion, agitation, and depression can also be symptoms of anemia. People with heart disease may notice worsening chest pain and swelling of the ankles. None of these symptoms is specific to anemia, and any of them can be produced by other conditions.

Evaluation of Anemia

There are many conditions that can cause anemia in an older individual, and a chance exists that several of them will occur simultaneously. This makes it difficult for a physician to decide how far to take an investigation into possible causes. Once the decision is made to investigate the cause of low hemoglobin in an older person, the principles involved in the assessment are similar to those used in any age group.

The physician's evaluation of an older person with anemia generally begins with an interview, followed by a complete physical examination, and a complete blood count to evaluate red blood cell size and to estimate how fast they are being produced.

Treatment of Anemia

The treatment of anemia will vary depending upon the underlying cause of this condition.

Bleeding and Clotting Disorders

Blood clotting involves three simultaneous and overlapping processes: the formation of a plug from platelets in the blood; binding the platelet plug to the site of injury to form a clot; and confining the clot to the area of injury. Normal platelets and normal clotting factors are needed for effective clotting. The older person is more prone to bleeding disorders than the younger person, and the causes for the disorders are different and more complex. A simple classification are conditions that reduce the number of platelets in the blood, platelets that do not work properly, and abnormalities in the clotting factors.

Platelets are the cells in the blood that when activated will form a plug in the blood vessel. They resemble flakes of dry oatmeal as they circulate in the blood. When activated by a vessel-wall injury, they enlarge and clump together just as cooked oatmeal does. When platelets in the blood are reduced in number, the blood does not always form a plug.

Reduced Numbers of Platelets in the Blood

Causes of Reduced Numbers of Platelets in the Blood. The most common cause of a reduced number of platelets in the blood (assuming normal numbers of both red and white blood cells) is an excessive removal of platelets by the scavenging cells in the spleen and liver. These scavenging cells are triggered to destroy the platelets when these latter become covered with antibodies. In older people, this condition occurs with malignancies of the lymph glands, chronic lymphocytic leukemia, systemic lupus erythematosus, and the use of drugs such as penicillin, heparin, and diuretics. In fact, the list of drugs is so extensive that all medications taken by the person should be taken into consideration when a physician is determining the cause of a low platelet count.

Symptoms and Treatment of Bleeding and Clotting Disorders Due to Reduced Platelet Count. People with this condition usually bleed from the mouth, the gastrointestinal tract, or the urinary system. The treatment of the low platelet count is directed at the cause. In most circumstances, corticosteroid therapy is used. If the person does not respond to this, the spleen may have to be surgically removed. When the low platelet count is caused by infections or cancer, especially cancer of the prostate, then restoration of a normal platelet count is dependent on effective treatment of these primary disorders.

Platelets That Don't Work Properly

The most common bleeding problem due to platelet abnormalities (when no reduction in the normal number of platelets is evident) is a disorder called von Willebrand's disease (named for the Finnish physician E. A. von Willebrand). This disorder occurs when the amount of the proteins required to form von Willebrand's factor is reduced. Von Willebrand's factor is a substance that makes it possible for platelets to stick to the blood vessel walls. Von Willebrand's disease is congenital and causes bleeding from the mouth, gastrointestinal tract, or urinary system, and abnormal blood-clotting tests but normal numbers of platelets. Other causes of platelet abnormalities include cancer, kidney failure, having a cardiopulmonary bypass as part of surgery, and a large number of medications (most commonly, aspirin).

Acquired Clotting Disorders

Deficiency of vitamin K is a common cause of bleeding problems in older people. The deficiency can result from not taking in enough vitamin K, from decreased ability to absorb this vitamin, or, most often, from the administration of coumarin anticoagulants (blood thinners). Anticoagulants inhibit blood clotting by interfering with the amount of vitamin K, which helps to activate the production of clotting factors by the liver. Vitamin K deficiency can be diagnosed through specific blood tests.

Another common cause of a clotting problem in elderly people is liver disease, which disrupts blood clotting by a number of mechanisms. The production of substances required for clotting (clotting factors) can be decreased as the result of liver damage. Alternatively, clots break down more easily because blood factors responsible for clot removal are not broken down rapidly enough to stop their clot-removing activities. Frequently, liver disease uses up substances required for clotting in the liver's blood vessels. Treatment for clotting disorders includes administration of vitamin K and, for the actively bleeding patient, replacing platelets and blood.

Blood Poisoning

The medical term for blood poisoning is septicemia, and it is caused by the continued and infecting presence of microorganisms or bacterial products in the blood. The implication of this is serious; the body can no longer contain the infection. People over the age of 60 account for between 40 percent and 60 percent of all cases of septicemia. Generally, the mortality rate increases with age.

A sudden change in mental function is often the first clue to septicemia. Additional symptoms are rapid, shallow breathing, a rapid pulse, a flushed face, and fever. These clues may not be present, though, and any older person with a sudden change in function should be promptly evaluated. Suspected blood poisoning is a medical emergency and calls for urgent attention.

Symptoms of Blood Poisoning

The site of infection is usually the urinary tract, lungs, gall bladder, gastrointestinal tract, or skin.

Causes of Blood Poisoning

Because many different organisms may be implicated, intravenous antibiotics need to be given promptly. In addition, the physician will search for the source of the infection and monitor carefully the function of the heart, lungs, and kidneys.

Treatment of Blood Poisoning

Leukemia (from the Greek roots meaning "white blood condition") is the malignant proliferation of abnormal white blood cells. Leukemias are subdivided into acute and chronic.

Leukemia

The incidence of acute leukemia increases with age, with half of the cases occurring in people who are older than 60. Risk factors appear to be radiation exposure, benzene exposure, and previous treatment of cancer with chemotherapy. Acute leukemia usually produces signs of infection (sudden high fever, change in mental function), progressive weakness, fatigue, pallor, or easy bruising and bleeding. The physician's evaluation usually consists of a complete blood count and a bone marrow examination.

Acute Leukemia

Treatment of Acute Leukemias. Unfortunately, increased age is associated with a poor outlook in terms of response to treatment. It is not clear whether the poor prognosis is due to decreased sensitivity of the leukemia cells, to the drugs, or to an increased risk of death from treatment complications. Age-related changes in the biology of the disease that might explain a poor prognosis are involvement of more than one type of cell in the leukemic process;

rapid growth of cells in the laboratory; preexisting problems in the bone marrow; and leukemia cells with a high number of chromosome abnormalities.

The management of acute leukemia involves treatment to induce a remission and then maintenance treatment. Remission is characterized by having no leukemia cells appear in the blood and having less than 5 percent leukemia cells in the bone marrow. In general, remission is accomplished with high-dose chemotherapy; maintenance therapy usually involves prolonged treatment with low doses of the same drugs used in the chemotherapy. In most cases, cytarabine is the cornerstone of initial and follow-up treatment. High doses of this drug, however, can cause problems in the cerebellum, the part of the brain that controls body coordination. Furthermore, it cannot be used when kidney function is poor.

While treatment for acute leukemia is generally aggressive, less aggressive therapy is indicated for those over age 65 because of the very high toxicity and side effects of the treatments.

Chronic Leukemias

Chronic leukemias have a more benign course than the acute leukemias. They are classified by the type of white cell involved: Myeloid cell involvement, the type of cells that mature to become granulytes, produces chronic myelocytic leukemia whereas lymphoid involvement, the cells that mature to become lymphocytes, is called chronic lymphocytic leukemia.

Chronic Myelocytic Leukemia

Chronic myelocytic leukemia is usually a disease of middle age but does occur in elderly people. The hallmark of the condition is a change in the chromosomes, which produces an abnormal chromosome called the Philadelphia chromosome. This abnormal chromosome is produced by joining parts of chromosomes 9 and 22. This change may have a role in the development and progression of the disease. The drug hydroxyurea is the standard treatment for this condition; however, the medication does not eliminate the cells carrying the Philadelphia chromosome and, ultimately, its impact on overall survival has been minimal. More promising results have been found by using moderate daily doses of alpha interferon, a drug that affects the immune system. Alpha interferon causes the disappearance of the Philadelphia chromosome in 15 to 25 percent of people; it may provide a more prolonged control of the problem. However, alpha interferon is more expensive and more toxic than hydroxyurea.

Chronic lymphocytic leukemia is the most common malignant disease affecting the blood system of older people. The most common symptoms are loss of energy, fatigue, decreased activity, and a reduced sense of well-being. Many people with the condition have no symptoms.

Chronic Lymphocytic Leukemia

Management of Chronic Leukemias. The management depends upon the extent of the disease. If the disease has reached an advanced stage (meaning it has spread extensively throughout the body), the prognosis is not good. When these factors are not present, it is generally not necessary to treat less extensive diseases. However, treatment is always necessary for extensive disease, usually with a drug like chlorambucil combined with prednisone. More aggressive chemotherapy has been reported to improve survival.

The lymph nodes and spleen form a major part of the immune system. Lymphoma is a malignancy of the lymph nodes and frequently involves the spleen. When lymphoma spreads to the blood it can manifest as leukemia. It is diagnosed by lymph node biopsy.

Lymphoma

Lymphomas are classified into Hodgkin's disease and non-Hodgkin's lymphoma. Hodgkin's disease spreads in a predictable way from one lymph node to another in a continuous manner. Non-Hodgkin's lymphomas are more widespread and can involve other body organs.

Hodgkin's disease is a type of lymphoma involving the lymph nodes (often in the neck) that spreads throughout the lymph tissue and forms nodular growths in body organs. (It is named after Thomas Hodgkin, who described it in 1832.) It appears to be more common in men and woodworkers.

Hodgkin's Disease

Symptoms and Treatment of Hodgkin's Disease. The disease produces painless, asymmetric enlargement of the lymph glands, usually in the neck, which sometimes feel rubbery. Other symptoms are more variable, including fever, weakness, itching, or weight loss. Anemia is often present. In a small percentage of patients, ingestion of alcohol produces pain in the tissues involved with Hodgkin's disease. The cause of the condition is not known.

Although the outlook for Hodgkin's disease worsens after age 40, advanced age should not by itself constrain treatment, and durable remissions are obtainable even in older patients.

Treatment involves radiation therapy and chemotherapy, alone or in combination, depending upon the extent of the disease.

Non-Hodgkin's Lymphoma

Non-Hodgkin's lymphoma is divided into low-grade (not very aggressive), intermediate-grade, and high-grade (aggressive) lymphomas. High-grade lymphomas are not common in elderly people, but the incidence of low-grade lymphomas increases with age.

Symptoms and Treatment of Non-Hodgkin's Lymphoma. Most people with non-Hodgkin's lymphoma notice large painless lymph glands in their neck or groin. Lymph nodes around the elbow suggest the disease. However, problems in the skin, liver, gastrointestinal tract, bones, and nervous system can be present.

While non-Hodgkin's lymphoma is usually managed with chemotherapy, the treatment for low-grade non-Hodgkin's lymphoma is controversial. People usually survive seven to ten years, and treatment does not appear to change these survival figures significantly. Generally, treatment is started only if a person has significant symptoms or has rapidly progressing disease. Sometimes low-grade non-Hodgkin's lymphoma may evolve to a more aggressive form. Any rapid change of disease progression suggests the need for another lymph node biopsy.

Intermediate-grade non-Hodgkin's lymphoma is the most common form in adults; the median survival rate for people without treatment is approximately 18 months. However, several different combinations of chemotherapy are capable of producing complete remissions in 50 to 80 percent of cases and about half of these people remain free of disease at least five years. Nevertheless, the most effective regimen remains a matter of controversy. The treatment of intermediate-grade lymphoma with full-dose combination chemotherapy has been associated with significant toxicity and disability in people older than 65.

Multiple myeloma (from the Greek roots meaning "marrow swelling") is a form of cancer involving the bone marrow not usually encountered in people under the age of 50. In multiple myeloma there is an uncontrolled growth of one family (clone) of cells that make antibodies. In most cases these cells make large amounts of a single protein called myeloma protein. The effects of multiple myeloma on the body usually result from the protein they produce or from the invasion of body tissues by myeloma cells.

Multiple Myeloma

People with the condition may experience weakness, loss of appetite, and weight loss. In more advanced disease the person may have bone pain, anemia, kidney problems, neurologic difficulties, or repeated infections. The outlook for people with multiple myeloma depends upon the extent of the disease.

Symptoms of Multiple Myeloma

The assessment of the severity and extent of the disease is determined by four factors: the amount of myeloma protein in the blood, the level of hemoglobin in the blood, the amount of calcium in the blood, and the presence or absence of bone lesions. More recently, a simple assessment system based on the level of a compound in the blood called beta$_2$ macroglobulin has been proposed.

Evaluation of Multiple Myeloma

Treatment may be delayed in older people who do not have symptoms of early multiple myeloma. In a small number of these people, the disease may remain stable for many years and will not require chemotherapy. Fluid intake should be increased to two to three quarts a day to help protect kidney function. Because multiple myeloma can accelerate bone loss, people with the disorder should remain active to help promote healthy bones. People with multiple myeloma are usually evaluated three or four times a year and chemotherapy is generally started if there is any evidence of disease progression. Complete remissions in multiple myeloma are rare. However, more than half of patients experience a partial remission, which entails a 50 to 75 percent decrease in the concentration of circulating myeloma protein. After the level of myeloma protein has

Treatment of Multiple Myeloma

stabilized, treatment with oral medications is continued for about six months. Recent evidence suggests that newer medicines such as alpha interferon may prolong treatment of multiple myeloma. Chemotherapy also provides effective relief of symptoms and is well tolerated even in the oldest patients.

Reduced White Blood Cells

The white blood cell plays an essential role in combating bacterial infection. It is also an essential component in the body's handling of inflammation. An abnormally low number of white blood cells due to the effects of certain drugs is the most common problem with this part of the immune system.

Causes of Reduced White Blood Cells

The three major causes for white blood cell reduction are shown in Table 29. The production of white blood cells by the bone marrow may be impaired. This occurs if the bone marrow is affected by a tumor or its activities suppressed by drugs or poisons. Severe malnutrition can also decrease the production of white blood cells. The second cause is ineffective production of white cells. In this setting, white blood cells that are abnormal in structure or functional capacities may actually increase in the marrow. These abnormal white blood cells cannot enter the circulation and are destroyed in the bone marrow. The ultimate result is a reduction in the number of mature white blood cells in the blood. Deficiencies of vitamin B_{12} and folic acid are the classic causes for this ineffective white blood cell production. Finally, normal, well-functioning white blood cells can be increasingly destroyed as a consequence of immune prob-

Table 29. Causes of Reduced White Blood Cells in Older People

DECREASED PRODUCTION	INEFFECTIVE PRODUCTION
Drugs	Folic acid deficiency
Infection	Vitamin B_{12} deficiency
Irradiation	INCREASED DESTRUCTION
Malignancy	Drugs
Severe malnutrition	Immune disease
	Severe septicemia
	Trapping in the spleen

lems, such as those associated with rheumatoid arthritis, medications, severe infections, or through a disorder of the spleen. A severe infection may both suppress the functioning of bone marrow and simultaneously destroy white blood cells. In the case of a spleen disorder, the spleen traps white blood cells, becoming enlarged while depleting the rest of the body's store of the cells.

The most common causes of a low white blood cell count in older people are chemotherapy for cancer, ionizing irradiation, and ingestion of toxins. In some cases, the decrease in white blood cells is dependent on the dosage of chemotherapy, irradiation, or toxins, and in other cases the decrease of white blood cells is thought to be due to allergic or immune reactions unconnected to dosage. Furthermore, various drugs can reduce white blood cell numbers in elderly people.

There are no specific symptoms of a reduced white blood cell count. If the white blood count declines below 1,000, the likelihood of infection increases. The types of infections depend upon which white cells are affected. For example, bacterial and fungal disease is more common if one type of white blood cell is reduced (neutrophils).

Symptoms of Reduced White Blood Cells

The evaluation of reduced numbers of white blood cells generally includes an examination of the blood marrow to determine the underlying cause of the low white blood cell count. Treatment depends upon the underlying cause.

Evaluation and Treatment of Reduced White Blood Cells

CHAPTER 21

LUNG AND BREATHING PROBLEMS

Overview   The basic function of the lungs is to exchange oxygen in the air we breathe in and carbon dioxide dissolved in the blood. The inspired air and the blood in the lungs are separated by a very thin membrane ideally suited to exchange these gases. As we age the total airflow into and out of the lungs (vital capacity) decreases and the lungs become less elastic. These and other changes increase the likelihood that we will experience age-related lung conditions.

SYMPTOMS Cough   The cough is part of the body's normal respiratory defenses. Coughing is usually caused by respiratory infections that resolve in a short time. If the cough lasts more than three to four weeks, however, it is considered a persistent cough.

Smokers are most likely to have a persistent cough, but, unfortunately, older smokers are less likely to seek medical attention for it. Persistent cough in people with no previously known lung disease and whose lungs look normal on chest X rays is usually discovered by careful examination.

A persistent cough is usually due to one of four things: airways that are very reactive (asthma), postnasal drip, chronic bronchitis, and the regurgitation of liquids and other materials from the stomach into the lungs (aspiration). Less common causes include heart failure, lung disease, and drugs.

Causes of Cough

Cough has been associated with some drugs, specifically those widely used for treating high blood pressure and heart failure, called angiotensin-converting enzyme inhibitors. Individuals who develop a cough while taking these medications should notify their physician for a substitute medication. Another class of drugs, called beta-adrenergic blockers, also used for treating high blood pressure may provoke coughing as a result of mild airway obstruction, but this is relatively uncommon.

Causes for a persistent cough can best be identified through a physical examination and interview with the primary physician. Additional testing, such as looking into the lungs with an instrument called a fiber-optic bronchoscope, is not usually necessary but can sometimes provide useful information. The treatment of cough depends upon its cause. Stopping smoking is also very important. Medication adjustment can be helpful.

Evaluation and Treatment of Cough

The air we breathe normally passes through flexible little tubes with thin muscular walls in our lungs. These little airways can contract when they are irritated, which makes it more difficult to exhale (see Figure 33). When we try to force air through these constricted passages, we produce a sound called a wheeze. Wheezing implies a spasm of the muscles in the airways, which causes a temporary obstruction of airflow.

Wheezing and Breathing Difficulty

Breathing difficulty refers to a shortness of breath with very minimal activity or an inability to sleep flat in bed without becoming breathless.

Causes of Breathing Difficulty

Whereas wheezing can be due to lung problems, such as allergic asthma and chronic obstructive pulmonary disease, not all causes of wheezing or breathing difficulty are due to disease in the lungs. Congestive heart failure is an important exception. In heart failure, the fluid pressure in the lungs increases, causing water and salt solutions to leak into the lungs. This can overwhelm the lungs' ability to drain themselves and narrow the airways by pushing on them. People with this condition may have symptoms resembling that of a person with asthma—wheezing, chest tightness, sweating, and a gray complexion, but it is important to remember that these symptoms are more apt to be caused by heart failure in older people. Recurrent aspiration of stomach contents can cause intermittent wheezing that also mimics asthma. In addition, blood clots in the

Figure 33. The Lungs and Chronic Lung Problems

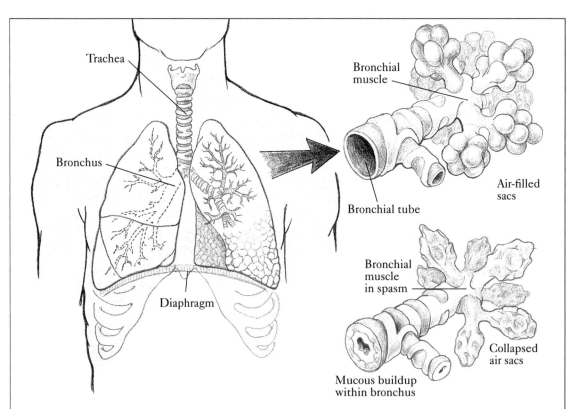

lungs can produce shortness of breath and sometimes wheezing (see Figure 34). Because these other conditions are also potentially life-threatening, any older person with wheezing should ask a physician to undertake a careful evaluation.

The physician's evaluation includes an examination of the lungs and heart. An X ray of the chest is sometimes obtained, and blood tests and an electrocardiogram are frequently ordered.

Evaluation of Breathing Difficulty

The basic treatment of wheezing caused by asthma is to open the airways with medications chemically related to adrenaline and to reduce the reactive nature of the airways. Wheezing and breathing difficulty due to other causes, such as congestive heart failure, respond to appropriate treatment of the underlying condition.

Treatment of Wheezing and Breathing Difficulty

Difficulty in expelling air from the lungs is a common element of a number of disorders known as chronic obstructive pulmonary disease (COPD). These disorders include emphysema, chronic bronchitis, and asthma. In elderly people, it may be very difficult to distinguish the symptoms and physical signs of asthma from those of the less treatable disorders, emphysema and chronic bronchitis.

**CONDITIONS
Chronic Lung Disease**

Emphysema is a condition where the small air spaces in the lungs are destroyed, leaving the lungs with large holes like Swiss cheese (see Figure 33). Chronic bronchitis is the clinical description of a condition wherein a person coughs up sputum (mucus or phlegm) every day for at least three months during two consecutive years. If strictly applied, this description applies to 50 percent of smokers. In a small proportion of people with chronic bronchitis there is difficulty in removing air from the lungs. This is caused by the thickening of the lining of the airways and the presence of secretions, which are often colonized with bacteria. While all these conditions seem clear-cut, most people have combinations of emphysema and chronic bronchitis; relatively few people have pure cases of one or the other.

Smoking is the primary cause in the overwhelming majority of people with COPD. Hereditary factors and certain occupations may also play a role or can also predispose a person to COPD.

Causes of Chronic Lung Disease

**Figure 34. Blood Clot in Lung That
Traveled From Elsewhere**

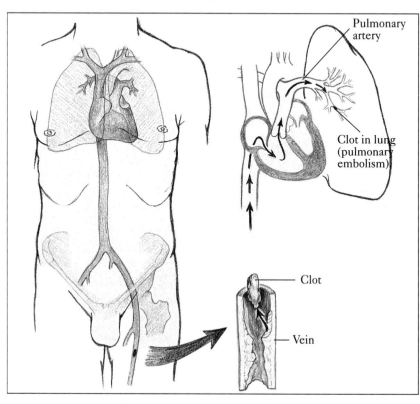

Pulmonary
artery

Clot in lung
(pulmonary
embolism)

Clot

Vein

**Symptoms of
Chronic Lung
Disease**

The person with COPD usually has a history of cigarette smoking, complains of being short of breath on exertion, and has higher levels of coughing and sputum production. The onset of these symptoms is hard to pinpoint, and the progression of symptoms is usually slow. The degree of airflow limitation may go undetected until another illness adds an additional burden on the respiratory system. Sometimes people with COPD develop a very large barrellike chest and it takes them a long time to empty their lungs of air with each breath.

**Evaluation of
Chronic Lung
Disease**

There are a number of tests available to detect COPD. The most useful and one of the simplest testing devices is called a spirogram. As a person breathes in and out of the spirogram, it measures the amount of air in the lungs as well as the emptying rate of the lungs. Additional tests include taking blood samples from an artery (usually in the wrist) to determine the amount of oxygen, carbon dioxide, and acid in the blood.

A person can be diagnosed as having asthma if the physician can demonstrate that the breathing difficulty can be corrected (reversed). This normally involves using the spirogram before and after the patient has inhaled medication that opens up the airways. An improvement of about 15 percent on the spirogram test indicates that the airways are responding to the medication, and therefore the breathing condition is asthma. There is also a test to attempt to provoke asthma, where the patient inhales a substance known to constrict the airways. If the lung function falls by 20 percent, the airways are reacting—in this case by constricting—and can therefore be treated. These different tests of airway responsiveness do not completely overlap, and a person may show that breathing capacity can be affected by one test but not on the other. Asthma occurs much more commonly in older people than originally thought. Recent studies have documented that between 15 and 50 percent of older people may have airway obstruction that can be successfully treated.

Treatment of Chronic Lung Disease

The treatment of COPD aims to maintain independent function of the person by avoiding infections and additional lung injury. Stopping cigarette smoking is very important. Drug treatment can reduce wheezing, cough, and sputum production, and can improve shortness of breath.

With an increasing number of new medications available for the treatment of COPD, one would expect that the disability and death rate of the disorder would decline. In fact, the death rate due to COPD has increased not only in the United States but throughout the world. The reasons for this increase are unknown, but some people feel that the marked increase in cigarette smoking following World War II may play an important role. Other environmental pollutants such as ozone, other gases containing nitrogen, sulfur dioxide, carbon monoxide, and small particles of dust also have an effect on lung function.

Aspiration

Aspiration of liquid and other materials into the airways can be a serious problem. When substances such as bacteria from the mouth, stomach contents, or foreign bodies are aspirated, they may produce local irritation of the air passages or progress to pneumonia (see page 346). Actually, everyone aspirates small amounts of saliva and oral bacteria, but the body's immune system usually prevents infection. When the amount aspirated is too great for the immune system to deal with, or when the body is already weakened, the resulting lung infection can be serious.

Risk Factors of Aspiration

Important predisposing factors for serious aspiration include recent stroke, seizure disorder, alcohol abuse, general anesthesia, any chronic illness that produces debilitation, and tubes placed in the airways or stomach for breathing or feeding.

Symptoms of Aspiration

The symptoms of aspiration can be subtle, but may include rapid breathing, fever, wheezing, or breathing that is more difficult at night (as aspiration is more common while lying down).

Treatment of Aspiration

While aspiration is not entirely preventable, one can decrease the chances of significant aspiration by keeping the head and shoulders slightly elevated at all times, especially at night, and minimizing drugs that decrease the level of consciousness such as alcohol, antihistamines, or other sedatives.

Lung Cancer

At the turn of the 20th century a leading scientist could find only 374 reported cases of lung cancer in the entire world. Today, lung cancer is the leading cause of cancer death in the United States; half of all lung cancers occur in elderly people. Lung cancer can arise from the cells that line the lung's airways (the bronchi and bronchioles) or the cells that form the lung tissue.

Causes of Lung Cancer

Cigarette smoking causes 80 to 90 percent of all lung cancers. Other risk factors include exposure to ionizing radiation and numerous occupational hazards, including exposure to asbestos and uranium. People who stop smoking immediately lower their risks and can eventually reduce their cancer risks to that of nonsmokers.

Lung cancer usually produces symptoms that are not immediately noticed, but lead to its eventual detection. Most of the symptoms are not very specific and are sometimes ignored or inappropriately considered to be part of another illness. For example, a persistent cough may be initially attributed to bronchitis. Any new symptom in an elderly smoker raises the possibility of lung cancer (see Table 30).

Symptoms of Lung Cancer

For practical purposes, lung cancers are divided into two major groups based on the way they appear under the microscope. Small-cell lung cancers constitute about one-fourth of cases while the remaining three-fourths are called non-small-cell cancers.

Classification of Lung Cancer

Surgery is the only form of life-prolonging treatment for non-small-cell lung cancers; therefore, any evaluation of the severity and extent of the disease is aimed at establishing whether or not the tumor can be removed surgically. To determine this, the physician considers the combined results of a physical examination, blood analysis, a bone scan, and special X rays of the chest to determine the spread of the tumor. Sometimes special X rays of the brain are also taken, because this type of cancer frequently spreads to the nervous system and brain.

Management of Non-Small-Cell Lung Cancer

For small-cell lung cancer, the physician's first goal is to take X rays of the brain in order to establish whether the disease is limited to one area or is widespread. This distinction is important because it determines both treatment options as well as the person's likely sur-

Management of Small-Cell Lung Cancer

Table 30. Symptoms of Lung Cancer

BASIC SYMPTOMS	SIGNS OF CANCER SPREAD
Cough	Abdominal pain
Fatigue and weakness	Bone pain
Fever and chills	Changes in mental function
Loss of appetite	Chest pain
Loss of weight	Hoarseness
Shortness of breath	Swallowing difficulty

vival. In limited disease spread, all of the detected cancer is confined to a single part of the chest that can receive radiation therapy. In extensive disease spread, the tumor cannot be effectively irradiated. Radiation therapy appears to work by producing chemical substances in the radiated tissues called free radicals. These chemicals interact with the cell DNA, leading to cell death. A problem with radiation therapy is that normal cells as well as tumor cells are affected. Another form of cancer treatment is to use anticancer drugs (chemotherapy) that kill cancer cells, but they also can cause problems for normal cells. Although chemotherapy alone or in combination with radiation therapy to the chest is the standard treatment for small-cell lung cancer, these two regimens can be difficult for an older person to tolerate. It is controversial whether radiation of the brain can help reduce the spread of the tumor. In individuals with lung cancer who are over the age of 65, brain irradiation has been associated with progressive dementia.

Pneumonia

Pneumonia, an infection of the lungs, is the fifth leading cause of death by disease in the United States. It is the most common cause of death in very elderly people and is found in about half of elderly individuals at autopsy. Pneumonia is 50 times more likely to develop in a person who is hospitalized or in a nursing home compared with a person living at home.

The symptoms and causes of pneumonia, the course of the illness, and the mortality rate of pneumonia are significantly different for old people compared with young people. Table 31 summarizes

Table 31. Contrasting Features of Pneumonia Between Young and Older People

YOUNG PEOPLE	OLDER PEOPLE
Chest pain common	Chest pain uncommon
Chills often present	Chills usually absent
Cough present in two-thirds	Cough present in one-half
Death rate: 10 percent	Death rate: 30 percent
Fever usually present	Fever frequently absent

some of the contrasting features between young and old pneumonia patients. Older people are more likely to have unusual symptoms, a more rapid decline, and a higher death rate. It is important for you to know that vaccinations for influenza and pneumonia caused by pneumococcus are available. (Prevention of pneumonia is discussed on page 44.)

The organisms that produce pneumonia in older people are not always the same as those responsible for pneumonia in younger people. No single organism can be identified as the cause of pneumonia in half of the cases of pneumonia.

Causes of Pneumonia

Infectious organisms reach the lungs either by inhalation or by aspiration of liquid from the mouth or stomach. Examples of pneumonia caused by breathing in the infectious organisms are tuberculosis, influenza virus, and legionella (the organism producing Legionnaires' disease). Most organisms producing pneumonia get to the lungs by aspiration (see page 344 for a discussion of aspiration).

The typical symptoms of pneumonia are fever, cough, and sputum production; these occur in older people but may be subtle or even absent. A sudden change in mental function can be an early clue.

Symptoms and Treatment of Pneumonia

Initially, most older people with pneumonia require hospitalization. Antibiotic therapy is usually given without knowing specifically which organisms are causing the pneumonia. Appropriate changes are made when laboratory data suggest a particular organism. Individuals can be managed in the nursing home if (1) they are stable, (2) there is 24-hour-a-day monitoring by experienced nursing personnel, (3) a laboratory is readily accessible, and (4) a physician is available on a regular basis to see them.

Tuberculosis is an infection caused by mycobacterium tuberculosis. This has lived with man throughout history as evidenced by findings in Egyptian mummies and prehistoric remains. Tuberculosis (from the Latin, meaning "swelling") was named because it forms hard nodules (tubercles). The infection most often involves the lungs but other body organs can be affected.

Tuberculosis

People who are over the age of 65 account for approximately 30

347

percent of the newly diagnosed cases of tuberculosis each year in the United States. In this age group, 85 to 90 percent of the tuberculosis cases are to be found among community-living individuals and about 10 to 15 percent are among nursing home patients. However, institutionalized older people have an increased likelihood of developing tuberculosis.

The majority of cases of active tuberculosis occurs in people over age 65 that were infected 50 to 70 years ago when 80 percent of people were infected before age 30. Most of these people carry the tuberculosis organism in their bodies where it remains dormant until changes in the immune system reactivate it. Conditions leading to this reactivation include malnutrition, diabetes mellitus, smoking, alcohol abuse, malignancy, or other serious illness.

Symptoms of Tuberculosis

The older person with tuberculosis often has very vague symptoms, such as weakness, fatigue, cough, and weight loss.

Evaluation of Tuberculosis

The infection is often discovered only when the physician or health care personnel suspect that it is present and attempt to confirm this suspicion with a series of tests. A skin test is extremely helpful in determining if the infection is present, but its application and interpretation may not be conclusive for the older person. A chest X ray is usually obtained to check for any abnormalities that are consistent with tuberculosis. Sputum is sent to the laboratory for testing. If the results of these procedures are inconclusive, other tests may be necessary.

Treatment of Tuberculosis

The treatment of active tuberculosis in the older person is the same as that for the general population. Isoniazid and rifampin is the combination of medication usually given for six to nine months. There are, however, other medications used to treat tuberculosis.

Overview

The digestive system consists of one continuous tube from the mouth to the rectum (see Figure 35). Its basic role is to digest and absorb food so that it can be converted into energy. On the whole, the digestive system shows fewer age-related changes in function than most of the other organ systems. The lining cells of the gut

Figure 35. The Gastrointestinal System

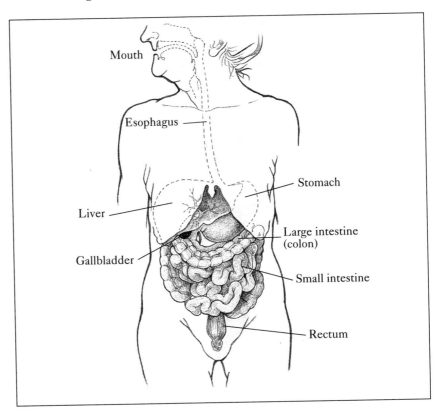

Mouth

Esophagus

Stomach

Liver

Large intestine
(colon)

Gallbladder

Small intestine

Rectum

maintain an extraordinary capacity to reproduce themselves and to absorb nutrients efficiently.

Older people experience the same bowel and digestive symptoms and conditions that younger people do. The effects of stress often lead to gastrointestinal symptoms. Constipation and diverticular disease are associated with aging, but generally digestive problems do not begin in old age. However, gastrointestinal malignancies occur more commonly in elderly people, and any change in bowel or digestive function warrants further evaluation.

SYMPTOMS
Abdominal Pain

Abdominal pain is a challenging condition to evaluate because it can be a sign of a serious illness or a relatively minor problem. Abdominal pain with bleeding or that becomes progressively worse can be a medical or surgical emergency.

350

Any of the structures in the lower chest, abdomen, or pelvis can cause abdominal pain. The location of the pain may not always indicate the location of the problem (see Figure 36). For example, stomach problems may cause pain in the middle of the upper abdomen; gallbladder and liver problems cause discomfort in the upper right side of the abdomen; the appendix in the lower right side. The nature of the discomfort can help identify the cause. Pain from the bowel or gallbladder tends to be sharp and intermittent like a gas pain. Pain caused by other structures tends to be more constant. Relatively common causes of progressive pain include a gallbladder attack; severe infection involving the gallbladder or liver; obstruction of the bowel; a twisting of the bowel, called volvulus; an infection

Causes of Abdominal Pain

Figure 36. Common Sites of Abdominal Pain

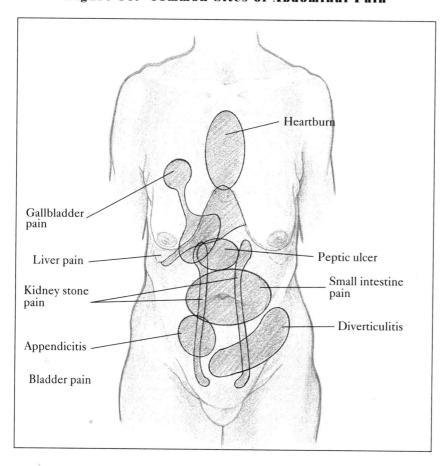

within the abdominal cavity due to a hole (perforation) in the large intestine. Inadequate circulation of blood in the bowel or gastrointestinal tract can produce severe pain.

Severe abdominal pain can also be caused by a variety of problems not involving the digestive system, for example, heart attack, shingles, kidney infection, and an expanding (or tearing) abdominal aortic aneurysm. These conditions are discussed elsewhere.

Evaluation of Abdominal Pain

Older people with abdominal pain and bleeding, fever, or any change in function require urgent medical attention. Although there is a mortality rate of 15 to 50 percent for emergency surgery in such cases, the survival rate is not related to age itself but rather to the associated medical problems and the timeliness of surgical intervention.

Treatment of Abdominal Pain

The treatment of abdominal pain depends upon its cause. Fortunately, minor problems are more common than major ones.

Loss of Appetite

Causes of Loss of Appetite

The loss of appetite is caused by medical or psychiatric diseases. Underlying illnesses such as infections, liver and kidney disease, or cancer can affect appetite. Various medications such as digitalis preparations may also have an impact on appetite. Depression can be another contributing factor and is discussed in detail on page 192. The reason for this association is not entirely clear, but some studies have shown that depressed people have elevated levels of corticotropin releasing factor (CRF) in their spinal fluid. As CRF is a potent inhibitor of food intake in animals, this small protein may play a role in the development of loss of appetite in depression. Although they are rare, classic cases of anorexia nervosa and distorted body image have been reported in elderly people. This suggests that in some cases weight loss may be caused by pathologic attitudes toward eating.

Evaluation of Loss of Appetite

Physicians generally evaluate loss of appetite by clinical interview, a physical examination, and specific laboratory tests. A report of weight loss is the most important information to be obtained from the interview. Other important clues are weakness, changes in smell or taste, abdominal pain, nausea, vomiting, diarrhea, constipation, difficulty swallowing, problems chewing food or in using dentures, changes in mental function, and the presence of other significant diseases. In the nursing home, diseases or conditions that affect appetite include hip fracture, pressure ulcers, depression, dementing illness, and cancer. Other important items to know about include all medications taken (both prescription and over-the-counter drugs) and any alcohol use.

The objective of general treatment is to maintain body weight, and it should begin while the underlying cause is still being investigated. It is important to be able to identify foods with high nutritional value and, if necessary, to be taught to improve shopping and food preparation techniques, and to be encouraged to make snacks of fruits and vegetables. (See Chapter 23 for more on nutrition.) The specific treatment depends upon the underlying condition.

Treatment of Loss of Appetite

Normal swallowing involves a complex coordination of muscles in the mouth, throat, and esophagus. A disturbance in this delicate coordination may result in decreased food intake. Difficulty in swallowing must always be thoroughly evaluated because it is never normal and may represent a treatable condition. Swallowing difficulty is the most common symptom of cancer of the esophagus.

Swallowing Difficulties

Swallowing difficulty is usually caused by either a problem in the upper third of the esophagus or in the lower two-thirds. Problems in the upper part of the esophagus make it difficult to initiate swallowing, so that people with this condition complain of food sticking in the back of the throat, but usually not of pain on swallowing. Regurgitation of food through the nose or aspiration of food into the lungs may occur. The disorders that often cause the difficulty—myasthenia gravis (a condition where the facial muscles fatigue excessively), hypothyroidism, or Parkinson's disease—usually affect the muscles in the upper esophagus. Sometimes a person who has abnormal relaxation of the upper part of the esophagus will have difficulty swallowing. This disorder is sometimes caused by a Zenker's diverticulum (named for the 19th-century German pathologist Friedrich Albert Zenker, who first described it). A Zenker's diverticulum occurs when the lining of the upper esophagus is squeezed through a portion of the outer esophageal wall, creating a little pouch that can fill with food (see Figure 37). Tumors of the throat and upper

Figure 37. Esophageal Diverticulum

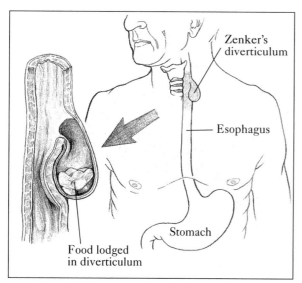

Zenker's diverticulum

Esophagus

Stomach

Food lodged in diverticulum

esophagus also cause swallowing problems. Certain strokes can produce damage to the brain's swallowing center or affect the nerves that control swallowing. The weakness of the tongue and facial muscles can be so severe that the person is unable to move food to the back of the throat.

People with swallowing difficulties in the lower esophagus complain either of food getting stuck in their throat or pain on swallowing. Progressive difficulty in swallowing only solid foods suggests that something is obstructing or narrowing the passage. Difficulty in swallowing both solids and liquids suggests a problem in coordinating the swallowing reflex. Intermittent symptoms without any progression suggest the presence of a constricting muscular ring, called a Schatzki's ring. When heartburn is present, long-standing irritation of the esophagus with severe narrowing may be responsible, but cancer in the esophagus may cause similar symptoms.

People who have problems with coordinated swallowing in the lower esophagus often have pain on swallowing or chest pain. Sometimes the esophagus can spasm due to simultaneous contractions. Occasionally people have a disorder where the opening between the lower esophagus and the stomach fails to relax properly (a condition called achalasia). People with this condition generally do not have pain but have swallowing difficulty that is relieved by regurgitation.

Evaluation of Swallowing Difficulties. Special x-ray studies create a moving picture of a person swallowing to determine if any abnormalities in the upper esophagus are present. If muscle disease is not seen, a careful examination of the ear, nose, throat, and esophagus is usually necessary.

Treatment of Swallowing Problems. Specific treatment is available for only a few of these neuromuscular disorders, such as myasthenia gravis and Parkinson's disease. Sometimes people with neuromuscular disorders benefit from rehabilitation and additional, supplemental nutrition. Surgery may repair a Zenker's diverticulum.

When a person with swallowing problems has difficulty in the lower esophagus, the physician will examine the esophagus carefully to check for signs of a malignant tumor or other signs of inflammation. Treatment will depend upon the underlying cause of the swallowing abnormality.

Heartburn

Heartburn occurs in people of all ages. It is more common in older people, but precise rates are hard to determine because people with the condition have many different complaints. Heartburn can produce discomfort that ranges from a mild burning in the chest to very severe chest pain. Coughing and wheezing can occur at night as a result of reflux of stomach contents into the lungs. Sometimes people complain only of hoarseness.

Causes of Heartburn

Heartburn is caused by excessive exposure of the lining of the esophagus to stomach contents, the major irritants being hydrochloric acid and an enzyme called pepsin. Normally stomach acid does not regurgitate into the esophagus because a one-way valve keeps stomach liquids from traveling toward the mouth. When the valve does not close as tightly as it should, heartburn results.

Sometimes heartburn is caused by pills that severely irritate the lining of the esophagus if they do not pass completely into the stomach. Pills likely to do this include potassium, tetracycline, or quinidine. Contributing factors include not drinking enough water when swallowing these medications, taking these medications while lying flat, or having a condition within the esophagus that prevents its emptying easily into the stomach.

Treatment of Heartburn

Treating heartburn involves modifications in lifestyle, such as eating smaller meals, eating more than three hours before lying flat, avoiding tight-fitting clothing, and avoiding certain foods and drugs that relax the valve in the lower part of the esophagus. These include alcohol, coffee, tomato sauce, chocolate, and some medicines. People with the condition should elevate the head of their bed six to eight inches with bricks or blocks. Generally sleeping on two or three pillows is not helpful because of the changes of positions that occur during sleep. If these nondrug treatments fail or if the person is found to have an ulcer, then medication therapy is necessary.

Although heartburn usually disappears with lifestyle changes and antacids or other medications, it can sometimes lead to significant bleeding in the esophagus or stomach. In this case, as in all circumstances involving active bleeding, the person needs prompt medical attention.

Constipation

Constipation is difficulty in forming or passing a bowel movement or a feeling of incomplete evacuation associated with a reduced number of bowel movements.

Causes of Constipation

As people age, the muscle tone of the rectum relaxes, which can disrupt the normal emptying of the colon and rectum. This in turn increases the likelihood of constipation. Constipation is usually painless and is related to the slowing down of the bowel, with most of the slowing occurring in the large intestine. Complications of constipation include the sense of not feeling right, intestinal blockage, a massively dilated bowel, and loss of bowel and bladder control. A new onset of constipation in an older person raises the possibility of obstruction of the colon from such conditions as a large amount of hard stool—called a fecal impaction—polyps or other benign tumors, and cancer.

Prolonged constipation over many years can lead to a condition called megacolon, a massively dilated colon that contracts very poorly. This megacolon can be seriously worsened by various medications, including those used for Parkinson's disease, iron supplements, and those that block the neurotransmitter acetylcholine (this blockade slows down bowel contraction). Older people who have developed megacolon are at increased risk for having the colon twist around itself, causing severe obstruction, a condition called volvulus.

Evaluation of Constipation

The physician's evaluation of constipation includes examination of the abdomen and rectum and often includes lower endoscopy. The lower endoscopy is an inspection of the lining of the rectum and large intestine using a flexible tube called an endoscope. Occasionally an X ray of the lower bowel (a barium enema) is obtained.

The treatment of constipation in older people begins with stopping any medications that slow down the bowel such as narcotics. The diet should be changed to increase the amount of dietary fiber intake to between 6 and 15 grams per day. Bran is the most effective source of fiber; somewhat less effective but useful sources include apples, cabbage, lettuce, and raw vegetables. Additional ways to prevent constipation include regularly scheduled mealtimes, drinking plenty of liquids to ensure adequate hydration, and regular physical activity. Stool softeners are commonly prescribed, and some people respond to lubricating the rectum with a glycerine suppository. The regular use of stimulant-type laxatives such as castor oil, cascara, or phenolphthalein is strongly discouraged for people who are otherwise physically active because these stimulants can damage the delicate nerve supply to the intestines and end up worsening the condition in the long run. Stimulant or saline laxatives, however, may be required to manage constipation in those people who have severely limited mobility or who have specific diseases that affect the intestines, such as Parkinson's disease.

One treatment for fecal impaction involves increasing the size and fluid nature of the stool with bulk-forming agents (such as Metamucil) or poorly absorbed sugars (such as lactulose), intermittent suppositories, or large-volume enemas.

Treatment of Constipation

Diarrhea is the body's way of rapidly getting rid of bacteria or toxins in the digestive system. It is usually defined as the passage of loose stools with a greater than normal water content, but some people equate the urgent desire to pass a bowel movement with diarrhea. Diarrhea can cause disabling loss of bowel control in elderly people.

Diarrhea

A list of causes of diarrhea is shown in Table 32. Overflow around a fecal impaction is found in almost 20 percent of people with diarrhea. Infections that produce diarrhea include those caused by bacteria such as *Campylobacter*, *Salmonella*, and *Shigella*. Drug-induced diarrhea is also common. Any medication should be

Causes of Diarrhea

considered a potential cause. In fact, infections and drugs (antibiotics) cause about one-third of the cases of diarrhea. Antibiotic-caused diarrhea is particularly common in elderly people. Up to one-third of people in a chronic care facility (nursing home) may have *Clostridium difficile*, a disease-producing bacterium that may be found in the stools of people with diarrhea who have been on antibiotics. Factors in the diet also need to be looked for, especially diarrhea caused by milk and dairy products. This can occur because of intolerance to lactose, a sugar found in milk. Underlying illnesses such as thyroid disease and diabetes mellitus must be considered when seeking the cause of diarrhea.

Evaluation of Diarrhea

The initial evaluation by a physician usually includes an interview and physical examination and examination of the stool to look for signs of inflammation. Stool samples are often sent to the laboratory to look for bacteria, toxins, and parasites. If these tests do not reveal the cause, a lower endoscopy is performed. This is an examination using a special tube to examine the lining of the rectum and large intestine.

Severe diarrhea can be prominent in people with long-standing diabetes, especially if the diabetes affects the nervous system. This type of diarrhea is generally worse at night and is characterized by watery, brown stools.

Treatment of Diarrhea

An important complication of diarrhea is dehydration. Fluid intake needs to be maintained, usually with clear liquids. It is a good idea to avoid milk for a few days because it can temporarily worsen diarrhea. Diarrhea lasting more than a week should receive medical evaluation. Severe diarrhea or the presence of any bloody stools

Table 32. Causes of Diarrhea in Older People

Colon cancer	Irritable bowel syndrome
Drug-induced diarrhea	Lactase deficiency
Fecal impaction	Laxative abuse
Inflammatory bowel disease	Malabsorption
Intestinal infection	Thyroid disease

warrants immediate medical attention. Specific treatments for diarrhea are available depending on the underlying cause.

Older people complain of passing excess gas, but it is hard to determine the extent of the problem since the complaint is so common in other age groups; no one knows if an increase in gas production occurs with aging.

Causes of Excess Gas

The two main causes of intestinal gas are swallowed air and gas production by bacteria in the bowel. Some people swallow large amounts of air, which they eventually return to the environment. These people can often be trained to avoid air swallowing. Sugars that are not absorbed in the small intestine can be chemically broken down by bacteria in the colon with significant gas production (hydrogen, carbon dioxide, and methane) as a result. Some older people have difficulty absorbing the milk sugar lactose, which can cause diarrhea, abdominal bloating, and gas.

Treatment of Excess Gas

Dietary modification, the use of yogurt, and low-lactose milk can be helpful. Effective dietary strategies include eliminating beans, cabbage, legumes, raisins, and nonabsorbable sugars (such as some artificial sweeteners). A product called Beeno is available to break down the nonabsorbable sugars in these foods that stimulate gas production. It appears to be safe, although it can cause mild elevations in the blood sugar. Unfortunately, there is no accepted treatment for foul-smelling gas.

CONDITIONS
Gastrointestinal Bleeding

Bleeding in the gastrointestinal tract is a significant cause of disability and mortality in elderly people. Bleeding can occur spontaneously or it may be related to disease in other organ systems.

Causes of Gastrointestinal Bleeding

Important causes of gastrointestinal bleeding in the esophagus, stomach, and small intestine include peptic ulcers, an irritated esophagus or stomach, and cancer. These gastrointestinal bleedings stop on their own in about 80 percent of people.

Hemorrhoids, diverticulosis, various tumors, and small abnormalities in the blood vessels lining the colon constitute the important causes of bleeding in the colon and rectum. In most circumstances, this lower gastrointestinal bleeding stops on its own.

Diverticula, tiny pouches that form in the intestinal lining, increase in number in the colon with age and are present in more than half of people over the age of 70 (see Figure 40 on page 371). Active bleeding occurs in only about 5 percent of people with diverticula. Generally when diverticula bleed, the person does not usually feel pain but notices bright red rectal blood. The bleeding usually stops by itself in 80 percent of people. About one-fourth of older people who have had bleeding diverticula will have another bleeding episode. Diverticular disease is common in older people, but it is not always the source of lower gastrointestinal bleeding. Other causes must be looked for in every person. It should never be assumed that significant bleeding from the lower tract is automatically due to hemorrhoids or diverticula, and a thorough evaluation by a physician is always warranted. Diverticulitis and hemorrhoids are discussed in more detail later in this chapter.

Evaluation of Gastrointestinal Bleeding

Delays in discovering the source of bleeding can result in a greater risk of mortality. As a result, it is crucial to have the physician identify the bleeding source rapidly in order to initiate prompt treatment.

The physician will want to know if the person has a history of peptic ulcer disease, liver disease, previous bleeding episodes, surgery in the abdomen, alcohol use, or uses NSAIDs or other drugs. Bleeding from the stomach or upper intestine usually produces dark tar-colored bowel movements. The patient may vomit blood, which may be bright red or look like coffee grounds. Bright, red blood passed from the rectum suggests that the bleeding is occurring in the colon or rectum. A recent history of severe abdominal pain suggests that something in the abdomen has been perforated or that there is poor blood flow to the intestines. For bleeding in the upper gastrointestinal tract, it is important for a gastroenterologist to look at the esophagus and stomach by means of a procedure called an upper gastrointestinal endoscopy in order to identify the bleeding site. Appropriate treatment can then begin immediately for those people with actively bleeding lesions who do not stop bleeding promptly. If this procedure does not identify the bleeding site, additional studies may be necessary. If lower gastrointestinal tract bleeding continues, the physician can perform special tests (sigmoidoscopy, special X rays) to identify the bleeding site and to determine the rate of bleeding.

Chronic or occult (invisible to the naked eye) blood loss through the intestines sometimes occurs in older people. People may see small amounts of blood in the stool, have a positive laboratory test for blood in a stool sample, or have unexplained iron-deficiency anemia. Iron-deficiency anemia without a known reason or the discovery of any blood in the stool requires prompt evaluation. This evaluation is necessary to detect and remove early gastrointestinal tumors and to diagnose and treat any underlying conditions. A test of a stool sample for blood will detect active blood loss from any site in the gastrointestinal tract. More commonly the source is located in the colon. As in more rapid bleeding in the intestines, the site responsible for the bleeding should be identified and treated.

More Subtle Bleeding in the Intestines

Treatment for gastrointestinal bleeding depends upon the source of the bleeding. Fortunately, most bleeding stops on its own. Active bleeding must be treated as a medical emergency. Surgery is the definitive treatment for persistent bleeding.

Treatment of Gastrointestinal Bleeding

The medical term for loss of bowel control is *fecal incontinence*. The term is applied to an inability either to hold or to pass fecal matter through voluntary muscle action. Its prevalence in the community is not known, but various studies have reported it to range from 17 to 66 percent in the hospital setting. Between 10 and 15 percent of people in long-term care facilities may have the problem.

Loss of Bowel Control

Loss of bowel control can have devastating consequences, significantly increasing the burden on caregivers and frequently resulting in institutionalization. It is a source of discomfort for the person with an intact mental function. It often occurs with urinary problems, including loss of bladder control.

The anal canal is approximately two inches long and its junction with the large intestine is maintained at a right angle (90 degrees) by a muscle that forms a powerful sling that helps support the pelvic structures (see Figure 38). The weight of the abdominal organs

Normal Bowel Control

Figure 38. The Large Intestine

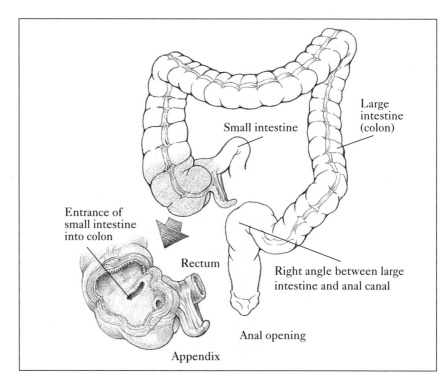

pushes down on the large intestine and closes the opening at the point of the right angle. This flap valve helps to prevent any leakage of stool into the anus, and any increases in abdominal pressure tend to make the valve more effective.

The normal anal muscles and lining perform two functions that are essential for bowel control. The first is the ability to discriminate between solid, liquid, or gas in the rectal area. The second is the ability to postpone a bowel movement to a convenient time and place. The nerve endings that line the anal canal normally enable people to tell gas from solid or liquid, but such exquisite anal sensation appears to diminish with age. The muscles forming the bowel control mechanism are influenced by the nervous system. In the resting state, the muscles maintain closure of the anal cavity by keeping maximally contracted.

An increase in abdominal pressure is followed by relaxation of the muscles that form the sling. This relaxation straightens the

Table 33. Causes of Loss of Bowel Control

FECAL STASIS AND IMPACTION

LOSS OF NORMAL CONTROL MECHANISM
Local nerve damage
Impaired neurologic reflexes
Surgical or obstetric damage

PROBLEMS THAT OVERWHELM THE NORMAL CONTROL MECHANISM
Diarrhea
Poor access to toileting facilities

PSYCHOLOGIC AND BEHAVIORAL PROBLEMS
Dementia
Severe depression

Source: Adapted from Goldstein M, Brown EM. Fecal incontinence in an elderly man. *Journal of the American Geriatrics Society.* 1989;37(10):994. Reprinted with permission.

right angle and allows the anal canal to distend and open. The contents of the bowel can then pass out through the anus.

Causes of Loss of Bowel Control

The causes of loss of bowel control are shown in Table 33. When hard stool collects and remains in the bowel for a long time, it creates a fecal impaction. This is the most common cause of loss of bowel control in elderly people. It is often associated with reduced mobility and commonly occurs in people who are hospitalized or in nursing homes. Physical inactivity is also an important factor. People with fecal impaction frequently have a history of constipation and of taking laxatives. They may also have diseases that slow the nervous system, such as Parkinson's disease, or take medications that reduce bowel contractions. In these people, the time that it takes for the stool to reach the rectum is usually prolonged (for normal people it may take three days for material to pass from the mouth to the rectum). This reduced bowel activity can progress to constipation, and eventually to impaction with a large mass of stool in the rectum. Other factors include a lack of fiber in the diet and changes in the gastrointestinal hormones that stimulate bowel motility. Most impactions can be easily found by the physician or nurse by inserting a finger into the rectum and feeling the unpassed stool in the rectal vault.

Damage to the nerves around the rectum, with resultant changes in the muscles, has been noted in people who have loss of bowel control. Such nerve loss can be caused by compression and stretching of the nerves due to prolonged straining. Nerve damage has also been shown in people who have decades of excessive laxative use. In addition, prolonged laxative use can produce a brown staining in the lining of the colon that is visible on examination. Local nerve damage can impair the efficiency of the flap-valve bowel control mechanism.

In older people, loss of bowel control due to neurological problems in the brain or spinal cord is more common than that due to damage to nerves around the rectum. Pinched nerves in the back, tumors, and abnormalities in the spinal cord can disrupt normal bowel contractions, cause loss of sensation, and produce incomplete bowel emptying. People with strokes or Alzheimer's disease sometimes have a loss of bowel control. People with these conditions may pass a formed stool following a cup of coffee or a meal. The bowel control mechanism can also be impaired by surgery or, in women, by trauma after labor and delivery; both of these can produce a loss of muscle tone and a disruption of the flap-valve mechanism.

Diarrhea overwhelms the normal bowel control mechanism. Diarrhea is caused by medications, bowel infections, and inflammation of the bowel. It is especially important to check for infectious causes if people have been treated with antibiotics, because organisms resistant to usual antibiotics may be causing the diarrhea. (Diarrhea is addressed more completely earlier in this chapter.)

Psychological and behavioral problems can also be responsible for loss of bowel control. They may be the signal of dementing illness or depression. Loss of bowel control may occur, for example, when a severely depressed person is unable to reach the toilet in time or when a demented person is unwilling to do so.

Evaluation of Loss of Bowel Control

The primary goals of the clinical evaluation are to identify the cause of the loss of bowel control and the effect on a person's ability to function (see Table 34).

**Table 34. Important Factors in the Evaluation
of Loss of Bowel Control**

CHARACTERISTICS OF THE LOSS OF CONTROL	
Onset: time and circumstance	Other gastrointestinal problems
Timing of accidents and normal stools	Other medical problems
Duration and frequency	Medications (prescription and over-the-counter)
Volume and consistency of stool	
Relation of food ingestion	Neurologic problems
Previous bowel pattern	Obstetric history
Associated symptoms	Diet
Urgency	Environmental factors
Deferral time (ability to reach commode or bathroom on time)	Restraints or bedrails that inhibit mobility
Pain	Location of bathroom or commode
Bleeding	Clothing
Abdominal cramps	Functional impact
Rectal sensation of fullness	Caregiver burden
Sensation of passing stool or gas	

Source: Goldstein M, Brown EM. Fecal incontinence in an elderly man. *Journal of the American Geriatrics Society.*
1989;37(10):996. Reprinted with permission.

The presence of other symptoms such as urgency, pain, bleeding, or abdominal cramps suggests problems in the anal area. Any obstetric history or record of previous surgery can also provide important clues. Bleeding indicates the need for prompt evaluation to look for infection, inflammation, or cancer.

The presence of any neurologic disease is especially relevant. Stroke, for example, can limit the person's access to the toilet, and Alzheimer's disease or other dementing illness can cause a number of difficulties. All medications should be reviewed. The amount of fluid and fiber intake and the timing and size of meals are also important. A person should be aware of constipating foods, such as foods with high fat content and refined breads. It is also important to understand the person's means of toileting, including access to a toilet and any difficulties in making use of toilet facilities. It is also helpful to consider the ease with which they can remove garments and the degree of privacy available.

The basic components of the physician's examination usually include determination of neurologic function and a careful examination of the abdomen and rectum. X rays and other special tests are sometimes ordered.

Management of Loss of Bowel Control

Loss of bowel control caused by fecal impaction is treated by addressing all conditions that increase difficulty in passing a bowel movement. If possible, all constipating medicines should be stopped and a thorough emptying of the bowel should be undertaken. Enemas are often administered until there is no return of stool, indicating that the bowel is clean. For hard stool, oil-retention enemas using olive oil are recommended.

To prevent recurrence, a maintenance program of exercise and diet is needed that includes increased exercise, increased water intake, and increased dietary fiber. The person should be encouraged to walk; people who are bedridden should be encouraged to perform simple exercises in bed to stimulate large bowel function. Daily intake of at least two quarts of liquid is desirable. Fiber in the diet needs to be increased to between 20 and 40 grams per day. Dietary fiber is important because it increases the stool bulk, speeds up the bowel motility, increases bowel contractions, and improves muscle tone. One nursing home documented that by adding bran cereal every morning, the need for laxatives in the facility was totally eliminated. A person must receive plenty of fluids with the fiber to prevent recurrence of constipation.

People with neurologic causes of loss of their bowel control experience frequent soiling with formed stools; their examination may be normal. The goal of treatment for these people is to have the bowel movement occur at predictable times to reduce both soiling and caregiver burden. This goal is usually accomplished by having bowel movements scheduled at the same time every day using simple behavioral therapies. A glycerin suppository is given to provide local stimulation of the anal sphincter and thereby enable the person to have a planned bowel movement. Usually the best time for this is just after the person wakes up or shortly after eating to utilize the normal bowel reflexes.

Bowel control can be maintained in people who have had damage to the pelvic muscles by avoiding constipation. Biofeedback therapy by an experienced professional can be helpful for most people who cannot otherwise achieve good bowel control. Successful conditioning using biofeedback consists of the person being able to tell when the rectum is full and learning how and when to contract the sphincter.

The treatment of diarrhea, which can overcome the continence mechanism of people at any age, is directed at the underlying problem. A common cause of poor bowel control when diarrhea is involved is inadequate access to toilet facilities. Obviously, the treatment of this problem should focus on providing adequate facilities and improving the person's mobility. People with mobility problems who cannot get to the bathroom on time can often benefit from a bedside commode. Clothing with elastic waistbands or Velcro fasteners may be used to simplify undressing. By using these approaches, bowel control can be achieved in up to 60 percent of people with the problem.

There is limited experience with surgical treatments for poor bowel control in older people. Individuals who are candidates for this type of surgery often have a history of previous pelvic or abdominal surgery, pelvic injury, or obstetrical trauma such as forceps delivery or significant muscle tears. Even after surgery, a majority of people will continue to have urgency, and three-quarters still experience some involuntary leakage.

Peptic Ulcer Disease

Peptic ulcer disease refers to erosions and craters in the lining of the stomach and duodenum, the first part of the small intestine. The incidence of peptic ulcer disease and the complications of ulcers is rising in elderly people.

What Causes Peptic Ulcers?

Ulcers generally occur when the normal defense mechanisms of the lining of the stomach and intestines become defective and no longer provide protection from stomach acid. Three important predisposing factors for peptic ulceration are infection with a bacterium called *Helicobacter pylori*, the use of nonsteroidal anti-inflammatory drugs (NSAIDs), and cigarette smoking. *H. pylori* is found in the stomachs of more than 95 percent of people with ulcers in the duodenum area, just beyond where the stomach joins the small intestine, and in two-thirds of those with ulcers in the stomach, called gastric ulcers. *H. pylori* is also present in about 60 percent of people who are older than age 60. The treatment for this particular bacterium requires three drugs, metronidazole, tetracycline, and bismuth subsalicylate—the best regimen is still being established.

NSAIDs are clearly implicated in the development of gastric ulcers but not duodenal ulcers. NSAIDs include aspirin, ibuprofen, indomethacin, naproxen, and several others. Ulcers caused by these drugs occur more frequently in older people because they use these drugs more than younger persons do. NSAID use increases the death rate due to complications of peptic ulcer disease. Among people using NSAIDs, 2 to 4 percent will develop a significant ulcer within a given year. In people who are older than age 65, the use of NSAIDs causes about one-fourth of all cases of upper intestinal hemorrhaging (which has a mortality rate of at least 10 percent). A history of peptic ulcer, cigarette smoking, and alcohol-related disease increases the risk for a NSAID-related ulcer complication. Age, however, is not a risk factor.

Symptoms of Peptic Ulcer Disease

Older people with peptic ulcer disease may experience a variety of discomforts. Up to one-third of elderly persons with peptic ulcer disease experience no abdominal pain and have no symptoms until a complication such as bleeding, perforation, or obstruction develops. Some people have the classic complaints (more common in younger people with peptic ulcer disease) of a hunger pain or burning in the upper part of the abdomen that is relieved by antacids or food. More often elderly people have vague abdominal discomfort, poor appetite, vomiting, or weight loss. Sometimes the appearance of blood in the stool is the first indication of an ulcer. A bloody stool often appears black and tarry and is usually foul smelling.

Evaluation of Peptic Ulcer Disease

People who suspect they have a peptic ulcer need prompt evaluation. Usually a physician will use an instrument called an endoscope to inspect the inside of the gastrointestinal tract. This enables the physician to look at the lining of the esophagus, stomach, and small intestine for ulcers or signs of irritation and bleeding. The physician may also use the endoscope to treat any bleeding sites, and biopsy any suspicious-looking areas to check for cancer or infection. In people with significant pain in the upper abdomen, the chance of finding evidence of illness through an endoscopic procedure is about 60 percent for those who are 65 and older. (In contrast, endoscopy reveals evidence of disease in only 30 percent of people ages 40 through 65 who complain of stomach pain.) An alternate but less precise procedure is a barium x-ray, which will show most gastric and many duodenal ulcers.

The treatment of peptic ulcer disease includes antacids, drugs to coat the surface of the ulcer, and drugs that decrease stomach acid production called histamine receptor antagonists. As a result of drug therapy, 80 to 90 percent of duodenal ulcers heal in 8 weeks. A similar percentage of gastric ulcers heal at 12 weeks. If after 12 weeks of treatment gastric ulcers are still present, the ulcer margins are usually biopsied to check for malignancy. The rate of healing is related to the size of the ulcer not to the age of the person; very large ulcers tend to heal slowly. Ulcers in the stomach and duodenum that are not associated with NSAID use tend to recur in about four months on average. Because of this, the need for maintenance therapy and the length of treatment remains controversial. Treatment of *H. pylori* bacteria may significantly reduce the rate of ulcer recurrence.

People who develop an ulcer while they are receiving NSAID therapy are best treated by stopping the NSAIDs; the ulcers then heal rapidly.

Treatment of Peptic Ulcer Disease

Stones are found in the gallbladders of about 20 percent of people who are 60 years and older, and the prevalence of gallstone disease increases with age. The gallbladder concentrates and stores the bile that is made in the liver. When the bile gets too concentrated, it crystallizes to form a stone.

Gallbladder Disease

Problems begin when stones move from the gallbladder and create severe pain (see Figure 39). The pain of a gallbladder attack is usually felt in the right upper part of the abdomen just below the ribs. The discomfort can be either sharp and crampy or steady and consistent. The person may feel nauseated and vomit, with fever and chills. If a gallstone obstructs the opening of the bile duct into the

Symptoms of Gallbladder Disease

Figure 39. The Gallbladder, Showing Gallstones

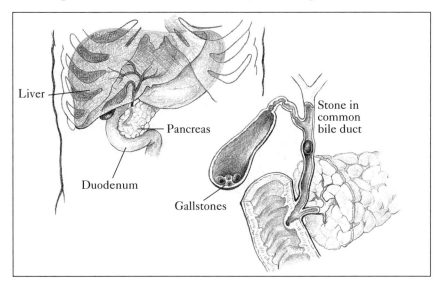

intestine, the person will develop intense fever, chills, and jaundice (a yellow discoloration of the skin and eyes).

Gallbladder inflammation without gallstones is also encountered in elderly people. The reason for this appears to be poor blood flow to the gallbladder. This condition tends to smolder, causing very minimal symptoms or signs of gallbladder problems. A physician may suspect and discover this condition before it causes the gallbladder to perforate or becomes a site for blood poisoning (septicemia).

Evaluation of Gallbladder Disease

Any new abdominal symptoms in an older person should warrant a very careful evaluation by a physician. Generally, the evaluation of someone suspected of having a gallbladder attack includes blood tests to check the function of the liver and an ultrasound, a noninvasive procedure using sound waves, which can detect gallstones, an enlarged gallbladder, bile duct enlargement, or, possibly, a localized abscess.

Treatment of Gallbladder Disease

The management of gallstones that do not cause symptoms (usually discovered by coincidence) is usually conservative because most people will not develop complications (people with diabetes mellitus are an important exception). In persons 60 years and older, removal of the gallbladder is the most commonly performed intraabdominal operation. In part, this is because the rate of septicemia, perforation, gangrene, and deaths associated with sudden gallbladder infection increases with advancing age.

Treatment options for gallstones that cause symptoms have expanded. Surgery remains the standard treatment, and new surgical techniques reduce the amount of discomfort after the operation. Some nonsurgical options include trying to dissolve the gallstones and trying to remove the stones by passing a tube into the stomach and through the small intestine to the site where the bile drains from the liver.

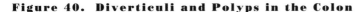

Diverticulitis

Diverticula are small outpouchings in the muscular wall of the large bowel that become more common with age (see Figure 40). Diverticulitis is the inflammation of one or more diverticula, and is often initiated by a small piece of hard stool becoming stuck in the "neck" of the diverticulum. Diverticulitis occurs in up to one-quarter of those people who have diverticulosis.

Figure 40. Diverticuli and Polyps in the Colon

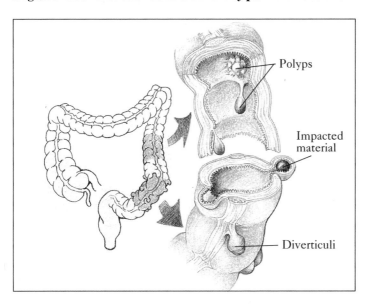

Symptoms of Diverticulitis　Older people with diverticulitis may have either very few symptoms or may feel a painful spasm in the lower abdomen, severe abdominal pain, or show signs of blood poisoning. Diverticulitis may lead to small perforations in the bowel wall, causing complications such as abscess formation, inflammation of the lining of the abdomen called peritonitis, or blood poisoning. Diverticulitis can produce many symptoms depending upon its severity. Other conditions with symptoms similar to diverticulitis include colon cancer, fecal impaction, poor circulation to the bowel, appendicitis, and urinary tract infection.

Evaluation of Diverticulitis　Because of the potential severity of these other conditions, prompt medical attention is necessary.

Treatment of Diverticulitis　Medical treatment for diverticulitis consists of intravenous fluids and antibiotics. Surgery may be necessary for recurrent episodes, large abscesses, obstruction of the bowel, or other conditions.

Appendicitis　Appendicitis is often not considered when an older person becomes ill. However, in people who have not had their appendixes removed, appendicitis remains a risk throughout life. Approximately 5 percent of all cases of appendicitis occur in people who are 60 years or older, but it is more important to note that the majority of appendicitis-related deaths occur in the older age group. This increased mortality is due in part to difficulty in identifying the condition, which in turn leads to complications such as perforation and gangrene of the appendix. The high mortality is also increased by the presence of other diseases and postoperative complications.

Symptoms of Appendicitis　Since the older person may not exhibit the usual signs and symptoms of appendicitis, the condition must be considered in any older person who has not had an appendectomy and who has unexplained abdominal pain of recent onset or who exhibits signs of infection such as fever or chills. These symptoms should receive prompt, immediate medical evaluation.

Treatment of Appendicitis　The treatment for appendicitis is surgery to remove the inflamed appendix (see Figure 36 on page 350).

Colon and rectal cancers are the second most common cancers in the United States, and their incidence increases with age.

Colon cancer seems to occur more commonly in people who eat diets that are low in fiber and high in refined sugar and animal fat. Other factors that increase the risk of colon cancer are having polyps in the colon, having a close relative with colon cancer, having breast cancer or other malignancy involving the female organs, having inflammatory bowel disease such as ulcerative colitis, and long-standing infection with parasites.

Risk Factors of Colon and Rectal Cancer

Polyps in the colon are thought to be precancerous and can usually be removed with an endoscope. If the polyps have cancer cells in their stalk or if many polyps are found, then surgical removal is recommended.

Early colon cancer does not produce symptoms, so the tumor must be discovered either by testing the stool for blood (which usually is not visible to the naked eye) or by inspection of the lining of the colon using a flexible tube called an endoscope.

Symptoms of Colon and Rectal Cancer

The symptoms of colon cancer depend upon where the cancer is in the colon. Rectal cancers often produce pain when passing a bowel movement, a sense that the rectum has not emptied completely, or rectal bleeding. Cancers in the colon above the rectum (on the left side of the body) tend to cause abdominal cramps and bleeding. Cancers even farther up the colon, near the appendix, can grow into large masses that can sometimes be felt. People with these cancers may experience fatigue, weakness, and loss of energy due to subtle blood loss and iron-deficiency anemia.

Colon cancer can be identified through endoscopy or X rays (barium enema). A biopsy of the area can be used to confirm the presence of colon cancer.

Evaluation of Colon and Rectal Cancer

Treatment of a tumor of the colon is surgical removal. This involves leaving margins that are free of any sign of cancer. Usually, this involves the placement of a temporary colostomy—a surgical creation of an opening of the colon on the outside of the body, usually on the surface of the abdomen. The bowel contents empty into a

Treatment of Colon and Rectal Cancer

plastic pouch that surrounds the opening. A colostomy is considered temporary if it can be reconstructed at a later time to restore normal elimination of stool through the rectum.

An abdominal operation may be required to treat primary rectal cancer; this is more likely to be needed in tumors that involve the middle or upper part of the rectum. Other surgical procedures that can be considered are lasers and freezing. Laser surgery may also offer some improvement in symptoms for people who are not candidates for very extensive procedures.

The outlook for people with either primary colon or primary rectal cancer is related to the extent of the disease. When the disease has spread to local or regional lymph nodes, chemotherapy may prolong survival for the afflicted person.

Figure 41. Rectal Problems

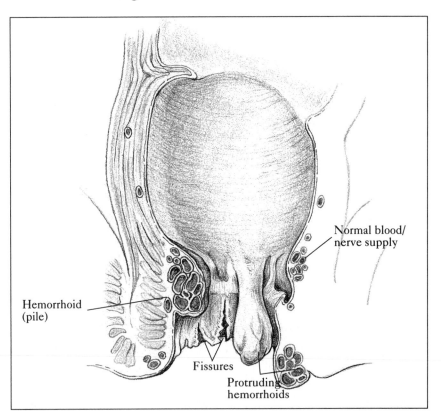

Normal blood/
nerve supply

Hemorrhoid
(pile)

Fissures

Protruding
hemorrhoids

Hemorrhoids are swellings of rectal tissue that are caused by dilated veins often produced from straining to pass a bowel movement. The complications of hemorrhoids, which are common in older people, include bleeding, enlargement, and pain.

Hemorrhoids and Other Rectal Problems

Prolapsed hemorrhoids appear as reddish masses protruding from the opening of the rectum (see Figure 41). They may spontaneously go back into the rectum or they may need to be pushed back in place by the finger. Although pain is not a frequent symptom, hemorrhoids that have clotted, called thrombotic hemorrhoids, can cause severe pain around the rectum.

Symptoms of Hemorrhoids and Other Rectal Problems

Tears along the anal lining, called fissures, usually cause pain while passing a bowel movement. Fissures can be treated with sitz baths, stool softeners, and pain-relieving ointments. However, tissues that do not heal may require surgical treatment. People who have abscesses around the rectal area often have pain that increases when trying to pass a bowel movement. Abscesses usually require surgical drainage.

Hemorrhoids and fissures can be detected through a rectal examination as well as through an examination of the lining of the rectum. This procedure is performed with a tube that is called a proctoscope.

Evaluation of Hemorrhoids and Other Rectal Problems

The treatment of hemorrhoids begins with the use of dietary fiber, stool softeners to reduce straining, pain-relieving ointments, and sitz baths. This may be all the treatment that is necessary for the early stages of hemorrhoids with either no prolapse or prolapse occurring with bowel movements that spontaneously resolves. However, if the hemorrhoids do not respond, more aggressive medical therapy is indicated. The goal of more aggressive treatments is to produce inflammation and scarring, which causes the hemorrhoids to adhere to the underlying muscle tissues. Surgery is often necessary for clotted hemorrhoids.

Treatment of Hemorrhoids and Other Rectal Problems

CHAPTER 23

NUTRITION CONCERNS

Nutritional Requirements

Malnutrition

Loss of Weight

Obesity

Nutritional Requirements

No one knows for sure what the absolute nutritional requirements are for older people. So there are no universal, age-related reference values. A decrease in nutrient reserves probably occurs in between 9 to 15 percent of older people seen in outpatient clinics, 5 to 12 percent of home-bound people with various chronic problems, 35 to 65 percent of people hospitalized for acute illness, and 25 to 60 percent of people living in institutions.

The lack of data on people who are over age 70 makes it difficult to establish separate recommended dietary allowances (called RDAs). Table 35 lists the 1989 suggested RDAs. The current RDA continues to separate old from young people at age 51 and extrapolates many of the values for the older age group from the younger group. In addition, blood levels of nutrients such as vitamin B_{12} may not accurately reflect the amount in the tissues, which makes it difficult to set effective treatment guidelines. Finally, nutrient requirements need to be adjusted to reflect various interactions that affect older people whether disease-nutrient, drug-nutrient, or economic-nutrient interactions.

Table 35. Recommended Nutrient Intakes for Men and Women Ages 51 Years and Older (1989)

NUTRIENT	RDA, PER DAY
Energy	Men: 2300 cal (calorie) (based on 77 kg [kilogram])
	Women: 1900 cal (based on 65 kg)
Protein	Men: 63 g (gram) (based on 77 kg)
	Women: 50 g (based on 65 kg)
Calcium	Men: 800 mg (milligram)
	Women: 800 mg
Iron	10 mg
Zinc	Men: 15 mg
	Women: 12 mg
Vitamin A	Men: 1000 µg (microgram)
	Women: 800 µg
Vitamin D	5 µg (as cholecalciferol)
Vitamin E	Men: 10 mg
	Women: 8 mg
Vitamin K	Men: 80 µg
	Women: 65 µg
Vitamin C	60 mg
Thiamin	Men: 1.2 mg
(B_1)	Women: 1.0 mg
Riboflavin	Men: 1.4 mg
(B_2)	Women: 1.2 mg
Pyridoxine	Men: 2.0 mg
(B_6)	Women: 1.6 mg
Cobalamin (B_{12})	2.0 µg
Niacin	Men: 15 mg
	Women: 13 mg
Folate	Men: 200 µg
	Women: 180 µg

RDA, recommended dietary allowance.

*Especially in malnourished people.

Source: In part from *Recommended Dietary Allowances*. 10th ed. Washington, DC: National Academy Press; 1989. Reprinted with permission. Comments reflect the views of the author.

Energy Requirements

Total energy requirements in men decrease from about 2,700 kilocalories per day at age 30 to around 2,100 kilocalories per day at age 80. About a third of this decrease is due to the decrease in metabolic rate caused by a decline in lean body mass, and the remaining two-thirds of the reduced energy requirements are probably due to decreases in energy expenditures. Recent studies have suggested that approximately one-fifth of people over the age of 60 consume fewer than 1,000 calories per day. No one is sure whether this decrease in energy intake places older people at risk for nutrient deficiencies.

Protein Requirements

It's unlikely that healthy older people suffer significant protein deficiency. The decrease in lean body mass associated with aging causes a decrease in the amount of amino acids, the building blocks for proteins. This decrease reduces the body's capacity to adapt to demands for increased protein use. As a result, protein consumption should be increased during periods of metabolic stress when, for instance, there is an infection or a broken bone. Then, the intake of protein should be increased to 1 to 1.5 grams of protein per every kilogram of body weight. This means that an elderly woman weighing 50 kilograms (110 pounds) might need to eat between 50 and 75 grams of protein each day if she develops a severe infection such as pneumonia or falls and breaks a hip. In the absence of stress, protein should make up between 10 and 15 percent of the total daily diet.

Fluids

Inadequate fluid intake is one of the most common causes of salt and water disorders (electrolyte disorders) in the older age group. A common cause includes metabolic stress such as an infection, which may increase fluid requirements and impair intake, causing dehydration (see page 404). In addition, there is an age-associated decrease in the thirst sensation, a very important regulator of fluid intake. Other changes occur in the secretion of hormones such as vasopressin, which are primarily concerned with water regulation. A general goal for fluid intake should be at least two liters (about two quarts) per day.

Vitamins and Minerals

Although uncommonly seen in noninstitutionalized elderly people, individual deficiencies of vitamins and minerals may occur. They

Table 36. Clinical Manifestations of Deficient Vitamins and Minerals in Older People

NUTRIENT	REPORTED CLINICAL MANIFESTATIONS	COMMENTS
Calcium	Increased risk of fracture (osteoporosis, osteomalacia)	Adequate intake (>800mg/day) throughout adulthood demonstrates greatest protection
Folate	Loss of appetite; anemia; malabsorption; fatigue; diarrhea; painful tongue; low platelets and white blood cells	Institutionalized patients are at risk
Iron	Apathy; decreased exercise tolerance; pallor; painful tongue; swallowing difficulty	
Niacin	Dermatitis; diarrhea; dementia	Called pellagra
Selenium	Poor heart function	Touted to be preventive against cancer
Vitamin A	Anemia; poor appetite; decreased wound healing; night blindness; dry skin	Second most commonly used supplement
Vitamin B$_1$ (thiamin)	Weight loss; malaise; fatigue; decreased reflexes; nervous system problems	Patients may exhibit mental status change; may contribute to heart problems
Vitamin B$_2$ (riboflavin)	Magenta tongue; dry cracks on the lips	Decreased reliability of assay in older people
Vitamin B$_6$	Nausea; vomiting; confusion; loss of appetite; dermatitis; motor weakness; depression; dizziness; sore tongue	May be associated with carpal tunnel syndrome
Vitamin B$_{12}$	Nausea; poor appetite; fatigue; constipation; depression; decreased memory; psychosis; anemia; malabsorption; clouding of consciousness in dementia; neurologic disease	Deficiency may be due to lack of intrinsic factor or stomach atrophy; can occur without anemia
Vitamin C	Weakness; irritability; skin changes; dry mouth	Most commonly used supplement
Vitamin D	Weakness; bone pain; gait disturbance	Decreased skin production
Vitamin E	Clinical manifestations of deficiency in humans are uncertain	Antioxidant; touted to be preventative against cancer
Zinc	Delayed wound healing; impaired immune function; loss of taste acuity; dementia; impotence; lethargy; decreased libido; poor appetite; skin changes	Supplementation might augment healing of pressure ulcers; possibly protective vs. muscular degeneration

Source: Modified from Silver AJ. Malnutrition. In: Beck JC, ed. *Geriatrics Review Syllabus: A Core Curriculum in Geriatric Medicine*, 1st ed. New York: American Geriatrics Society; 1989:102. Reprinted with permission.

are sometimes discovered when a physician recognizes the signs and symptoms as shown in Table 36, asks specific and detailed questions about the diet, or, more commonly, analyzes blood samples for particular nutrients. This final approach assumes that nutrient levels in the blood reflect nutrient levels in the tissue, which is not always the case.

A much more common and serious problem is taking too much of a vitamin (hypervitaminosis). In one study, investigators found that 10 percent of elderly men were consuming ten times the RDA for vitamins C, D, E, and B-complex vitamins, and that 10 percent of women were consuming ten times the RDA for thiamin and iron. Many older people believe that such megadoses can prolong life, cure ailments, improve their ability to deal with stress, improve sexual function, and enhance the immune system. Regretfully, the truth seems just the opposite: hypervitaminosis can result in significant toxicities. Megadoses of vitamin C can produce kidney stones and gastrointestinal problems; too much vitamin A can produce fatigue and weakness, cause liver dysfunction, headache, produce high calcium in the blood, and reduce the number of circulating white blood cells; megadoses of vitamin B_6 can cause significant damage to nerves in the arms and legs.

Malnutrition

Many factors increase the risk for malnutrition in older individuals (see Table 37). Malnutrition, in turn, places older people at risk for subsequent illness, disability, and even increased mortality. With

Table 37. Causes of Malnutrition in Older People

Decreased feeding drive	Medical illness
Decreased thirst	Medications
Dementing illness	Poverty
Dental problems	Social isolation
Depression	Swallowing difficulty
Early satiety	

Source: Modified from Silver AJ. Malnutrition. In: Beck JC, ed. *Geriatrics Review Syllabus: A Core Curriculum in Geriatric Medicine*, 1st ed. New York: American Geriatrics Society; 1989:100. Reprinted with permission.

appropriate replacement of nutritional deficiencies, most if not all of these processes can be reversed. Therefore, maintaining an adequate nutritional status is a cornerstone of preventive medicine in caring for older people.

Protein Energy Malnutrition

There is no readily agreed upon definition for protein energy malnutrition in elderly people. One classification system uses body measurements and blood tests to produce two categories: inadequate intake of calories and protein (marasmus) and malnutrition in response to biologic stress (low-albumin malnutrition).

In marasmus a person loses weight while maintaining a normal level of albumin in the blood. Marasmus is also characterized by decreased amounts of body fat and muscle and a mild decline in the body's immune function. This condition is more likely to occur in older people living in the community and institutionalized elderly people. It is less likely to occur in acutely ill hospitalized elderly people.

The low-albumin form of malnutrition occurs almost exclusively as a response to infection or injury and therefore is usually seen in the hospital setting. Other causes include a very low intake (when protein makes up less than 3 percent of the total calories) or liver disease, bowel disease, or kidney disease.

The Assessment of Suspected Undernutrition

Physicians generally evaluate undernutrition by clinical interview, a physical examination, and specific laboratory tests. A report of weight loss is the most important information to be obtained from the interview since this finding is the strongest predictor of death one year after hospitalization for acute illness. Weight loss during a nursing home stay is also predictive of increased disability and death. Other important clues are weakness, changes in smell or taste, abdominal pain, decreased appetite, nausea, vomiting, diarrhea, constipation, difficulty swallowing, problems chewing food or in using dentures, changes in mental status, and the presence of other significant diseases. In the nursing home, diseases or conditions that occur with undernutrition include anemia, hip fracture, pressure ulcers, depression, dementing illness, and cancer. Other important items include all medications taken (both prescription and over-the-counter drugs) and any alcohol use.

Social influences include who lives at home with the person, the person's cooking facilities, the distance from the home to the store, and the person's income. In this context, a home visit by a health professional (nurse, occupational therapist, or physician) may be extremely helpful in evaluating a person's capacity to feed himself and his ability to obtain food easily. It is also important to explore the possibility of depression and impairment of mental function.

Treatment of Undernutrition

The treatment of undernutrition should begin while the underlying cause is still being investigated. It is important for older people to be able to identify foods with high nutritional value and, if necessary, to be taught to improve their shopping and food preparation techniques, and to be encouraged to make snacks of fruits and vegetables. If necessary, the person should be given actual meal support by enrollment in such programs as Meals on Wheels or Congregate-Meals. At least once a week the calorie intake should be measured, and the weight should be taken every three to seven days, with adjustments made for periods of stress. Family members and other caregivers should be encouraged to participate in the treatment.

The treatment for institutionalized or hospitalized older people is generally oriented toward stabilizing any acute disease processes, determining the amount of calories needed, and aiming for a high intake of calories, up to 35 kilocalories per kilogram of body weight (women over 50 kilograms [110 pounds] would need 1,750 kilocalories each day). Individuals taking oral supplements such as milk shakes should be encouraged to use them as snacks rather than meal substitutes, particularly in the evening. For individuals with severe malnutrition, oral supplements may not improve the clinical situation, and tube feedings or intravenous feedings may be required. Following initial treatment with tube feedings, an increase in body weight may occur. Generally, tube feedings (or intravenous feedings) should be continued until the person has gained within 10 percent of his ideal body weight based on weight-adjusted tables, or until adequate oral feedings can be tolerated.

Ethical Considerations

A number of court cases have concluded that feedings can be withheld or withdrawn in individuals whose previous wishes for this

Table 38. Common Causes of Weight Loss in Elderly People

Alcohol and drug abuse
Chronic medical illness (especially gastrointestinal diseases, tuberculosis, thyroid disease, and cancer)
Dementing illness
Dental problems
Depression
Limited access to food
Medication side effects
Poverty
Unpleasant eating environment

action were known. In addition, competent individuals may refuse intravenous or tube feedings. Difficulties arise when individuals are depressed or incompetent or refuse to eat and yet want aggressive medical interventions if the situation warrants. In the decision-making process that precedes tube placement, active participation by the older person and family members should be encouraged and respected. (See Chapter 11 for more information on ethical issues.)

Loss of Weight

A person's weight is made up of body water, lean muscle mass, and fat. Weight loss implies low lean muscle mass and loss of fat. In older people, low lean muscle mass causes weakness and difficulty in walking and performing daily activities; low bone mass increases the risk for fractures. Relatively low amounts of body fat represent no clear danger, but this condition may reflect an increased risk for protein energy malnutrition, especially in people who develop diseases that require surgery.

Causes of Weight Loss

Some of the common causes of weight loss in elderly people are shown in Table 38. Depression, lung cancer, other malignancies, and gastrointestinal problems are the major causes of unintentional weight loss. The greatest amount of weight loss occurs with tuberculosis and thyroid disease; however, weight loss can be an important clue to any major disease in older people. Any older person unintentionally losing more than five pounds in a six-month period needs a thorough medical evaluation.

Evaluation and Treatment of Weight Loss

Unexplained weight loss indicates an active problem, and it is easier to interpret weight changes when many weights over a period of time are available. The availability of many such weight records in nursing homes makes it easier to determine the degree of weight loss. For people who live in the community, it's important to obtain repeated weights. Often the physician will order blood tests to check the severity of the disorder; a blood test will reveal if the person has loss of vitality (no abnormalities) or cachexia (severe abnormalities). In either case, it's crucial to determine whether the problem is due to a loss of appetite or due to a significant medical problem. It is important to look carefully at the person's psychological state, functional ability, social situation, and mental function—it is also important to check for depression. Screening for vision and hearing loss as well as evaluating the person's ability to perform basic activities may reveal functional causes of weight loss. The person's social situation should be evaluated for clues to the cause of weight loss and for the effects of the social condition on the person's ability to deal with problems in general. Relevant social considerations include the number of immediate family members and friends who may be able to help, and determining whether there are financial or other barriers to obtaining adequate food and housing. Living alone is the most important social factor in predicting institutionalization. The elderly person who lives alone is at increased risk for medical, functional, and psychologic problems.

Treatment of Weight Loss

Weight loss is difficult to treat, and sometimes severe malnutrition occurs even when there is adequate social, functional, and psychological support. Usually, weight loss occurs when a person simply does not eat enough. Any existing medical problems such as infection, malignancy, depression, gastrointestinal disease, and medications need appropriate management. The person's optimal food intake is estimated to set appropriate goals; the advice of a dietitian can be helpful.

If the diet taken voluntarily by the person is not adequate to maintain weight, a major decision is whether to initiate additional feedings. These feedings are usually accomplished by placing a tube from the mouth or nose into the stomach. If the underlying health problem is reversible and the person agrees to it, then tube feedings are indicated. When the person is not competent to make decisions, advanced directives such as living wills can decide whether tube feedings should begin (see Chapter 11 for more on advanced directives). One approach is to establish goals with the person, such as a specific amount of weight gain or an improvement in certain blood values such as albumin. This allows a trial of a tube feeding to begin with the understanding that if there is no improvement, the feedings will be stopped. This may be especially appropriate in very old people in whom tube feedings have a high rate of complication and questionable efficacy.

The use of medications to treat weight loss has not been fully explored. The medicines of a century ago that improved appetite and caused weight gain were widely promoted, but many of them contained poisonous substances such as strychnine. If they worked at all they did so because of their effect on taste; strychnine, for example, is very bitter. Interestingly, the use of nonpoisonous bitters as appetizers continues to be popular. Appetite stimulants have not been evaluated even though investigation in this area is appealing. From time to time the use of insulin and a variety of steroids that help promote muscle growth has been advocated for people with cancer, but their efficacy remains unproven. Recently, studies of growth hormone suggest that it reverses some of the metabolic effects that are associated with aging. This treatment is very expensive and the potential benefits are not known. It seems likely, however, that growth hormone or growth hormone–like substances may be used to treat some people who have unexplained weight loss.

Obesity

In the United States approximately one-fourth of white men and one-third of white women between the ages of 65 and 76 are overweight. With advancing age there tends to be an increase in upper body (abdomen) obesity compared with lower body (hips and thighs) obesity. Upper body obesity increases the risk for diabetes mellitus, high blood pressure, and heart and blood vessel disease. In elderly people, obesity increases the likelihood of high blood pressure, diabetes mellitus, decreased functional ability, pressure ulcers, and significant sleeping problems. The risk of death increases as obesity increases.

The first step in weight reduction is an exercise program, which should be started immediately for people whose body weight is 30 percent above the average. For people with diabetes mellitus, exercise is especially important if they are 10 percent over their ideal weight. Walking is popular because it encourages socialization and can be done in an indoor environment such as a shopping mall. A physical therapist can help devise an appropriate exercise program.

Food intake should not be fewer than 1,000 calories per day. Nutritional education may be helpful to the overweight person to improve food choices (low-fat, low-calorie foods). Although there is very little information on dieting in elderly people, sudden death has been associated with various weight-reduction schemes in younger people. Because of this, fad diets, such as grapefruit diets, should all be avoided. Behavioral modification or support groups may be useful for some people.

CHAPTER 24

BLADDER, URINARY, AND KIDNEY CONDITIONS

Overview

Symptoms

    Blood in the Urine (Hematuria)

    Loss of Bladder Control (Urinary Incontinence)

Conditions

    Urinary Tract Infection

    Bladder Cancer

    Kidney Problems Caused by Blood Vessel Disease

    Problems with the Kidneys' Filtering Apparatus (Glomerulonephritis)

    Sudden Kidney Failure

The kidneys are responsible for a number of activities, including monitoring and maintaining a normal balance of body salt and water. The kidneys become smaller and filter less blood as we age. These changes increase the vulnerability of the kidneys to damage caused by diseases and toxins. Nevertheless, aging kidneys usually maintain adequate function even in extreme old age.

In general, the signs and symptoms of kidney disease in older people are similar to those in younger people. A few of the many signs of kidney disease are increasing fluid accumulation, swelling in the extremities, blood in the urine, and high levels of various compounds in the blood normally filtered and removed by the kidney.

Overview

SYMPTOMS
Blood in the Urine (Hematuria)

Blood in the urine, or hematuria, has been documented in approximately 10 percent of men 50 years or older who had no other symptoms. Microscopic hematuria means that there is a small amount of blood in the urine that is not visible to the naked eye. Hematuria cannot be diagnosed if a special tube called a catheter was used to obtain the specimen by passing it up the urethra into the bladder because the catheter itself can cause enough injury to produce temporary bleeding. If an older person is catheterized when the hematuria is found, the catheter must be withdrawn and the urine reexamined several days after the catheter has been removed.

Causes of Hematuria and Their Symptoms

Conditions causing hematuria can be categorized according to (1) diseases that affect the kidney, (2) diseases in the bladder or urethra, or (3) problems that cause blood-clotting abnormalities. Some prescription and over-the-counter medications can also cause blood in the urine.

Hematuria in association with fever, pain on urinating, or frequent urination may suggest a urinary tract or prostate infection. Many elderly people do not experience all these symptoms, so their absence does not mean that an infection is not present. A sense of burning, urgency, or dribbling, and a narrow urinary stream suggest obstruction or prostate disease. If hematuria is associated with high blood pressure, swelling of the legs and sometimes around the eyes, and signs of reduced kidney function on blood testing, it suggests disease within the kidney. The combination of hematuria, changes in blood pressure, and pain in the flank may indicate a blood clot or an embolus that has traveled to the kidney. In this setting, an embolus could be a piece of debris that has broken off from a cholesterol deposit occurring within the wall of the aorta.

Evaluation of Hematuria

To help identify the cause of hematuria, the physician examines a freshly voided urine specimen. A doctor may perform additional procedures, such as culturing the urine to look for infection and having the person collect all of their urine over a 24-hour period to determine the overall kidney function more precisely. Blood tests will make sure that the person's blood clots normally and determine additional aspects of kidney function. Special x-ray procedures are sometimes required to look for masses within the kidney. Occasionally a urologist may be consulted to look within the bladder to see if a bleeding source can be identified.

After a thorough evaluation, the cause of blood in the urine can be identified in approximately 85 percent of cases. Various growths within the kidney account for between one-fourth and one-third of all hematuria in elderly people. Of these, prostate cancer and cancer involving the kidney are the two most common types of growths discovered. If no cause for hematuria is discovered after initial evaluation, periodic follow-up is appropriate; most people in this category, however, will not discover the reason for their hematuria even after a period of up to five years.

Urinary incontinence is the involuntary loss of urine that can cause a social or hygienic problem.

Approximately one-third of community-living people over the age of 60 experience some degree of urinary incontinence; its prevalence is twice as high in women as in men. Approximately 5 percent of this age group have very severe incontinence, with urinary accidents occurring weekly or more often. In the nursing home setting, the prevalence of incontinence approaches 50 percent. Clearly, incontinence can have significant psychological, social, medical, and economic consequences. If not effectively treated, it increases social isolation, frequently resulting in a loss of independence through institutionalization, and predisposes the person to infection and skin breakdown.

The degree of incontinence may change over time. Over the course of one year, incontinence may affect 20 percent of women and 10 percent of men, but within these groups it may disappear spontaneously in about 12 percent of the women and 30 percent of the men. The factors associated with the development and remission of incontinent symptoms are under investigation. Fewer than half of older adults affected by urinary incontinence consult a health professional about the condition. Because the majority of people with incontinence can be cured, there is room and need for considerable education about the availability of treatment options.

Loss of Bladder Control (Urinary Incontinence)

**The Urinary
System: How It
Works**

Stretch receptors located in the bladder wall communicate to the brain how full the bladder is—they play a key role in maintaining continence. When a critical degree of bladder distention is reached, bladder contractions of increasing force occur; these contractions must be inhibited by the brain to avoid the abrupt and unwanted emptying of the bladder.

In order to hold the urine in the bladder, the pressure within the bladder must always be less than that in the urethra. Bladder pressure is affected by three factors: abdominal pressure, the amount of urine collected in the bladder, and the bladder muscle tone.

The pressure within the urethra is maintained through skeletal muscle (muscle that contracts voluntarily) that lines the urethra, smooth muscle (muscle that contracts involuntarily) of the urethra and bladder neck, and the thickness of the urethral lining. The thickness of the urethral lining in women is maintained by estrogens and thins significantly after the menopause due to estrogen deficiency.

**Figure 42. Normal Urinary Anatomy in
a Man and Woman**

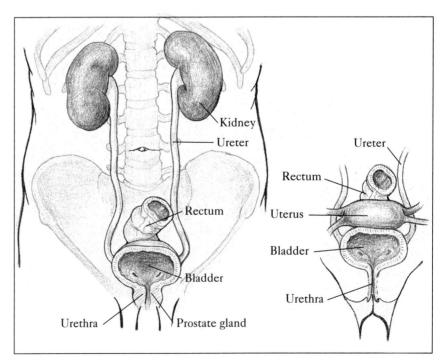

Table 39. Causes of Urinary Incontinence

CLINICAL CONDITION	MECHANISM	SYMPTOMS
Detrusor overactivity	Bladder contracts when it shouldn't	Difficulty holding urine
Stress incontinence	Urethral resistance is too low	Difficulty holding urine
Overflow incontinence	Bladder does not contract or urethral resistance is too high	Difficulty emptying the bladder
Functional incontinence	Problem not in urinary system; usually musculoskeletal or psychiatric illness	Other difficulties

The Causes of Urinary Incontinence

Urinary incontinence occurs when the bladder pressure overcomes the urethral resistance. Whereas a bewildering array of terms have been proposed to classify urinary incontinence, in reality there are only five basic mechanisms that can occur singly or in combination to produce incontinence: (1) the bladder contracts when it shouldn't (this goes under the clinical name of detrusor overactivity), (2) urethral resistance is too weak to hold urine (stress incontinence), (3) the bladder doesn't contract when it should (overflow incontinence), (4) the urethral resistance is too high (overflow incontinence), or (5) the problem is not in the urinary system at all (functional incontinence). (See Table 39).

Detrusor Overactivity. Detrusor overactivity occurs when involuntary bladder contractions overcome the normal resistance of the urethra. This is also referred to as unstable bladder, spastic bladder, uninhibited bladder, or urge incontinence. This is generally the most common type of incontinence, occurring in up to 70 percent of all people with incontinence. The three basic underlying causes of this condition are: (1) defects in the brain's inhibitory mechanisms; (2) increased excitability of the bladder from such causes as infection, irritation, or a fecal impaction; and (3) a loss of the normal voiding reflexes. This loss of normal reflexes can be self-induced or can be unintentionally caused by physicians. For example, embarrassment over a single episode of incontinence may lead a person to void frequently in an attempt to keep the bladder empty to avoid another accident. Or the person may cut back on fluids in an attempt to decrease urine. Both strategies, however, eventually cause the bladder wall to contract and lose its capacity to stretch, thereby reducing bladder capacity and increasing bladder muscle tone. The ultimate result is further episodes of incontinence. Loss of bladder reflexes caused by physicians can result when toileting becomes associated with uncomfortable equipment such as cold bedpans or toilet seats, or when the increased physical or verbal attention brought on by the incontinence makes the incontinent person feel rewarded.

Stress Incontinence. Stress incontinence is very common in elderly women and occurs when the urethral resistance to flow is reduced. The probable causes are the changes in the lining in the urethra after the menopause, related to the decline of estrogens, combined with an earlier weakening of the pelvic muscles following childbirth. In addition, urinary tract infections may precipitate stress incontinence. Stress incontinence in men usually occurs only with urinary tract infections, after surgery, or as the result of severe disease of the nervous system (see Figure 42).

The features of stress incontinence include the loss of urine following coughing, laughing, straining, sneezing, or any other condition that causes an abrupt increase in the abdominal pressure. Simply pushing on the abdomen may cause the passage of urine. People with stress incontinence usually stay dry at night. For a woman, the pelvic examination by a physician may reveal signs of decreased estrogen. For both women and men, testing may reveal signs of a urinary tract infection.

Overflow Incontinence. Overflow incontinence occurs when the bladder cannot empty properly. This is generally the result of either very poor bladder contractions or an elevated resistance to urine flow. The bladder that cannot contract is sometimes called an atonic bladder or neurogenic bladder, and usually occurs in connection with severe diabetes mellitus, or disease of the spinal cord. Resistance to urine flow is usually due to an obstruction of the bladder outlet caused by an enlarged prostate, a stone, or cancer. A third mechanism is an impaired ability to sense that the bladder is full and requires voiding. Generally, people with overflow incontinence have the feeling that their bladder has not emptied completely, experience difficulty starting to void, and note that their urinary stream is weak and dribbly. Examination by a physician may reveal an enlarged bladder; if the bladder is drained with a catheter, large amounts of urine are obtained, confirming that the bladder was, in fact, not successfully emptied.

Functional Incontinence. Functional incontinence occurs in people who have a normal urinary system but who cannot or will not reach the toilet in time. Generally, this is due to problems in the musculoskeletal system and/or environmental limitations that can be identified. People with dementia may not be able to recognize the need to void or to locate and use toileting facilities. Sometimes incontinence is part of a psychiatric condition. This "spiteful" incontinence is intermittent and usually does not occur at night. There is often an element of depression, hostility, or anger. Drugs and other factors may aggravate or unmask any of these problems. The use of diuretics or physical restraints may make it difficult for an older person to stay continent. In addition, strong sedatives can create a loss of attention to bladder cues. Medications can also directly affect the bladder contractions and the urinary outlet.

An evaluation of urinary incontinence has three objectives: (1) to identify and manage the factors that may be contributing to the incontinence, (2) to determine if further diagnostic evaluation is indicated, and (3) to develop a management plan, which may include further evaluation or a trial of therapy. The overall goal of this evaluation is to determine how bladder pressure is overcoming the urethral resistance. Useful information includes the onset, duration, and pattern of the incontinence; the amount of urine lost; all medications used; and any associated symptoms such as straining or burning while trying to void. It is helpful to know the amount of fluid a person is taking in. It is also important to know about any existing medical or surgical conditions such as diabetes mellitus, recent surgery, or the presence of any neurologic illness.

Evaluation of Urinary Incontinence

Detrusor overactivity often has associated symptoms of urgency where there is an intense need to void. Overflow incontinence is sometimes associated with symptoms of incomplete bladder emptying. Stress incontinence is associated with urine leakage uniquely associated with situations that increase abdominal pressure, such as coughing, jogging, laughing, sneezing, and bending over. Identification of the various types of incontinence can be simplified if the following points are kept in mind: (1) an enlarged bladder signifies overflow incontinence, (2) the absence of any signs of any overflow or stress incontinence suggests detrusor overactivity, and (3) if stress incontinence is present, particularly in older women, it may be the only condition or it may be mixed with other forms of incontinence.

Generally, the physician's physical examination is oriented toward identifying changes in the nervous system or in the genital, pelvic, and rectal areas. A urinalysis helps to check for infections and other local problems in the bladder. Sometimes the bladder is catheterized to determine the amount of urine left in the bladder after the person has tried to void. Other diagnostic procedures may be helpful in certain cases. The use of a particular diagnostic procedure depends upon whether the result will change the way the person is managed and whether not using a procedure could cause a physician to miss a particular condition. For example, since there is evidence that behavioral treatments are effective for both stress incontinence and detrusor overactivity, expensive testing to document stress incontinence or detrusor overactivity may be unnecessary if the person is going to be treated with behavioral therapies. On the other hand, looking within the bladder may be critically important if a bladder cancer is suspected. Additional studies may be needed if surgery is being considered.

Treatment of Urinary Incontinence

The first considerations in treating urinary incontinence are that *most people can be substantially improved or cured* and that family members and other caregivers should provide supportive measures when possible. A number of simple interventions have produced favorable results. For elderly women living in the community who have either detrusor overactivity or stress incontinence, bladder training—where the voiding interval is progressively lengthened—has proven to be highly effective. Pelvic muscle exercises are also very helpful for women with stress incontinence. Special techniques using biofeedback to help a person become aware of muscle contractions can be used—in some cases to train a person in the use of pelvic muscle exercises and other behavioral interventions. All of these behavioral interventions require a highly motivated person and multiple sessions with a skilled and enthusiastic trainer; however, they may not be appropriate or possible for everyone. There have not been any good comparisons made between behavioral treatments and drug treatments. People with incontinence are usually offered a choice of one or a combination of both approaches. Prompted voiding (asking the person if he or she needs to urinate) and similar techniques work well for people in nursing homes who have urinary incontinence.

For detrusor overactivity the goal of treatment is to decrease the bladder contractions and to improve bladder capacity. As mentioned, treatments that do not require drugs include bladder training programs, pelvic floor exercises, and biofeedback. In general, medications used to treat detrusor overactivity work by decreasing bladder contractions. Sometimes medications are given to improve the resistance of the urethral sphincter. The doses of all medications used must be carefully monitored, as they sometimes result in incomplete voiding or even the inability to void. Side effects such as confusion, agitation, a drop in blood pressure upon standing, dry mouth, and various irregularities of the heart rhythm can occur.

The goal of treatment for stress incontinence is to increase the urethral resistance. For mild to moderate stress incontinence in women, using medication to reinforce urethral resistance is about as effective as doing exercises that strengthen the pelvic floor muscles. Estrogens offer beneficial effects on the tissues around the urethra and are often part of the regimen; but the extent of their helpfulness is not clear. In addition to strengthening the pelvic floor muscles through specific exercises, increased walking is helpful. Walking improves a person's ability to sense that the bladder is filling. In cases that do not respond to any of these treatments, surgical procedures may be necessary—for instance, to support a sagging or prolapsed bladder. Surgical techniques are improving. Injection of substances into the tissues surrounding the urethra is an option in some cases when the older woman does not want or cannot tolerate a full surgical procedure.

The goal of treatment for overflow incontinence is to drain the bladder. Generally, a nondrug strategy works best in this condition. Surgery is preferred in those cases where there is obstruction to outflow caused by a large prostate, cancer, or a stone. When the overflow is the result of a bladder that contracts poorly, it can then be decompressed for a period of about two weeks with an indwelling catheter. If bladder function is not restored, placing a tube (catheter) into the bladder may be required for adequate drainage. Sometimes the obstruction can be overcome by the use of drugs that relax the urethral sphincter; these drugs may be helpful to delay or avoid surgery.

Functional incontinence is best managed by a simple approach. Physical and environmental impediments to effective toileting should be recognized and corrected. To avoid inadvertent conditioning toward incontinent behavior, the person should not be asked to go to the toilet or to use other unpleasant stimuli, such as bedpans or cold toilet seats immediately after an episode of incontinence. A toileting program can be established based on an evaluation of the person's voiding pattern. To accomplish this, the person is checked every two hours over a two-day period and a record is kept of whether the person is wet or dry. The optimal toileting schedule can then be established to allow toilet use at a time when the bladder is most likely to be full. Successful toileting should be positively reinforced.

A variety of products that are not excessively bulky under the clothing are available to keep incontinent people dry and to control odor. These items include rubber or plastic pants with absorbent pads, intermittent catheterization, and external catheters or collecting devices. Generally, these are used only as last resorts and only after careful evaluation and treatment have failed to resolve the incontinence. Because the vast majority of people with urinary incontinence can be successfully managed or cured, these items should be used very sparingly if at all.

CONDITIONS
Urinary Tract
Infection

Urinary tract infections occur in up to 10 percent of elderly people each year. A large proportion of these infections are in elderly women. However, urinary infections become increasingly common in older men because of prostate enlargement.

Compared with younger people, older people with urinary tract infection may have a much more diverse set of bacterial organisms causing the infection. People with catheters in for a long time always have bacteria in their urine, which often contains many different types of organisms. In addition, these organisms are often highly resistant to antibiotics. People at high risk for this infection include those who have had catheters or other objects in the genitourinary tract; those who have abnormalities of function such as kidney stones, urinary incontinence, or decreased bladder emptying; or those with indwelling urinary catheters.

Causes of Urinary Tract Infection

Urinary tract infection should be suspected in any older person with pain, frequency or urgency of urination, or in the presence of any recent unexplained change in general function. Nonspecific complaints of urinary tract infection include fever, chills, poor appetite, or weakness. Urinary incontinence or change in mental function can also be early clues. Many older people may have a large number of bacteria in their urine, although they have no symptoms at all and appear to be well.

Symptoms of Urinary Tract Infection

In older people, the treatment regimens for urinary tract infection vary depending upon the severity of the infection. If a person is highly functional with an uncomplicated urinary infection, then simple oral antibiotics may be used. These people are generally healthy, functionally independent, have no bladder catheter, have not been recently taking antibiotics, and have no history of recurrent urinary tract infections. Cultures ten days to two weeks later help guide the physician in knowing whether or not to change the antibiotic regimen. For people with more complicated infections, such as those who have kidney stones, have been recently taking antibiotics, or have been in the hospital, the treatment usually begins with stronger antibiotics. Again, culture results help guide the prescribing physician in deciding on the need for any changes in medications. Older people with urinary tract infections who require hospitalization usually need to be treated with medications that can only be given intravenously.

Treatment of Urinary Tract Infection

For many older people, bacteria in the urine that do not cause discomfort or other symptoms do not need to be treated with antibiotics. Sometimes these individuals are treated, however, if there is a history of recurrent symptomatic infections or of chronic obstruction of the urinary tract (as with prostate enlargement). People with indwelling catheters will have persistent bacteria in their urine and should be treated when symptoms develop or when there is a decline in function that cannot be explained by other factors.

Bladder Cancer The incidence of bladder cancer increases with age. It is also more common in male cigarette smokers and people exposed to chemical dyes used in manufacturing. Worldwide, bladder cancer occurs more commonly in areas infected with the schistosome parasite. Most people with bladder cancer have bloody urine without pain or other symptoms.

Treatment of Bladder Cancer Bladder cancer that does not extend beyond the bladder lining can be controlled for a long time with local treatments, which include simple surgical removal of the tumor and instilling chemical agents or biological agents by placing a tube into the bladder. A special preparation called BCG is the most effective form of instillation therapy for the bladder. For more advanced bladder cancer, the standard treatment is removal of the bladder and surrounding tissues. With newer chemotherapeutic agents such as cisplatin, it may not be necessary to remove the bladder for individuals with advanced bladder cancer. The combination of chemotherapy and radiotherapy is comparable, in terms of survival, to complete bladder removal. However, some people who have initially been treated with medical therapies may eventually require surgery because of recurrent disease. Even people treated surgically have a 40 to 80 percent chance of having the bladder cancer recur. In two-thirds of people with cancer that has spread throughout the body, the condition can be treated but not cured by a drug regimen containing cisplatin. Even patients who are older than 80 have tolerated these aggressive treatment regimens well.

Kidney Problems Caused by Blood Vessel Disease In about half of those people over age 60 with no symptoms for kidney disease, X rays have revealed narrowing of at least one of the large arteries supplying blood to the kidneys. (See Chapter 19 on heart and circulation problems for more information on blood vessel disease.) While this condition may be asymptomatic, it can cause high blood pressure, sudden shortness of breath, long-term kidney problems, and even serious kidney failure.

The clues that would lead one to suspect underlying vascular disease involving the kidneys in an older person include the onset of high blood pressure, worsening of preexisting high blood pressure (especially if medications do not seem to control it), or unexplained loss of kidney function, especially in people who have blood vessel disease elsewhere.

Symptoms of Kidney Problems Caused by Blood Vessel Disease

Several procedures will determine if the large artery supplying a kidney with blood (the renal artery) has narrowed. The most informative is an arteriogram, but it is also the most invasive and the most risky. This highly specialized test involves passing a catheter into the large artery in the leg (the femoral artery). It is threaded upstream toward the heart until it reaches the section through which blood flows to the kidney. The physician then injects a small amount of dye to outline the blood vessels supplying the kidney. An x-ray is then taken of the arteries, which reveals their thickness or narrowness. This test is usually needed prior to any surgical treatment.

Evaluation of Kidney Problems Caused by Blood Vessel Disease

Vascular disease of the kidney, if not treated, will continue to reduce blood flow to the kidney, leading to progressive elevations of blood pressure and further compromises of kidney function. Procedures to open the blood vessels have been developed. One method requires passing a small balloon attached to a catheter into the narrowed artery and then inflating the balloon to open up the narrow area. This is called angioplasty (from the Greek, meaning "to form a vessel"). An alternative approach involves surgery. While both angioplasty and surgery relieve the high blood pressure, surgery may also preserve kidney function. Treatment of high blood pressure with medications is helpful, but it does not prevent the progressive kidney damage caused by loss of circulation.

Treatment of Kidney Problems Caused by Blood Vessel Disease

Cholesterol embolization is another blood vessel problem of the kidney that frequently goes unrecognized in older people. In this condition, small fragments of cholesterol plaque break off from the wall of the aorta, travel downstream, and lodge in the kidney. Older people are predisposed to this because they frequently have

Figure 43. The Kidney, with Common Problems

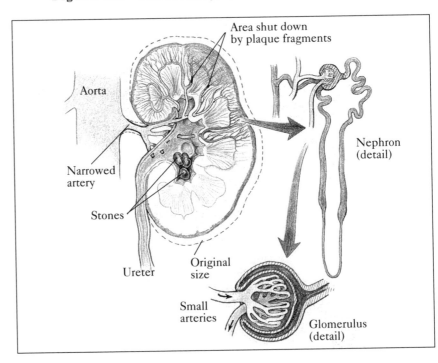

advanced stages of blood vessel disease. People in this situation may have blood pressures that fluctuate. They may also show changes in their mental function, an abrupt decline in kidney function, and signs of embolization to other parts of the body. Treatment for this condition is basic supportive care. There is no specific treatment for the disorder.

Problems with the Kidneys' Filtering Apparatus (Glomerulo-nephritis)

The part of the kidney that filters the blood is called the glomerulus (see Figure 43). Diseases involving this structure occur in all age groups. Although these diseases are similar in young and older people, there is a tendency for physicians to overlook them in people over age 50. The two major ways that glomerular diseases show up are described below.

Symptoms of Glomerular Disease

Typically, the person with sudden inflammation of the glomerular units (acute glomerulonephritis) has the rapid onset of an elevated blood pressure, edema (fluid retention), decreasing kidney function, and blood in the urine. The condition is usually confirmed by a biopsy of the kidney. In this procedure a small needle is inserted through the skin of the flank to obtain a sample of kidney tissue. The most common form of acute glomerulonephritis in people over the age of 65 is characterized by lack of deposits of immune material (antibodies) within biopsied section of the glomerulus. Although the cause of this condition is not known, it may represent a form of blood vessel inflammation called vasculitis. Generally, the outlook for this disease is not good. However, some people have experienced improvement or even resolution of the condition after high-dose corticosteroid treatment. Other more aggressive therapies may be useful in some cases.

The other way glomerular disease shows up is when there is too much protein in the urine, a condition called the nephrotic syndrome. It is estimated that about 25 percent of adults with nephrotic syndrome are over age 60. Usually a person with this condition has edema, a very high amount of protein in the urine, and a very low amount of albumin in the blood. Sometimes the blood pressure is high and the kidney function is impaired. Occasionally only the abnormalities in the urine are present without any symptoms at all. The treatment for nephrotic syndrome often involves corticosteroids to help relieve the condition causing the glomerular problem. The decision to use corticosteroids is difficult because of their side effects. Additional treatment includes controlling blood pressure and restricting the amount of protein in the diet.

Types of Glomerular Disease

A kidney biopsy is sometimes performed to determine the type of problem causing the glomerulonephritis. The five types most common in people over age 60 based on biopsy findings include membranous glomerulonephritis, minimal change glomerulonephritis, focal-segmental glomerulonephritis, amyloidosis, and multiple myeloma.

Since membranous glomerulonephritis occurs with cancer in up to 70 percent of instances, people whose kidney biopsies indicate this condition are often evaluated for the presence of malignancy. About half the time this condition progresses to kidney failure. This progression can sometimes be prevented with medications.

Minimal change glomerulonephritis usually does not progress to kidney failure and is usually treated with corticosteroids. This condition is sometimes seen with Hodgkin's disease.

Most people with focal-segmental glomerulosclerosis have a slow progression to complete kidney failure. There is no consistent therapy for this condition.

Amyloidosis, a condition where a silklike substance is deposited around blood vessels, is found in up to 20 percent of people over the age of 65 with nephrotic syndrome. Amyloidosis can involve just the kidneys or involve other organs as well. In people with involvement of other organs, a drop in blood pressure with standing or sitting is common. Amyloidosis is usually progressive, and the long-term outlook is not good.

Multiple myeloma is another cause of increased protein in the urine in elderly people. Typically a large amount of a single protein is found in the person's blood or in the urine. Other clues to this condition include anemia or low back pain. Myeloma can cause kidney failure in several ways, including toxicity of the myeloma protein to the kidney, severe dehydration, kidney stones, and damage to other portions of the kidney.

Sudden Kidney Failure

Because of the normal changes that occur in the kidney with aging, older people are especially predisposed to sudden kidney failure.

Causes of Sudden Kidney Failure

Sudden kidney failure can be caused by disease within the kidney, severe dehydration, problems in regulating the kidney blood flow, and urinary tract obstruction. These circumstances can cause either sudden or gradually progressive kidney failure.

Kidney Failure Caused by Problems Within the Kidney. Many diseases and medications can injure the kidney and cause kidney failure. An allergic reaction involving the kidney is occasionally caused by a medication. A person with this situation often feels fever and malaise. High levels of a type of white blood cell called eosinophils (because they take up a chemical dye call eosin) are seen when the blood and urine are examined under a microscope. These cells are sometimes increased in allergic conditions. Usually the treatment involves very conservative care and discontinuing the offending medication.

Sometimes changes in kidney function are due to problems within the kidney tubules. The tubules help adjust the concentration of acids and salts in the urine. Tubular dysfunction can be caused by poor blood flow or by specific kidney poisons.

In some cases, the older kidney is more sensitive to contrast material (dye) used for various diagnostic X ray procedures to identify problems in the circulation. Sometimes the people who have these X ray procedures are dehydrated at the time of testing. They may also have diabetes mellitus or other conditions that can compromise the kidney. This combination predisposes the individual to kidney failure. If kidney failure occurs, the management consists of careful monitoring and watching for complications such as heart failure or infection, although dialysis (a technique using the abdominal cavity or a machine to filter the blood) is sometimes needed for purifying the blood. The loss of kidney function is usually temporary unless the person has had significant kidney disease before the X ray study. The most important form of management is to anticipate and prevent this condition. Commonsense ways to do this include carefully evaluating the need for an X ray test and making sure the person is well hydrated if such testing becomes necessary.

Medications can also produce sudden loss of kidney function. Certain antibiotics can be especially toxic to the kidney. In addition, drugs used to treat arthritis, such as nonsteroidal anti-inflammatory drugs (NSAIDs), can cause kidney problems with certain diseases such as congestive heart failure, liver failure, and dehydration. NSAIDs seem to reduce the ability of the kidney to regulate its own blood flow. This can result in creating areas of the kidney that do not receive enough blood. Sometimes kidney failure can occur within days. Kidney function is usually checked when these medications are first started in very old people. If no change in kidney function is noted in three weeks, it is unlikely to occur at a later time unless other factors interfere.

Usually the sudden kidney failure reverses once the medications are stopped. Not all NSAIDs affect the kidney to the same degree, but if a person has had kidney failure caused by these medications, it seems wise to avoid them. In addition to kidney failure, these drugs can cause increased amounts of protein in the urine, an increased potassium in the blood, retention of salt and water, and other forms of kidney damage. They may also reduce the effectiveness of some high blood pressure medications.

Kidney Failure Caused by Dehydration. Many diseases reduce blood flow to the kidney, which in turn decreases the kidney's ability to produce urine (dehydration is one of the most common causes). Elderly people are predisposed to developing salt and water depletion because of age-related changes in the kidney. In addition they are often taking diuretic medications. In the hospital they are not allowed to eat or drink by mouth before having many medical and surgical procedures. Low blood pressure, congestive heart failure, and blood vessel disease involving the kidney and other conditions can worsen the situation.

For the person who is dehydrated, the treatment involves replacing the lost fluid. If, however, the problem is one of poor circulation, such as congestive heart failure, treatment is directed toward the underlying disease.

Kidney Failure Caused by Severe Muscle Damage. Extreme damage to muscles can cause kidney failure in elderly people. This may develop in a person who is immobilized because of illness or who has fallen and been unable to get up for an extended period of time. During this time, components of the dying muscles are released into the bloodstream and excessive amounts of them can poison the kidney. The treatment involves correcting any dehydration that is present and increasing the urine flow by forcing fluids to help wash the material from the kidney.

Kidney Failure Caused by Obstructed Urinary Flow. In people who are 65 and older, obstruction of urine flow is a frequent cause of kidney failure and therefore must be considered in any elderly person with new or worsening kidney disease. The flow of urine can be blocked either because changes in body structures obstruct the flow or because certain valves within the urinary system do not open properly. In men, an enlarged prostate is by far the most common cause of obstruction. In women, a change in the position of the uterus or uterine or ovarian cancer is a likely cause. Neurological disorders affecting the bladder's ability to contract can cause urinary obstruction in people with diabetes mellitus. Sometimes bladder cancer, enlarged lymph glands, kidney stones, and other conditions obstruct the urinary flow. In addition, medications can cause an obstruction by disrupting delicate neurologic reflexes. A procedure called kidney ultrasound is one way to look for obstruction. This test sends sound waves from a microphone placed on the abdominal wall and uses the echoes to produce pictures of the underlying tissues. This test is especially helpful in kidney disease because it avoids the use of potentially toxic intravenous contrast agents. The treatment of urinary obstruction is often surgery to remove the blockage. Other treatments depend upon the cause of the obstruction.

CHAPTER 25

SEXUALITY AND SEXUAL CONCERNS

Overview   The normal changes in sexual behavior in older people are not well known, although surveys of sexual activity in older age groups suggest decreases in sexual interest and frequency of sexual intercourse in both men and women. Across all age ranges, women report having less sexual interest and lower rates of intercourse than their male peers. However, these findings must be interpreted cautiously because these surveys cannot distinguish between effects that are due to aging, social customs and values, and gender differences in marital status. There are more elderly widows than widowers, and husbands tend to be several years older than their wives. One study done over a six-year period suggests that men and women have stable patterns of sexual activity: No aging effect was seen.

Diseases common in older people, such as arthritis, can have an important impact on sexuality. And any medical illness, especially if it engenders anxiety about sex or physical discomfort during sex, can be a barrier to healthy sexual enjoyment. Depression is another common condition that can affect sexual function. Because any sexual problem can be a symptom of a problem within the relationship, the quality of the partnership may also be an issue.

Sexuality in Relation to Coexisting Illness

Various forms of heart disease, including congestive heart failure, recent heart attacks, and angina pectoris, can interfere with sexual function. For example, ordinarily anxiety after a heart attack can cause a decrease in sexual desire and lead to impotence. However, elderly people who can tolerate mild physical exertion, such as walking up two flights of stairs, are capable of sexual intercourse. Even people who have had a recent heart attack can safely engage in routine sexual activity if they can tolerate mild or moderate activity. Clearly, it is important that these fears be alleviated and normal sexual activity encouraged if appropriate.

Arthritis

Sexual activity can also be reduced in people who have arthritis and suffer from pain, limited joint movement, and impaired mobility. (Chapter 17 contains more information on arthritis.) About half of the people who have osteoarthritis of the hip report that there is some interference with sexual activity. In addition to interventions that include adequate management of the underlying arthritis and counseling, specific advice on the selection of positions for sexual intercourse that reduce the stress on the affected joints is available.

Prostate Surgery

Few men who undergo surgical removal of all or part of the prostate, an operation known as transurethral resection of the prostate (TURP), experience difficulties with potency. Therefore, other causes need to be considered if impotence does occur. Before surgery, however, a counselor should discuss with the patient a common complication called retrograde ejaculation into the bladder. This complication, wherein the seminal fluid goes into the bladder rather than out the urethra with orgasm, occurs in as many as 90 percent of men who undergo TURP. Erectile capability and the potential for orgasm, however, are not impaired. Men who must have very extensive prostate surgery for cancer are often concerned that the surgery will result in incontinence or impotence. However, when a nerve-sparing procedure is used, the chance of this happening is usually less than 5 percent.

Breast Cancer

Although men have been known to have breast cancer, by far the greatest incidence is among women. In relation to sexuality, women who have had newly diagnosed breast cancer commonly develop fears of mutilation and anxiety about rejection by their sexual partners. According to one study, only 4 out of 60 women reported having any initial discussion with their physician or nurse about how mastectomy might affect their sexuality, yet more than half of these women expressed the desire for such a discussion. While one-half of these women resumed regular intercourse within one month after their discharge from the hospital, a third had not resumed sexual intercourse six months after hospitalization. In addition to adjusting psychologically to the mastectomy, problems may arise from various treatments and complications that may place physical limitations on sexual activity.

Other Malignancies

Although the emotional responses to cancer cannot be separated from the biomedical conditions that evoke them, terminally ill people may also have sexual needs or sexual problems. Some people may want to push others away, but more typically, people who are affected by malignancy want closeness and reassurance from their sexual partner.

Counseling

Counseling can be a part of any therapeutic plan for older people with sexual concerns. This counseling usually involves evaluating the person's expectations and knowledge of age-related changes in sexual activity. Active communication between the sexual partners is generally encouraged, and, for individuals who do not have an available sexual partner, masturbation is an option. In the nursing home setting, the staff and person's family need to be counseled to address negative feelings about sexual activity between residents. It may be possible for the physician to encourage changes in the nursing home that could facilitate privacy and also promote a better understanding of sexual activity in older people.

The determinants of sexual behavior in older women are complex and interrelated, but we can begin by considering three aspects: motivation and desire, changes in the body's response, and social and cultural influences. The sources of sexual desire have been sought in both biologic and psychologic studies. Biologic research has focused mainly on hormones and transmitter substances between nerves, but the role of these substances remains difficult to determine. Estrogens, because of their beneficial effect on the sense of well-being and other menopausal symptoms, may indirectly have a positive effect on motivation and desire. Psychological investigations have measured sexual thoughts and fantasies as indirect ways to understand motivation and desire. In women who have had their ovaries removed surgically, their sexual fantasies and thoughts are increased by receiving male hormones, but their physical responsiveness and frequency of intercourse are not affected by the surgery.

FEMALE SEXUALITY AND WOMEN'S HEALTH CONCERNS

Sexual thoughts, urges, and desires decrease with increasing age, but again, it is not known how much of this can be attributed to aging per se. Regardless of the state of the woman's motivation, however, older men and women both report that the behavior of the male partner often determines the frequency of sexual activity.

The body's responses to sexual arousal include increased genital blood flow, vaginal expansion, and lubrication of the lining. Because estrogen stimulation is necessary to maintain the lining of the vagina and the tissues around the urethra, it probably also has a role in providing the necessary reactions for the arousal response. Although arousal occurs in healthy women who have very low estrogen levels, the response is slower and less intense. The actual mechanism of arousal is not clearly understood, but it seems to be under the control of very rudimentary parts of the central nervous system.

In older women, the low estrogen state that follows the menopause can lead to thinning of the external and internal genitalia. Pain with sexual activity is the hallmark of this altered anatomy, but reduced sexual function can also occur even if there is no discomfort. For example, women after the menopause may report that they feel less genital sensation, which may mean that they feel and respond less during the arousal phase of the sexual response cycle. Other changes include reduced secretions of the opening of the vagina, diminished vaginal lubrication, lessened vaginal expansion, and decreased swelling of the blood vessels in the lower vagina. These changes may not be perceived by the older women as discrete events or signs, but they may collectively reinforce her perception that she is less sexually responsive.

Social and cultural influences on sexual behavior in older women include age-related assumptions about appropriate gender-specific behaviors and acceptable sexual practices. For example, one assumption might be that men should be the initiators of sexual activity. Another belief might be that there is only one correct position for intercourse or that intercourse is the only way of expressing intimacy. These assumptions may persist even in the face of physical or emotional changes that come with age. Clearly, a broader definition of acceptable activities, responses, or expressions should be considered to accommodate the older self and the older body.

Addressing Female Sexual Concerns

Women have not traditionally been comfortable volunteering information about sexual problems, but as the past several decades have brought dramatic shifts of self-perception and general awareness of gender issues, both women and physicians, whether male or female, are perhaps feeling less reticent about discussing sexual problems and what can be done to treat them. This is not to say all reticence is gone, however. In one gynecologic practice, for example, only 3 percent of the women patients came to see a physician specifically because of a sexual complaint, but when all the women patients were questioned directly, 15 percent revealed that they did, in fact, have such concerns. Some women may require a long-term relationship with their doctor before they will disclose any sexual complaints, and some doctors may find it difficult to raise the subject of sexual activity. One way to approach the subject is to raise questions or include comments about sexual function in matter-of-fact discussions of overall health status, raising more specific concerns if necessary.

Your doctor's recommendations for treatment of various problems will depend upon the cause. A list of possible causes and treatments of sexual dysfunction in older women is shown in Table 40. Sexual counseling and educational strategies may be the most effective approach to resolving a sexual problem. Physicians have sometimes hesitated to offer such counsel because they felt it involved discussing a patient's intimate behavior and would offend their patients. Recent experience, however, suggests that people with problems are eager for advice or recommendations for solutions. For example, one interview conducted in an arthritis clinic found that 40 percent of the women expressed interest in hearing specific sexual advice from their physician. Encourage your doctor to share simple educational directives with you, as these are often all that is needed. For example, experimenting with various positions during intercourse to reduce discomfort, or considering alternative forms of intimacy such as hugging, caressing, and fondling can make a significant difference in sexual enjoyment for the older woman who has arthritic or other movement disorders.

Estrogen Therapy

While the overall relationship between estrogen supplementation and female sexual functioning is complicated and not well understood, some of the beneficial effects are clear. Estrogen reduces genital atrophy and can reduce the discomfort sometimes caused by sexual activity. It is likely that the improved genital tissue due to estrogen supplementation has a beneficial effect on arousal. Regardless of the precise mechanism, a relationship probably does exist between an improvement in the sense of overall well-being and mood and improvements in the desire and motivation of sexual functioning.

Because of the limits of current information, women and their physicians should have an open discussion about the benefits and risks of estrogen supplementation, wherein both parties are able to express their concerns. Several routes of estrogen administration are available, each with specific advantages and disadvantages.

For the older woman who is already taking estrogen but has a lowered interest in sex, there is no obvious solution. The question is whether androgens or male hormones could provide a little extra benefit. However, before considering the use of these compounds,

**Table 40. Possible Causes and Treatments of
Sexual Dysfunction in Elderly Women**

FACTORS AFFECTING DIMINISHED SEXUAL FUNCTION	POSSIBLE CAUSES*	THERAPEUTIC STRATEGIES†
Decreased motivation	Partner's decreased motivation/capability	Psychosocial evaluation
	Genital dysfunction with secondary loss of interest	Medical evaluation
	Perceived socially appropriate behavior for age and gender	Education and counseling
	Primary alteration in sexual drive	Estrogen/androgen
	Relationship dysfunction	Psychosocial evaluation
	Depression	Counseling/antidepressants
Genital changes	Vaginal atrophy	Oral or vaginal estrogen Lubricants
	Atrophy of the urethra (may contribute to incontinence during sexual activity)	Oral or vaginal estrogen
Changes in body response	Decreased arousal phase	Estrogen (to restore tissue integrity)
	Decreased hormonal mediators	Estrogen
Behavioral limitations	Established patterns of male initiation	Education and counseling
	Limited sexual script (range of acceptable sexual behaviors)	Explicit advice on sexual practices, with specific attention to limitations that may be operative

*More than one of these may be present.
†More than one modality may be required.

there are many other contributing factors that must be reviewed. One should also note that while male hormones do increase sexual fantasies and urges in women, this may not automatically translate into an actual change in the frequency of sexual activity or in an increase in the body's responsiveness.

A woman's reproduction system is affected by alterations in the pelvic structures and changes due to the menopause (see Figure 44). Other physical problems, such as arthritis of the hips, can make it uncomfortable for the woman to lie in the normal examination position.

Gynecologic Disorders

As women age, visual inspection of the external genitalia skin may reveal common changes: Usually, the pubic hair is quite thin; the vaginal opening may be smaller and the lining may be pale and thinned; or the vaginal vault may be shortened or narrowed. These changes may be due as much to vaginal disuse as to tissue atrophy caused by loss of estrogen. Women who have maintained

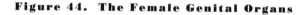

Figure 44. The Female Genital Organs

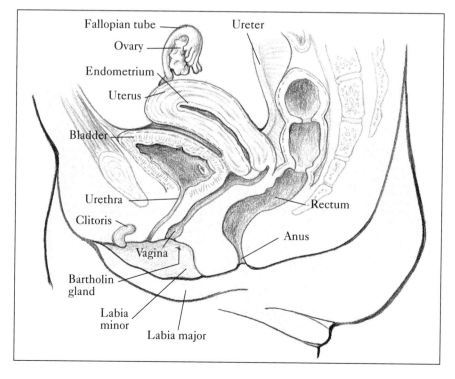

sexual activities do not show these changes to the same extent as women who have not been sexually active for a long time. These changes can make obtaining a Pap smear or an endometrial sample very difficult.

Pap smears should be obtained at least every three years until the age of 65. After that, there is little evidence for continuing them. However, older women who have not had regular Pap smears should have at least two tests, one year apart, before screening is stopped. Women who have had hysterectomies generally do not need further Pap smears.

Disorders of the External Genitalia

Disorders of the skin and labia increase in frequency with advancing age and can be caused by a number of conditions, including many benign skin growths and some malignancies. Approximately 3 to 5 percent of women with skin disorders have invasive cancer, and approximately 4 to 8 percent have premalignant conditions. Because of this, if you notice any changes in the area of the external genitalia, you should request a careful inspection by your physician who should biopsy any suspicious areas. Any enlargement of the Bartholin glands (located on either side of the vaginal opening) is considered to be caused by a malignancy until proven otherwise with negative biopsies.

It is important that any abnormalities in the external genitalia be evaluated because they frequently occur with other medical problems (usually metabolic disorders) and because the symptoms can often be uncomfortable and disabling. Moreover, most conditions generally improve dramatically with appropriate treatment.

Changes of the labia and skin may have pigmentation or may be white, depending upon local factors such as scratching and hygiene. As part of the evaluation, the physician may apply a small amount of a 1 or 2 percent acetic acid (purified vinegar) and then carefully inspect the area with a special magnifying glass or other instrument. This method offers the best chance for discovering abnormalities. The acetic acid causes suspicious areas to turn white. Biopsies are easily performed by using local anesthesia to numb the area and then removing a very small amount of tissue for testing.

Benign infections of the external genitalia, such as contact dermatitis, allergic reactions, and fungal, yeast, or bacterial infections, can occur in women at any age. Because the skin in this area perspires more than skin elsewhere, increased moisture and irritation contribute to these conditions. Older women will have the same symptoms as those experienced by younger women: redness, itching, swelling, or pain. A physician will likely prescribe a course of genital hygiene and possibly some medication.

Although cancer involving the external genitalia is rare, its incidence increases with age and peaks in people in their seventies. In the past, radical surgery with regional removal of lymph nodes was the treatment of choice for all invasive cancers involving the external genitalia. More recent studies have suggested that more conservative approaches may avoid the considerable changes in body image, sexual dysfunction, and prolonged recovery time associated with such radical surgery. Again, it must be stressed that biopsy must be done of every suspicious area of the external genitalia so that minimally invasive cancers can be treated early and with minimal surgical procedures to avoid or reduce disability.

For some people with recurring or advanced cancer, combined radiation therapy and chemotherapy may be effective. This combination is also used for principal treatment in people who are medically unable to withstand surgery.

Of all the gynecologic cancers that occur in women older than age 75, vaginal cancers constitute the smallest percentage (only 7 percent). Because the majority of women with cancer of the vagina have bleeding, any vaginal bleeding must be checked by an experienced physician. (See page 417 for more on vaginal bleeding.)

Treatment of the External Genitalia. An effective treatment for many skin and labial disorders is good hygiene and keeping the area clean and free from excessive moisture. Sometimes skin conditions are treated with corticosteroids, which unfortunately can cause atrophy of the skin if they are overused.

Disorders of the Vagina

Thinning, paleness, and loss of elasticity are some of the common changes seen in the vaginal lining of postmenopausal women. These changes significantly increase the overall chance of infection and irritation. Although the incidence of vaginal irritation is greater in younger women, the frequency of this problem may increase in older women because of changes that occur after menopause. The types of bacteria and fungi that cause vaginitis, however, are quite similar in younger and older women. The evaluation and management of the condition is essentially the same in both age groups.

Symptoms of Atrophic Vaginitis. Vaginal irritation caused by atrophy frequently produces symptoms of itching, burning, milky or creamy discharge, and discomfort when urinating or with sexual intercourse. Bleeding may also be an early symptom. Changes to the external genitalia become apparent only months or years after the first vaginal changes appear. The smaller labia shrink, and the vaginal opening may become narrow and rigid so that intercourse becomes impossible.

Treatment of Atrophic Vaginitis. While estrogens will usually resolve the symptoms of vaginal atrophy, several precautions must be exercised. Locally applied estrogen creams in the usual doses of 1 to 4 grams per day are readily absorbed through the vaginal lining with resulting effects all over the body. Lower doses of topical estrogens such as 0.5 gram every third day will provide significant relief from symptoms and produce fewer effects overall. However, even at these lower doses, many clinicians still recommend that other hormones such as progestins be used occasionally to protect the lining of the uterus against the effects of estrogen stimulation. Increased use of the vagina can also significantly improve atrophy.

Sagging Pelvic Structures

The pelvic structures are supported by a combination of muscles and ligaments. Injury during childbirth, complications of obesity, atrophy after the menopause, or strenuous activity may damage or weaken the supporting structures and cause the uterus to sag out of place. Some sagging, called prolapse (from the Latin, meaning "before the fall"), is classified according to its severity.

Prolapse of the Uterus

Prolapse of the uterus is termed "first-degree" if the cervix (the opening of the uterus) appears at the vaginal opening, "second-degree" if the cervix and half of the uterus protrude, and "third-degree" if the vaginal walls are turned completely inside out and the entire uterus is exposed.

416

Symptoms of Prolapse of the Uterus. Women with this condition may notice a sense of pelvic heaviness, a vaginal mass, back pain, urinary incontinence, or bleeding of the exposed organs.

Treatment of Prolapse of the Uterus. When the degree of relaxation is mild, intensive exercises may be beneficial to increase the muscle tone and support the base of the pelvis. Estrogens may also be helpful. However, surgery is usually necessary in instances of complete (third-degree) prolapse. The usual procedure is a hysterectomy. Other surgical repairs may be necessary if the bladder and rectum have also prolapsed.

Use of a vaginal pessary, a device inserted into the vagina that helps to support the uterus, may be an effective treatment for women who are unable or unwilling to have surgery. There are pessaries in the shape of a rectangle, a ring, or a doughnut. Insertion and removal of a pessary are easier if it is inflatable.

Bladder and Rectal Prolapse

The sagging, or prolapse, of the bladder against the opening of the vagina is called a cystocele. This can accompany or even precede uterine prolapse. The symptoms involve a sense of vaginal fullness or a palpable mass protruding from the top of the vagina. This condition may also cause recurrent urinary tract infections, due to incomplete bladder emptying, or urinary incontinence. Ulcerations in the vaginal lining can occur as the tissues dry out; these ulcers may indicate that surgical repair is necessary to treat the cystocele.

A rectocele is a bulging of the rectum up through the vaginal opening. A large rectocele may result in incomplete passage of bowel movements. With large rectoceles, surgery is the recommended treatment.

Vaginal Bleeding

About 20 percent of women who experience vaginal bleeding that occurs after the menopause have malignancies. The likelihood that malignancy will be the cause of bleeding increases with age; therefore, any episodes of bleeding after the menopause should be fully evaluated. Conditions that can cause this bleeding are shown in Table 41.

Generally, an evaluation of the condition involves a thorough examination to check for visual evidence of the conditions listed in

Table 41. Causes of Postmenopausal Vaginal Bleeding

VULVAR AND VAGINAL
Ulceration
Malignancy

CERVICAL
Irritation/infection
Malignant tumor
Polyp

UTERINE
Abnormal cell growth in endometrium
Swelling of glands in endometrium; polyps in endometrium
Tumor in endometrium
Other malignant tumor (sarcoma, etc.)

URINARY TRACT
Urethra (with irritation)
Bladder (infection, malignant tumor, polyp, stone)
Ureter (stone or malignant tumor)
Kidney (stone or malignant tumor)

OTHER
Tubal or ovarian malignant tumor
Bleeding tendency
Hormonal cause (estrogen replacement, adrenal or ovarian tumor)
Opening in vaginal wall to bowel

Table 41. Endometrial biopsy, Pap smear, and possibly additional studies are needed unless an obvious source of bleeding is discovered. Any abnormal-appearing areas are usually biopsied. Sometimes a progesterone challenge test is performed if the results of biopsies are unremarkable or no other cause for the bleeding has been found. In this test, the hormone progesterone is given for about two weeks. If bleeding occurs when this medication is stopped, this indicates an abnormality involving the lining of the uterus. Further medical evaluation is then required.

Breast Cancer

Breast cancer is the most common malignancy in American women, and its incidence increases with age. The survival time is shorter in women whose cancer is diagnosed after age 75 compared with younger postmenopausal women. This difference in survival is due in part to socioeconomic and cultural factors, such as limited access to health care and the unwillingness of some physicians to submit older patients to aggressive testing and intensive therapy.

Breast cancer screening by means of monthly self-examination, an annual examination, and mammography every one to two years is recommended for women over age 50. Although there is no reliable information on whether there should be an age limit to screening, it's also recommended that screening be discontinued at age 75. On average, breast cancer takes about ten years to grow to about the size of a large pea (1 centimeter, about ½ inch, in diameter). In older women, breast cancers are generally slower growing and less aggressive than they are in younger women.

The outlook for women with breast cancer depends upon a number of factors including the stage or extent of the disease, the presence of hormone receptors for estrogen and other female hormones on the cancerous cells, the degree of cellular maturity (immature cells are more aggressive), the pace of the tumor's growth, and the extent of expression of a special gene called HER-2. The risk of recurrence of cancer in women who have surgical removal of breast tumors (partial or complete mastectomies) is predicted by the presence of cancer cells in the regional lymph nodes, usually under the arm. Even in women with no signs of cancer cells in these lymph nodes, the likelihood of recurrence increases if there is a lack of hormone receptors, if there are very immature cancer cells, or if there is a high degree of rapid cell growth. Approximately two-thirds of cancers in postmenopausal women contain hormone receptors, a finding that generally signifies a more favorable course.

Evaluation of Breast Cancer

In addition to the physical examination, the initial assessment of the severity and extent of breast cancer usually includes blood tests and a chest X ray to look for involvement of other organs such as the bones, liver, or lungs. If these procedures show no specific symptoms or abnormal test results, the value of more extensive investigations remains controversial.

**Treatment of
Breast Cancer**

Surgery is the primary treatment for breast cancer. When the diameter of the primary tumor is 5 centimeters (about 2 inches) or less, removal of the tumor (lumpectomy) and the lymph glands under the arm, in combination with radiation treatment of the breast, is as effective as removal of the whole breast (mastectomy). A critical factor in deciding whether to perform a simple lumpectomy or a mastectomy is determining whether the breast tissue will allow an adequate surgical repair of the breast. An alternative to surgery for either women who have a short life expectancy due to other reasons or who have very small primary tumors may be treatment with a medication like tamoxifen.

Tamoxifen is also used to delay the recurrence of breast cancer and prolong survival for many older women. While the optimal duration of this treatment has not been established, a minimum of two years' treatment is necessary. Some experts have recommended lifelong treatment. The value of chemotherapy that is more extensive than tamoxifen in postmenopausal women with breast cancer is controversial. Many experts recommend that all women with breast cancer over the age of 65 have hormonal manipulation as first-line treatment, regardless of their hormone receptor status, and that chemotherapy be reserved for women in whom hormonal treatment has failed. Hormonal manipulation as single therapy is ineffective for women with such life-threatening conditions as extensive spread of cancer to the lungs or the liver. In these situations the addition of aggressive chemotherapy is an option to induce a rapid resolution of the tumor.

Tamoxifen is currently the most common form of hormone treatment. Although medications of the progesterone type are as effective, they are more toxic and therefore best reserved for patients in whom treatment with tamoxifen has failed. Commonly used chemotherapy regimens consist of a combination of medications including cyclophosphamide, methotrexate, and 5-fluorouracil.

Cervical Cancer

The overall incidence of cervical cancer that invades the surrounding tissues has decreased by approximately 80 percent, but it is increasing in older women. It is now clear that many subpopulations of elderly women, particularly those with limited access to continuing health care, were not adequately screened for this disease throughout their lives. Older women who have had normal Pap smears do not benefit from further testing. However, nearly half of women over age 65 have never had a Pap test at all and three-quarters have not had regular testing. Further screening of this group is important with two smears taken at least one year apart. If these smears are normal then no further screening is necessary.

The primary therapy for limited cervical cancer is surgical removal of the tumor and some of the surrounding tissue. At present, the management of advanced disease with chemotherapy is experimental.

Uterine or Endometrial Cancer

The most common gynecologic cancer in older women, endometrial cancer, involves the uterine lining. Predisposing factors include obesity, never having children, a family history of multiple cancers, diseases of the ovary, and the prolonged use of postmenopausal estrogens without the use of progesterone. For most elderly women, vaginal bleeding is the most common initial symptom, and this often allows uterine cancer to be discovered early. Because screening asymptomatic women has not been shown to decrease mortality of endometrial cancer, routine endometrial biopsies are not recommended unless a woman takes estrogens with progesterone. Surgery is the only curative treatment, but approximately 30 percent of women with widespread disease will respond to various hormonal medications, such as progesterone therapy and to tamoxifen.

Ovarian Cancer

Although it is much less prevalent than cervical cancer or endometrial cancer, cancer of the ovary is the most common cause of death from a gynecologic cancer, and its incidence increases with age. Ovarian cancer does not usually produce symptoms until it has widely spread to other organs. This diagnosis, usually late in the course of the illness, accounts for its high death rate.

The outlook of advanced ovarian cancer has been improved by the use of various combination chemotherapies. For advanced ovarian cancer, the optimum treatment consists of maximal surgical removal of the tumor followed by special courses of chemotherapy. The response rate obtained by this therapeutic strategy is better than 60 percent. The median survival period for this condition exceeds two years.

MALE SEXUALITY AND MALE GENITAL DISORDERS

Sexuality constitutes an integral part of the quality of life for older men. Older men usually notice, however, a distinct difference between their current level of sexual interest and that experienced during early adulthood. Not only is there less interest in the frequency of sexual contact but also the focus of sexual interaction may change from primarily physical to increasingly emotional. Nevertheless, even men who are over the age of 85 still have sexual interest, and intercourse remains the preferred form of physical sexual contact.

Impotence

Impotence, the most common sexual complaint in men, is the inability to maintain an adequate penile erection for successful sexual intercourse. Although information on erections and aging is incomplete, it appears that erection rigidity peaks in the late teens and then gradually declines throughout adult life. In the absence of disease, the older man's erections remain adequate for intercourse, but they require a greater amount of direct stimulation to be maintained. Some men may perceive this requirement for additional stimulation as a sign of impending failure, which it is not. When disorders involving the pelvic blood vessels and nerves are superimposed on these age-related changes in erections, inadequate rigidity for intercourse often results (see Figure 45).

The male hormone, testosterone, is responsible for maintaining genital tissues as well as inducing sexual interest. While it appears to play a role in facilitating fantasy-induced erections, the role of testosterone in maintaining erections produced by local stimulation appears to be minimal.

How Erections Are Produced

The neurologic stimulation for erection can either be caused by fantasy or local stimulation. Specific parts of the brain and nervous system mediate these various responses. Direct genital stimulation produces impulses that travel to the lower part of the spinal cord and then return to the penis, traveling each way through specific nerves. Substances are released that cause relaxation of the blood vessels. An erection occurs through a dilation of the blood vessels that increases inflow to the penis. As this blood flow increases, the venous outflow is also restricted. The increasing blood flow with relatively reduced outflow results in increasing pressure within the penis and produces

Figure 45. The Male Genital Organs

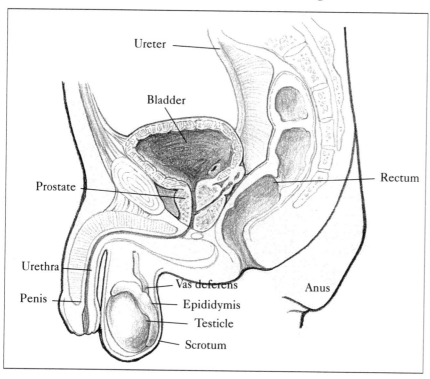

rigidity. Orgasmic release of chemical messengers allows for the out-flow of blood, and the tissue of the penis deflates.

Generally, when an older man who complains of impotence con-sults with his physician, the physician will need to determine whether an evaluation is needed. Most older men report a grad-ual increase in the amount of stimulation required to achieve an erection, and that both the rigidity and duration of erections decline with aging. If the physician concludes that an assessment is warranted, it generally includes a detailed medical interview and evaluation focusing on information that is shown in Table 42. Monitoring for erections that occur during sleep may help dif-ferentiate medical from psychological causes of impotence, al-though the validity of these observations in older men is not clear, and the results of any tests should be interpreted with extreme caution.

Evaluation of Impotence

Table 42. Information to Be Obtained During an Evaluation for Impotence

DEFINITION OF THE PROBLEM
  Is the dysfunction really erectile failure?
  Or is the dysfunction related to decreased sexual interest,
    orgasmic ability, mobility?

PRIOR FUNCTIONING
  Compare quality of best prior erections to that of current erections.

ONSET
  Acute onset suggests psychogenic cause or adverse drug reaction.
  Chronic onset suggests an underlying disease.

PROGRESSION
  Intermittent progression suggests psychogenic cause.
  Progressive progression suggests an underlying disease.
  Establish duration of erectile dysfunction.

ERECTIONS UPON AWAKENING
  Rigid erections suggest psychogenic cause.
  Nonrigid or absent erections suggest an underlying disease.

ASSOCIATED MEDICAL/SOCIAL DISORDERS
  Prescription or social drugs (e.g., cigarettes, alcohol).
  Diabetes mellitus, neurologic disease, vascular disease, pelvic or
    abdominal surgery.

Breast enlargement suggests endocrine disorder.

Poor circulation in the legs suggest vascular disease.

Penile size—enlarged abdomen and small penis may hinder the
  effectiveness of a suction device.

Neurologic disease in the pelvis or legs suggests penile neuropathy.

Testicular atrophy suggests hypogonadism, alcoholism.

The blood vessel supply to the penis can be assessed using ultrasound. Generally, the penile blood pressure is compared to the blood pressure in the arm. Blood tests are sometimes obtained to check for diabetes mellitus or low testosterone levels in the blood. Sometimes a very high level of the hormone prolactin can cause impotence even with normal testosterone levels. Because of this, physicians sometimes order a prolactin blood test if testosterone treatment is not effective. In most cases, the high prolactin level is due to the effect of medications or to kidney failure. A pituitary tumor can cause this condition.

As with most conditions, impotence is most likely to be successfully treated when therapy is based on the cause of the disorder. For example, the man whose impotence is related to drugs is unlikely to respond to sex therapy.

Treatment of Impotence

The advantages and disadvantages of various treatments for impotence are shown in Table 43. Of these therapies, the least invasive is the penile orthotic device, which is also referred to as a vacuum device. There are two types. The first is a hollow cylinder in which the flaccid penis is placed. The cylinder is then attached to a pump that generates a negative pressure, thus pulling blood into the penis and surrounding tissues. An erectlike state is created and can be maintained by placing a constricting band around the base of the penis before removing the cylinder. This constricting band should not be left in place for more than 30 minutes because of decreased blood flow to the penis. This approach has few adverse effects, but it does require good hand coordination and men with very severe blood vessel disease may not be able to achieve adequate rigidity. The treatment is best suited for men with nervous system problems or problems in the veins. On the positive side, the device is effective, noninvasive, and reversible. It is certainly a procedure men with impotence should consider.

The second type of vacuum device is condom-shaped and maintains rigidity during intercourse. It is connected to a small tube with which air is sucked out, thus creating a slight vacuum that helps draw the penis into the condom. The condom itself is relatively rigid so that the combined rigidity of the condom and the penis is usually adequate for penetration. This device can be

**Table 43. Treatment Options for
Elderly Men with Impotence**

TREATMENT	ADVANTAGES	DISADVANTAGES
Testosterone	Inexpensive Noninvasive	Rarely effective
Sex therapy	Noninvasive	Expensive Time-consuming
Vacuum erection devices	Noninvasive	Cumbersome Not effective in presence of severe vascular disease
Rigid condom devices	Noninvasive Effective regardless of cause	Decreases sensitivity Lacks aesthetic appeal
Papaverine or phentolamine	Erection looks normal	Cavernosal fibrosis (uncommon) Requires injection
Prostaglandin E_1	Erection looks normal	Burning sensation Requires injection
Malleable prosthesis	No mechanical parts that might malfunction	Permanent erection
Inflatable prosthesis	Erection looks normal	Often requires reoperation
Arterial bypass	Definitive therapy	Very invasive High failure rate
Venous ligation	Definitive therapy	Very invasive High failure rate

helpful in impotence caused by virtually any problem, but it may be especially useful for men with penile curvature. However, its use is associated with decreased sensitivity, and the lack of aesthetic appeal makes it an undesirable therapy except for couples who are very supportive in their relationship.

Self-injection of the penis is the treatment receiving the most attention today. It involves the direct injection of vasoactive substances, blood vessel activators, which chemically bypass the usual nervous system pathways to produce an erection. Because this process mimics that of a normal erection, injection-induced erections are natural in appearance and function. The substances injected usually include papaverine, phentolamine, and prostaglandin E_1. These are all effective agents for penile self-injection, but the person's response depends upon the cause of the impotence. For men with impotence caused by nervous system disease, there may be a hyperresponsiveness to these injections, while a person with very severe blood vessel disease or fibrosis may not be able to develop a completely firm erection. The self-injection technique represents a major advance to treating impotence but is associated with some short-term complications, such as prolonged erections, which need to be reversed if they last more than four hours. There are simple ways to do this under a physician's supervision. Studies have shown that prostaglandin E_1 causes a slight burning sensation in the penis for some men. There are also indications that papaverine and phentolamine can occasionally cause penile scar tissue.

Penile prostheses or implants are safe and effective but they should be reserved for individuals who have experienced failure with other treatments. The prostheses that are currently available include rigid, flexible, and multiple-component inflatable devices. The rigid devices have solid cylinders that are surgically implanted within the penis. Their major disadvantage is that they make the penis permanently firm. While the flexible prosthesis is similar, it can be bent for improved concealability. Both rigid and flexible prostheses can be inserted under local anesthesia. The inflatable prostheses have fluid-filled cylinders that are inserted within the penis and backed up by a pump placed near the scrotum and a reservoir placed in the abdomen. These control the movement of fluid. The pump controls the erection and requires manual skill to operate it, and mechanical problems frequently occur. The overall reliability of these devices is unknown.

The type of prosthesis chosen depends upon the preferences of the person and his partner. Satisfaction after prosthesis implantation has been good in short-term studies, but well-designed long-term follow-up studies that measure satisfaction have not been completed. A few accounts suggest that the inflatable devices produce greater satisfaction than the other devices. Taken together, the surgical complications of these implants are relatively few, and their success rate is high enough that the implant option is reasonable for older men.

While improving the blood supply of the penis through surgery to the arteries and veins has the potential for correcting the underlying causes of impotence, attempts to do this have met with only limited success. Such procedures have a very disappointing success rate of much less than 50 percent.

Prostate Problems

Prostate Enlargement

Benign prostatic hypertrophy (or BPH) is the gradual enlargement of the prostate gland. It is rarely identified in men under age 40, and its occurrence increases progressively with advancing age so that it is present in about 90 percent of 80-year-old men. A 50-year-old man has about a 20 to 25 percent chance of requiring surgery to reduce the size of the prostate gland. Development of BPH is believed to be caused by male hormones.

Symptoms of Prostate Enlargement. BPH usually begins to produce symptoms in men at about age 50. Because urine flows from the bladder through the prostate gland, prostate enlargement often begins to block the passage of urine. The common symptoms of BPH are caused by either obstruction or irritation. The most common obstructive symptoms are difficulty beginning to urinate, straining, decreased force and caliber of the urinary stream, dribbling after voiding, a sensation that the bladder has not emptied completely, and not fully emptying the bladder after urinating. A man with irritative symptoms might complain of frequent urinating, urinating at night, pain on urinating, and a sense of the urgent need to urinate. Men who complain of irritative symptoms may have a disease other than BPH, such as a urinary tract infection, bladder cancer, or the effects of neurological diseases on the bladder.

Evaluation of Prostate Enlargement. A rectal examination to feel the prostate gland does not reliably identify BPH or the possible obstruction caused by it. Therefore, if any of the symptoms listed above are present, the physician may recommend other studies, such as ultrasound (an examination of the bladder and prostate using sound waves), to obtain a clearer picture of the prostate size.

Treatment of Prostate Enlargement. Surgical removal of the obstructing tissue around the urethra is the usual treatment for BPH. It may be recommended if there is a change in kidney function, complete obstruction of the kidneys, recurrent urinary tract infections, or significant retention of urine in the bladder. In the absence of these indications, it is difficult to know whether surgery will help. Certainly, the severity of symptoms and the expected gains in the quality of life after surgery are important considerations. At times, urinary incontinence associated with a constant feeling that one needs to urinate suggests that surgery would very likely correct the problem. There are situations, however, in which the removal of obstructions may actually worsen incontinence.

If surgical therapy is selected, the size of the prostate gland determines the type of surgical approach. For relatively small prostate glands, a simple incision (or cut) along the prostate can be performed. This incision made through the urethra is usually a shorter operation with less frequent postoperative bladder neck scarring compared with the actual removal of prostate tissue (transurethral resection). However, since the incisional approach does not remove any prostate tissue, it is more likely to miss early stages of prostate cancer. For prostate glands of moderate size, the standard procedure is to core out the center of the prostate in a transurethral resection. For a very large prostate gland, surgery using an abdominal incision or an incision between the scrotum and rectum may be performed. Sexual potency is generally preserved after prostate surgery, but a common complication is retrograde ejaculation, where the seminal fluid prompted by orgasm is propelled into the bladder rather than out of the urethra. Despite the backward movement of seminal fluid, the pleasure of sexual activity is not affected.

A procedure involving balloon dilation of the prostate is not recommended since obstruction frequently recurs, and bleeding and incontinence frequently result.

For men who do not undergo surgery, medical therapy may be helpful but not curative. For example, certain medicines may decrease the muscle tone of the prostate and may benefit up to 20 percent of men, even though medication does not reduce the size of the obstructing prostate. In addition, drugs that block the action of male hormones have also improved urinary function in some men. These medications are very expensive, and therapy must continue indefinitely for the benefits to be retained.

Prostate Infection

Infection of the prostate (prostatitis) can occur as either a sudden or a smoldering infection. Although sudden prostatitis does occasionally occur in older men, smoldering infection called chronic bacterial prostatitis (CBP) is more common. More important, CBP may contribute to concurrent urinary tract infection. While older men with CBP may have no symptoms at all, common complaints include mid- to low-back pain, urinary urgency, frequency, need to void at night, and discomfort between the scrotum and rectum. The condition requires careful evaluation by a physician. The treatment for CBP is generally antibiotics taken orally, for at least four weeks.

Prostate Cancer

Prostate cancer is the most common cancer among men over the age of 65, and its management is related to the extent of the disease. Prostate cancer has an extremely variable growth rate and many men live a long time without any treatment. A lab test called PSA, or prostate specific antigen, is often used to follow the progression of the disease, and it is sometimes used as a screening test.

There is a lot of controversy about the treatment for prostate cancer; therefore, an older man may get varying opinions from different physicians. If a man is found to have a small amount of prostate cancer that has not spread outside the gland, then surgery to remove the prostate is often recommended. If the cancer is restricted to the prostate, there is a good chance that surgery (prostatectomy) will be curative. In this situation, some physicians may recommend radiation therapy rather than surgery, which is also acceptable. Each approach has its benefits and drawbacks, but both seem to be effective in early prostate cancer. Radiation therapy is more likely to cause problems with the intestines or bladder whereas surgery (prostatectomy) is more likely to cause impotence and urinary incontinence. The likelihood of impotence following surgery has markedly decreased with a special procedure that spares the nerves that produce an erection.

If the cancer cells have spread outside the prostate, there are several treatment options to try to inhibit the growth of the tumor. Hormonal therapy is often used in an attempt to deprive the tumor of male hormones, which are necessary for its growth. This can be achieved with castration, drug therapy, or combination therapies. Radiation therapy or surgery is sometimes used to decrease the amount of the tumor, and can relieve urinary obstruction or local pain. Widespread prostate cancer is not currently a curable disease, but there are many scientists investigating the use of chemotherapy. Bone pain is a major complication of extensive prostate cancer, and it is usually responsive to hormonal therapy, radiation treatments, corticosteroids, or pain medications.

CHAPTER 26

OTHER IMPORTANT CONDITIONS

Cancer (General)

Disorders of Salt and Water

Diabetes Mellitus

Heat Stroke

Hypothermia

Infections (General)

Loss of Vitality

Medication Problems (Polypharmacy)

Pain

Sleep Problems

Walking Problems, Immobility, and Falls

Cancer (General)

Abnormal cellular growths in the body are classified as either benign or malignant. An example of a benign growth is a wart. Malignant growths are called cancer, and incidence of these increases with age. Among people older than age 65 in the United States, cancer represents the second most common cause of death. (In Japan, cancer is the leading cause of death.) The prevention and early detection of cancer is critical in older people; if it is detected, then the effectiveness of cancer treatment and the older person's tolerance of cancer treatments need to be considered carefully.

The intricate mechanisms regulating the growth of cancerous cells have been partially unraveled by ongoing research. Growth factors activate the nuclei of cells and trigger them to grow and reproduce. This involves specific proteins called proto-oncogenes that help to regulate growth and repair normal tissues. In the normal situation, efficient mechanisms keep these proto-oncogenes under control. A failure of these controls can result in the unregulated growth of cells: neoplastic, or cancerous growth.

The discovery of some of the genes that are related to cancer has led to a multiple-step theory that helps to explain why the incidence of cancer increases with age. In older people, the effects of early exposure to various chemicals that promote cancer—i.e., carcinogens such as asbestos or uranium—have a longer period in which to act. Furthermore, when combined with the normal age-related changes that occur in the nuclei of cells, these cells may become more vulnerable to subsequent exposures with multiple carcinogens.

The goals of cancer treatment—to prolong life and to relieve symptoms—may be influenced by age-associated changes in life expectancy, the aggressiveness of the cancer, and the effectiveness and complications of therapy. Some malignancies may have a milder course in older people, such as lung cancer and prostate cancer, while other malignancies, including Hodgkin's disease and acute leukemias, may actually be more aggressive. Furthermore, the number of tumors resistant to chemotherapy may increase in the older age group.

The main forms of cancer treatment are surgery, radiation therapy, chemotherapy, and hormonal therapies that modulate the body's response to tumor cells. Elective surgery is relatively well tolerated in people of advanced age, and rarely is age alone a reason for rejecting elective surgical treatment of cancer. Emergency surgery in older patients has a significantly increased death rate. Surgery is offered to remove a tumor and possibly cure the condition to prevent future problems (such as obstruction in colon cancer) or to clearly determine how far the disease has spread.

Radiation therapy uses energy produced by machines or naturally occurring elements such as cobalt or radium to penetrate body tissues to affect body cells. This radiation energy can be focused to the site of the cancer to provide greater radiation exposure to the malignancy and somewhat less to the normal tissues. Radiation therapy may be combined with surgery or may be used in some cases as a single treatment for some malignancies, such as lymphoma. (See Chapter 20 for more information on lymphoma.) A major role of radiation is to control spread of cancer and to manage pain. Bone pain may respond dramatically to radiation.

While surgery and radiation have been used for over a century, chemotherapy for cancer is a relatively new treatment. Chemotherapy uses chemicals derived from plants or developed in laboratories to kill cancer cells. Unfortunately, other body cells are also affected, such as in the bone marrow, intestinal tract, or hair follicles. Because of this, chemotherapy may cause problems with blood counts; induce nausea, vomiting, or diarrhea; and cause loss of hair. These effects can usually be controlled. Chemotherapy is given by mouth or by intravenous line and circulates throughout the body. This circulation allows the chemicals to reach cancer cells anywhere in the body except the brain. The brain has a natural protective chemical barrier.

Modulating the immune response is an especially appealing form of cancer treatment in older people whose immune defenses may be weak or less effective. Hormonal therapy for cancer is generally safe in older patients. For example, the anticancer medication tamoxifen has remarkably few side effects in older people.

Adjuvant treatments are treatments used to boost the primary forms of cancer treatment in controlling or eliminating the cancer. Both bone cancer and colon cancer are examples of conditions in which adjuvant chemotherapy prolongs survival. Considerable research is under way to develop therapeutic agents.

Disorders of Salt and Water

Low Sodium

The sodium level in the blood reflects the relative amounts of sodium and water. A low sodium can mean either too much water or too little sodium. Older people are predisposed to develop low sodium in the blood for several reasons. Two of the most common are a decrease in kidney function and an increase in the levels of a hormone in the blood called antidiuretic hormone, or vasopressin. Several diseases that are especially prevalent in older people are associated with high levels of antidiuretic hormone, including cancer, lung disease, and nervous system disease. High levels of this hormone seem to keep the kidney from letting excess amounts of water in the body pass on to the bladder so that it can be excreted as urine. Thus, the extra water that cannot be eliminated dilutes the amount of sodium in the blood. This hormonal action can cause the urine to appear dark and concentrated. Furthermore, some drugs can cause low sodium in the blood, either by increasing the amount of antidiuretic hormone or by enhancing its action on the kidney.

Generally, the physician's approach to sorting out the causes of low sodium in the blood depend upon first confirming that the sodium is in fact low, and not just reduced because of very high blood sugar, fats, or proteins. The next step depends upon whether the person appears to be dehydrated, normally hydrated, or overhydrated. If the person is dehydrated, then the physician would look further for conditions that might cause loss of sodium and fluid from the gastrointestinal tract, skin, lungs, kidneys, or other sources. A person with a normal amount of fluid volume but a low sodium in the blood could have such conditions as kidney disease, severe loss of potassium, thyroid gland disease, adrenal gland disease, or be drinking too much water. People who have low sodium in the blood but who have an excess fluid volume usually have swelling in the skin, especially in the legs and feet. Conditions to consider in this situation include congestive heart failure, liver disease, and kidney disease.

The outlook for people with a low sodium depends upon many things, particularly the presence of any associated diseases, how rapidly the low sodium condition came about, and how low the level is. A low sodium level often reflects a serious problem because it occurs in advanced disease states. For example, people may develop a low sodium when they have significant heart, liver, or lung disease, or cancer that has spread widely. For people in the hospital, it means a poor outlook and a sevenfold increase in death.

Diuretic medications are one of the most common causes of a low sodium. Many people on diuretics become mildly dehydrated, with losses of potassium and magnesium. Apparently, the fluid loss caused by diuretics results in very high releases of antidiuretic hormone. This hormone and an increased sensation of thirst, which leads to drinking more and more water, combined with the inability to get rid of the extra water (because of the antidiuretic effects of the hormone on the kidney) causes the concentration of sodium to fall. Such a sequence of events frequently occurs in people who are hospitalized and given extra water by intravenous fluids.

The treatment of mild to moderate degrees of sodium loss involves restricting water to less than a liter per day, discontinuing any drugs that could aggravate the problem and treating underlying diseases. Severe symptoms include lethargy, seizures, coma, or other neurologic deficits, and require more aggressive treatment. Any treatment for sodium loss, particularly when a case is severe, should be given under the supervision of a physician because significant brain damage can occur if the sodium is corrected too rapidly.

An Elevated Sodium in the Blood

An elevated sodium in the blood is usually caused by defects in the body's ability to conserve water. This can occur through illnesses, immobility, and a reduced capacity to feel thirst—all common problems in elderly people. A high blood sodium level is also a marker of serious illness and carries a high death rate. As with the low sodium in the blood, if the adjustment of the sodium level is made too rapidly, it can cause serious deterioration of the central nervous system. Treatment of this disorder should be done under a physician's supervision and usually requires intravenous fluids.

Potassium Imbalance

Approximately 15 percent of hospitalized men over the age of 70 have a high potassium level in the blood. In many cases this is due to decreased excretion of potassium through the urine. This decrease in secretion is partly due to changes in kidney hormones aggravated by long-standing kidney disease and partly by diseases or treatments that inhibit potassium excretion, for example, many nonsteroidal anti-inflammatory drugs (NSAIDs).

A low potassium level in the blood is commonly due to gastrointestinal disease or the use of diuretics (fluid pills). Low potassium can produce serious heartbeat irregularities, especially in people who have underlying heart problems. Sometimes a low potassium level is also associated with a low magnesium level in the blood. The low potassium cannot be corrected until the magnesium deficit has been resolved.

Diabetes Mellitus

Diabetes mellitus (from the Greek and Latin, meaning "honey sweet siphon") refers to problems in regulating the blood sugar, and is usually identified by a high level of glucose in the blood.

The prevalence of diabetes mellitus increases with age. It is present in approximately 8 percent of people 65 and older and increases to 25 percent in those older than age 85. Usually, people in these older age groups have what is called Type 2 or non-insulin-dependent diabetes. This means that the problem is not due to the complete lack of insulin (Type 1 diabetes) but rather a relative unresponsiveness to normal or even high amounts of insulin.

Without a blood test, diabetes can be difficult to identify. People with diabetes mellitus usually have vague complaints of slowly resolving infections, weight loss, fatigue, weakness, loss of vitality, or neurologic changes such as numbness or tingling in their feet, acute confusion, or depression. In contrast to younger people, older people do not generally show increasing urination or fluid intake because both the kidney function and the thirst response tend to decline with age. In addition, glucose may not appear in the urine until the blood sugar reaches very high levels.

Symptoms of Diabetes Mellitus

Older people with diabetes are subject to all of the complications of advanced diabetes: cardiovascular disease, eye problems, problems of the nervous system, and kidney disease. Older people may be at greater risk for certain complications such as blood vessel disease in the eye and neurological changes. These nervous system changes can cause impotence, difficulty with the muscles that control the eyes, painful nerves in the arms and legs, and problems with bowel function. Some studies suggest that poor control of diabetes can cause abnormalities of mental function in older people.

The degree to which blood sugar levels must be controlled in older people is still a matter of controversy. Obviously the treatment for diabetes is directed toward decreasing the symptoms and reducing the chance of infections, coma, and other disorders caused by having too high a blood sugar. It is also very important to avoid having too low a blood sugar (a condition called hypoglycemia) because older people tolerate low blood sugar levels very poorly. The strategy for treatment is aimed, moreover, at controlling other risk factors for blood vessel disease such as smoking and high blood pressure, each of which seems to accelerate the complications of diabetes. Some medications, such as diuretics and corticosteroids, can increase the blood sugar, making it more difficult to keep it at

Treatment of Diabetes Mellitus

an appropriate level. Chronic conditions such as arthritis, decreased vision, and poor teeth may affect the person's ability to modify diet or exercise regimens.

As with younger people, the treatment for older people generally involves changing the diet. If the person is overweight, a loss of 10 to 15 pounds may improve the blood sugar control significantly. About half of the total calories in a diabetic person's diet should come from complex carbohydrates such as cereals, grains, pasta, and breads; less than 30 percent of the calories should come from fat (with an increase in polyunsaturated fats and a decrease in saturated fats), and the rest should come from protein. The diet should also be high in fiber. Despite its appeal, diet therapy is successful in only 10 to 20 percent of people. The next step in treating diabetes involves an exercise program tailored to the individual. Walking for about 20 to 30 minutes three times a week significantly improves the body's ability to utilize glucose.

If, after several weeks of conservative treatment the levels of fasting blood sugars continue to be high, oral medications are often recommended but their use is controversial. From what is known, these medications work by increasing the amount of insulin produced by the pancreas and by changing the body's receptors for insulin to make them more plentiful and more sensitive to stimulation. Medications that stay in the body for less than a day are preferred and reduce the chance of the blood sugar dropping too low. These oral medications do not appear to have an increased effect with increased dosage; thus, if an initial trial of treatment is not effective, the drug is unlikely to work.

The physician will most likely suggest insulin treatment if the levels of blood sugar remain high or are high initially, or if adequate control has not been achieved on oral medications. Usually the initial dose of insulin is low (about 15 units of an intermediate-acting insulin) as a once-a-day injection before breakfast. Older people often do not show early symptoms of a very low blood sugar. Because of this, blood sugar levels must be checked on an empty stomach, after eating, and at bedtime to be sure that no severe drops occur. Older people and care providers should learn how to use a simple machine to check blood glucose. The blood sugar should be checked every week even if the levels have stabilized.

Coma resulting from a very high blood sugar (hyperglycemic coma) is a complication of diabetes that is observed almost exclusively in older people. Blood sugar levels rise because of an age-related reduction in kidney function (which limits the kidneys' ability to excrete glucose in the urine) and an inability to feel thirst, which causes a progressive dehydration. The rising glucose in the face of dehydration increases the thickness of the blood, making it more like molasses. About one-third of people suffering a hyperglycemic coma have no previous history of diabetes. The situation may be precipitated by a sudden illness, particularly an infection, or by certain medications. People who are susceptible to hyperglycemic coma often show signs of physical weakness, lethargy, agitation, a sudden change in their mental function, or coma. Changes in the nervous system can be pronounced and can even mimic a stroke. Significant dehydration and kidney failure are usually also present.

The goal of treatment for this sort of coma is to replace the fluids that have been lost, thereby restoring blood volume and reducing the blood viscosity. This is normally done over a period of two days. Very small amounts of insulin may also be given. A search for the underlying cause leading up to the coma such as pneumonia or a heart attack is conducted while treatment begins for the dehydration and increased blood sugar. The changes in body chemistry may improve in one to two days, but changes in mental function, including confusion and agitation, may persist for several weeks. People are usually discharged from the hospital without the need for ongoing insulin treatment, although they are at risk for a recurrence of hyperglycemia and need to be followed carefully.

Heat Stroke

Heat stroke is a medical emergency characterized by high fever, no sweating, and severe nervous system problems.

Causes of Heat Stroke

In elderly people, heat stroke occurs because normal body heat is not effectively dissipated. A person's perception of heat decreases with advancing age. Furthermore, the older person's thirst mechanism is less likely to sense and respond to fluid loss, increasing the chance of dehydration. Other factors that predispose people to heat stroke include cardiovascular diseases, neurologic disorders, medications, and extreme old age.

439

Symptoms of Heat Stroke

The older person with heat stroke has a change in mental function, high temperature, rapid heart rate, rapid breathing, and low blood pressure. The death rate is very high (around 10 percent) and emergency medical attention is required.

Treatment of Heat Stroke

The treatment for heat stroke involves cooling the body as rapidly as possible using ice water or other appropriate measures and replacing fluids.

Older people taking psychotropic (neuroleptic) medicines may develop a very high body temperature (over 104°F), called the malignant neuroleptic syndrome. Fortunately this condition is uncommon and usually appears within the first month of therapy. In addition to the very high temperature, the person may have muscle rigidity, mental status changes, and extreme fluctuation in blood pressure and heart rate. Treatment requires stopping the neuroleptic drug and providing basic support. The death rate approaches 25 percent.

Hypothermia

Hypothermia is a medical emergency in which body temperature decreases to below 95°F. As might be expected, hypothermia is more common during the winter months and in colder climates.

Causes of Hypothermia

Older people are more likely to experience abnormal regulation of body temperature. The body's energy production is lower, as is heat produced by muscle activity, in part because of decreased muscle bulk. In addition, blood vessels in the skin of the older person are less able to constrict as a heat-conserving response. The perception of a drop in room temperature as well as body temperature becomes less acute with age, and the body's shivering response is blunted—these conditions reduce a person's awareness of a need to take self-protective measures.

Numerous other commonly occurring diseases also predispose older people to having a low body temperature. These conditions include thyroid disease, previous stroke, Parkinson's disease, diabetes mellitus, congestive heart failure, malnutrition, and septicemia and are discussed separately in other parts of this book. The use of alcohol and other drugs can diminish the body's ability to maintain a normal temperature. In people over the age of 75 the risk of death due to hypothermia is five times that of younger people.

The older person with hypothermia does not complain of being cold. One should suspect hypothermia when the older person wearing thin clothing does not appear to be cold especially if the temperature is low and other people feel cold. The skin is cold and the face is often pale and puffy. Mottled red and purple skin discoloration is often seen. Obviously, adding more clothing or blankets is appropriate. Rectal thermometers are used to measure core body temperature; a body temperature less than 95°F defines hypothermia.

Symptoms of Hypothermia

Management of any underlying medical conditions is critical to recovery. Active rewarming with inhaled heated mist is safe and can easily be instituted in a hospital emergency room. This is an urgent situation and medical supervision is necessary.

Treatment of Hypothermia

While various age-related changes do compromise the body's ability to resist and control infectious organisms, there is disagreement among experts as to whether aging alone weakens the body's resistance. Other factors that increase the likelihood of infections in older as well as younger people include underlying diseases, hospitalization, stress, poor nutritional status, drug treatment, and complications of medical therapies. These factors are, however, more significant in older people.

Infections (General)

The skin and mucous membranes are important barriers to infection. Microorganisms are always present on the skin and mucous membranes, but their activity varies according to the degree of dryness, the amount of acid on the surface, sweat gland secretions, and the presence of normal skin bacteria that help reduce the number of pathogens. Some of these barrier and antimicrobial properties of the skin may be impaired with age. In addition, certain skin conditions that predispose to infection, for example, pressure ulcers and blisters, are common in older people.

Barrier Defenses

The mucous membrane surfaces that form the lining of the

respiratory tract, gastrointestinal tract, and urinary system help prevent infection by trapping organisms in mucous secretions and removing them by transporting this mucous to a body opening where they are eliminated in sputum, urine, or vaginal discharge. Changes with aging may reduce the functioning of these barriers, thereby allowing increased numbers of potentially infectious bacteria to collect on the skin and mucous membranes. The mechanisms that keep bacteria from attaching to these surfaces may become less effective in older people due to changes in body hormones, such as decreased estrogen, and a decrease in the antibodies that attack the proteins used by bacteria to attach themselves to body surfaces.

Physical and Mechanical Defenses

Difficulty in swallowing, a common age-related change, predisposes older people to aspiration (see Chapter 21), which is a common cause of pneumonia. Aspiration together with the slowing of the mucous-transporting apparatus means that less material is cleared out of the lungs and airways. In addition, an older person may not be able to cough as vigorously as before. Changes in the breathing structures in the lungs, especially the collapse of small airways and the loss of lung elasticity, also increase the likelihood of infection.

Changes in the digestive system, such as reductions in the amount of gastric acid produced or reduced contractions throughout the bowel, alter the bacteria living in the gastrointestinal tract. Little pouches protruding from the wall of the lower intestine, called diverticula, can become inflamed when bacteria grow inside them. Changes in the urinary tract can produce any of the following: alterations in the composition of the urine; decreased prostatic fluid with reduced bacterial activity; a diminished flushing mechanism of the bladder; reflux of material from the bladder toward the kidney; and the potential for obstruction to urine flow by a prostate enlargement, displacement of urinary structures, narrowings of the urinary canals, or stones.

Changes in the Immune System with Age

The age-related change in the immune system may explain some of the increased likelihood of infections, tumors, and blood vessel and immune diseases in older people. Older bodies are less able to produce the substances collectively called antibodies necessary to fight infection. Older people show less vigorous reactions to chemicals injected into the skin to check for previous infection (skin test reactions) suggesting that the response is impaired and that immunological memory of previous exposures may be affected.

Three basic principles help an older person or that person's caregiver to suspect and recognize infection in the older person. First, infection may cause an unexplained and rapid decline in ability to function or in a sense of well-being. Second, serious infections will generally produce a fever. Any elevated temperature in an older person requires very careful evaluation. Finally, up to 20 to 30 percent of older people can have serious infections such as pneumonia, urinary tract infections, an abscess in the abdomen, or tuberculosis without manifesting fever.

Identifying Infection in an Older Person

While any bacteria, given the right conditions, can cause an infection, different patterns of infection are seen in different settings. Recognition of these patterns can be helpful in identifying the probable source of the infection, especially in people with non-specific symptoms.

In relatively healthy, functionally independent older people who live in the community, the most frequently seen infections are respiratory (influenza, bronchitis, and pneumonia), as well as urinary tract infections and intraabdominal infections (bladder infections, diverticulitis, appendicitis).

For people in the hospital, the major infections include urinary tract infection, which is often related to use of a catheter; pneumonia caused by aspiration; and skin and soft tissue infections such as infected pressure ulcers and postoperative wounds. Blood clots in the lungs and medications are also sources of fever in hospitalized older people.

When older people living in a nursing home are transferred to the hospital, it is usually because of fever or suspected infection. Pneumonia, urinary tract infection, and skin or soft tissue infection account for 70 to 80 percent of proven infections in this situation. Tuberculosis or infectious diarrhea should also be considered when an older person living in a nursing home appears to have an infection.

Treatment of Infections in General

The greatest overall reduction in human suffering and death has resulted from the treatment of infectious diseases. Sulfonamides, sulfur-containing drugs, were introduced into medical practice in the 1930s, quickly followed by penicillin in the 1940s. Since then, hundreds of chemical compounds have become available to treat a wide variety of viral, bacterial, fungal, and parasitic infections. These compounds are called antibiotics (from the Greek, meaning "destructive of life"). Antibiotics work by inhibiting the growth of the infecting organism. Somewhat surprisingly, they generally do not seriously damage normal body cells despite significantly destroying invading microorganisms.

Loss of Vitality

The severe loss of vitality in an older person represents a breakdown in overall biological and social function leading ultimately to institutionalization and death. Older people with this condition are typically frail and have difficulty in maintaining their independence. Clinically, loss of vitality shows itself as unintentional weight loss. The combination of severe weight loss along with various metabolic abnormalities on blood tests is sometimes called cachexia (from the Latin, "bad condition"). Both loss of vitality and cachexia impair body defenses and increase the susceptibility to the development of pressure ulcers.

Risk Factors for Loss of Vitality

Factors associated with increased mortality are low weight, diminished muscle mass, and physical weakness. Anemia and a low cholesterol in the blood are metabolic risk factors for death in elderly men living in nursing homes. Also well documented is the extreme decline in both physical function and the ability to conduct basic daily activities before death. The last activity to be lost is the ability to eat without assistance. People who require help with eating have an increased death rate. In addition, the loss of social interactions prior to death has been noted. Interestingly, there does not appear to be any precipitous decline in psychologic well-being immediately before death. As one might expect, loss of vitality frequently precedes institutionalization. The increase in risk factors that lead to institutionalization—decline in physical function, psychologic function, and social abilities—is significant but varies widely in individual circumstances.

Table 44. Causes of Loss of Vitality in Older People

MEDICAL	PSYCHOLOGIC	FUNCTIONAL	SOCIAL
Cancer	Depression	Immobility (e.g., disuse or arthritis)	Isolation
Endocrine disease (e.g., diabetes or hypothyroidism)	Dementia	Deafness	Poverty
	Psychosis		Caregiver fatigue
Organ failure (e.g., cardiac, hepatic, or renal)	Grief	Blindness	Neglect
	Intentional loss of vitality	Dental problems	Abuse
Infection			
Inflammation			
Neurologic disease (e.g., stroke or parkinsonism)			

In general, the diseases that lead to progressive weight loss, weakness, and, ultimately, loss of vitality are the same for people of all ages. These include cancer, heart failure, liver disease, and renal failure. Malignancies can lead to significant wasting of the body before they are discovered. Chronic infections can cause loss of vitality with very few other symptoms. The poor absorption of nutrients due to gastrointestinal disease can also reduce vitality.

Sensory conditions such as the loss of smell and problems with taste can lead to a loss of interest in foods. Loss of smell may be temporary if caused by an upper respiratory infection, and taste abnormalities are occasionally caused by reversible nutrient deficiencies such as zinc deficiency. Taste abnormalities can also be caused by medications including heart medicines and drugs used to treat psychiatric conditions. Adverse drug reactions are a common cause of loss of vitality in elderly people.

Difficulties in function can limit a person's ability to obtain food, cook it, or eat it. With advancing age, common conditions such as arthritis may affect both physical and social functions and are major sources of disability. Difficulties with hearing and vision can also produce progressive disability and social dysfunction. For example,

Causes of Loss of Vitality

Table 45. Treatment of Loss of Vitality in Older People

MEDICAL	PSYCHOLOGIC	FUNCTIONAL	SOCIAL
Disease-specific treatment	Counseling	Occupational therapy	Meals on Wheels
Visiting nursesPhysician visits	Support groups	Physical therapy	Support groups
	Drugs (e.g., antipsychotics, tricyclics)	Home health aids	Home health aids
	ECT*	Hearing aids	Assisted living
		Vision aids	Respite care
		Dentures	Nursing homes

*ECT, electroconvulsive therapy.

they can limit the use of the telephone or automobile. All of these difficulties are compounded by social isolation and lack of community support. A major cause of loss of vitality is the increased disability due to simultaneous difficulties in many areas; for example, the combination of arthritis, hearing difficulty, and declining social support. Finally, even when food is available, problems with the teeth or dentures, a very dry mouth, or problems with swallowing can interfere with food intake.

Psychologic problems such as dementing illness, depression, and prolonged grief reaction can be especially devastating in the elderly. Serious depression and other psychiatric problems can occur. In some cases, when an older person appears to give up, loss of vitality may be intentional.

A related problem that can result in loss of vitality is known as caregiver fatigue, which is caused by emotional and physical burnout. Poverty and isolation are other possibly reversible causes of loss of vitality.

Treatment of Loss of Vitality

A goal of effective care for older people consists of identifying and treating reversible causes of loss of vitality (see Tables 44 and 45). If they are not treated early, the condition can progress to such an extent that an irreversible loss of muscle mass occurs. As mentioned, this malnourished state is called cachexia. During the progression from loss of vitality to cachexia, people may demonstrate continued decline toward death. Elderly people in this situation are very vulnerable to acute events such as infections or falls. An acute event can then trigger further problems such as severe malnutrition or pressure ulcers, and these in turn can stimulate further declines in function propelling a vicious cycle that culminates in death. For an elderly person with the loss of vitality syndrome, a minor accident such as a fall can lead to death.

A key aspect of therapy is to have counseling on end-of-life decisions. Frank discussions between family members, your doctor, a religious counselor, and others can explore treatment preferences and alternatives. It is very important for as many caring people as possible to be clear about your wishes for care. (Chapter 11 contains more information on ethical issues and ways to make sure your decisions are respected if you can no longer participate in the decision-making process.)

Use of multiple medications, known as polypharmacy, places older people at increased risk of adverse drug reactions. (See Chapter 9 for additional information on adverse drug reactions.) The average older American uses 5 prescription medicines at any given time and fills from 12 to 17 prescriptions each year. Although comprising between 12 and 13 percent of the population, older Americans use over 25 percent of all prescription drugs. In addition, they use an average of 3½ over-the-counter medications. Frail older people tend to consume even more medicines. The average person in the nursing home takes more than 8 medications. In the nursing home setting, there is a particularly frequent use of medications that commonly lead to side effects, such as digitalis, diuretics, and drugs that affect the nervous system. The cost of prescription medications used by older people is well over $10 billion a year.

Medication Problems (Polypharmacy)

Older people are particularly vulnerable to adverse drug reactions because of the changes that occur with normal aging. Adverse drug reactions (ADRs) are defined as the development of unwanted symptoms, changes in blood or other tests taken, or death directly related to the use of a medication. The number of ADRs increases with the number of medications used and with the increasing age of the person (see Figure 46 and Table 46). Some studies suggest that there is no independent age effect on the rate of adverse reactions and that the risk of ADR may be increased in older people simply because of an increased prevalence of overall risk factors. In other words, adverse reactions probably occur more often in older people because they take more medicines, they have more illnesses, their illnesses are more severe, and there are changes in their bodies that affect the way medications are absorbed and eliminated.

Drugs that are used concurrently may interact with each other and these drug-on-drug interactions may have clinically significant consequences. One drug may either cause another to act more powerfully or may inhibit its action. Because of this, a sudden toxic reaction can develop when a seemingly safe medication is added to the medical regimen of a person who has been using another medication for a long time without any problems. For example, a person who has been taking stable doses of drug X may have a toxic reaction when given drug Y, if drug Y disrupts the metabolism of drug X. Even without changing the dosage level of a drug, drug-on-drug interactions can alter the effectiveness of a drug. For example,

Figure 46. Adverse Drug Reactions Increase with Age

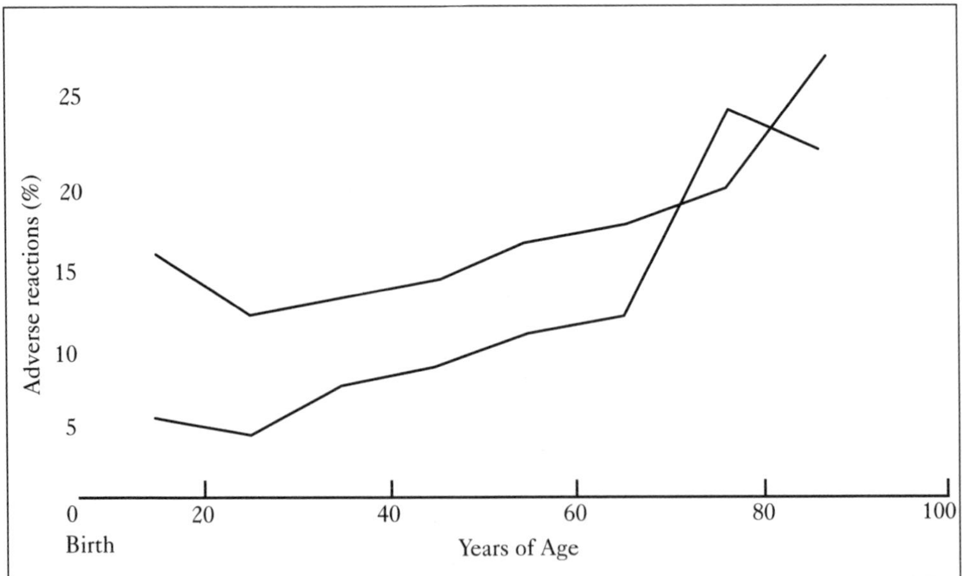

Source: Redrawn from Medication for the elderly. A report of the Royal College of Physicians. *The Journal of the Royal College of Physicians of London*. 1984:18(a):8. Reprinted with permission.

Table 46. Number of Drugs Used and Relationship to Adverse Reactions

NUMBER OF MEDICATIONS USED IN 1 YEAR	PERSONS WITH ADVERSE REACTIONS, %
1–2	2
3–5	7
6–10	13
>10	17

Source: Adapted from Hutchinson TA, Flegel KM, Kramer MS, et al. Frequency, severity and risk factors for adverse drug reactions in adult out-patients: a perspective study. *Journal of Chronic Diseases*. 1986:39(7):537. Reprinted with permission.

some antidepressant medications may inhibit the effect of certain drugs (like clonidine) given for high blood pressure.

Older people are at increased risk for what might be called a drug-disease interaction. This occurs when medications that are useful in treating one illness exacerbate another illness. For example, an older person given eyedrops for glaucoma may faint because of a preexisting heart disease. This happens because the eyedrops are absorbed into the body and cause the already susceptible heart to beat slower. Similarly, an older man with an enlarged prostate who is given an antihistamine for an allergic reaction may have difficulty urinating. Antihistamines inhibit nerve response in this case, making it difficult to pass the urine through the prostatic obstruction.

How Much Medication Is Enough and How Much Is Too Much?

Paradoxically, the increased prevalence of disease that makes the use of medications riskier in older people may also require that they use more medications. Because of this potentially vicious cycle, a concept of appropriateness of medication use has been developed among medical professionals. By the most commonly used clinical definition, the use of a medication is appropriate if its benefits significantly outweigh its potential risks. This means that medications may be correctly used, overused, underused, or misused. Medication is overused if it is prescribed without a good reason for doing so, underused if it is not prescribed when its use could be helpful, and misused if its use is appropriate but it is prescribed in an incorrect dose or for too short (or too long) a time, or in some other way that involves unnecessary risk.

By definition, inappropriate use of medications is associated with increased risk. An estimated 10 to 17 percent of hospital admissions for older people is directly attributable to inappropriate medication use. Older people break their hips twice as often while under the influence of some medications, such as long-acting benzodiazepines or drugs used to treat psychiatric conditions. One in 1,000 older people who are hospitalized dies because of the side effects of medications. As for underuse, it has been estimated that increasing the percentage of older people who are vaccinated against influenza to 50 percent would prevent more than 3,000 deaths each year. Clearly, inappropriate use of medication is a major health problem that could be avoided.

Compliance with Medications

Compliance means that the patient follows the physician's instructions. Noncompliance with prescriptions is a problem in all age groups and does not appear to increase with age. Noncompliance increases with the number of medications a person uses and is a common problem in elderly people because they use more prescription medications. Sometimes there may be good reasons to not always follow a physician's advice, such as the appearance of a side effect or an error in prescribing.

Nearly one in five people fails to fill a prescription. In addition, between 30 and 60 percent of those who do fill a prescription use the medication differently from the way it was prescribed. As a result, about half of all prescriptions fail to produce the desired effect.

Some of the factors that affect compliance are shown in Table 47. People are more likely to comply with treatment if they believe that their condition is serious, that they might be susceptible to disease, or that the medication prescribed is effective in treating or preventing the disease. When noncompliance is a concern, the reasons need to be explored. For example, the person might have stopped taking the medication because of toxicity or adverse side effects. Methods of improving compliance include clarifying written and verbal instructions about the purpose and use of the medications, reducing the number of medications to be taken, simplifying the

Table 47. Factors Influencing Compliance

FACTOR	EFFECT ON COMPLIANCE*
Belief by patients that the disease to be treated is serious	Increase
Belief by patients that the medication will treat or prevent the disease	Increase
Belief by patients that they are likely to have or develop the disease	Increase
Careful explanation by doctor for the purpose of the medication	Increase
Increased number of drugs used	Decrease
Belief by patients that the medication will cause toxicity	Decrease
Long duration of therapy	Decrease
Complex scheduling	Decrease
Safety-closure bottles	Decrease

*Age, gender, ethnicity, educational level, financial status, the actual severity of the diseases, and the actual toxicity of the drug do not seem to have an effect on compliance.

Source: Adapted from Stewart RB, Caranasos GJ. Medication compliance in the elderly. *Medical Clinics of North America*. 1989;73:1551–63. Reprinted with permission.

dosage schedules, and providing devices that make accurate self-administration more likely. On the other hand, long-term treatment, complex scheduling, increasing the number of medicines, and difficult-to-open containers, as well as the person's perception that the medication may cause side effects, reduce compliance.

Why a Person May Be Taking Too Many Drugs

More than 60 percent of all visits to physicians conclude with the physician writing out a prescription. Half of all visits to an emergency room result in a prescription being given for at least one medicine. Moreover, by the time older people are discharged from the hospital, half of their medications have been replaced with new ones. Medications proved to be ineffective for some diseases, such as Alzheimer's disease, are still frequently prescribed.

Many physicians are reluctant to stop medications, especially if the medications have been used for a long period of time and the person is clinically stable. Even when physicians cannot determine whether the use of a medication was appropriate or whether the conditions that indicated its use continue to exist, they may fear that stopping the medication will precipitate problems.

Another way people end up taking too many medications is that they often see more than one physician. While some consulting physicians communicate directly with the referring physician, others typically prescribe for and advise patients directly. Furthermore, communication with the referring physicians is often imperfect, or people may seek consultations without informing their primary physician. People often fail to tell their primary physicians about medications that have been added to their regimen by other doctors. The discharge process from hospitals may also contribute to a person's taking too many medications since the medications that are routinely ordered in the hospital, such as sedatives, laxatives, and pain relievers are often continued unnecessarily when the patient is discharged. Discharged patients are sometimes not given adequate instructions about the adjustments they should follow in their medication regimen.

Finally, physicians are sometimes hampered by the inadequacy of their own records, because outpatient medical records may not contain accurate information on medication use. Even in the hospital and nursing home, where record keeping about current medications is usually accurate, a medical record is generally an unreliable source of information about medications a person may have used in the past or about a person's history of allergic and adverse reactions to drugs, or failure to recover from a disease treated with medications.

Strategies to Decrease Polypharmacy

Clearly, physicians must keep accurate records of medication use as a basic medical responsibility. The medication listing must be updated at regular intervals so that medications prescribed by other physicians can be added to the list, ineffective medications can be stopped, and misunderstandings about how the medication should be taken can be detected and corrected. With medications used on a long-term basis it is important to review periodically whether they are still necessary, whether all medications currently being used are the safest and most effective ones available, and whether published evidence and expert medical opinion continues to support the use of each medicine. The older person's physician should not be complacent about continuing unnecessary medications since these may pose risks.

Any medication may cause side effects in older people, but certain drugs are more likely than others to cause problems. Examples of those that are best avoided are the long-lasting benzodiazepines and medications that powerfully affect the nervous system. If, for example, there is a need for these particular medications, safer alternatives are almost always available. A physician should prescribe other medications with extreme caution after taking note of any age-related body changes. (See Chapter 9 for more on age-related changes in the body's handling of medications.) Many physicians are not aware of these age-related changes.

Keeping up with all the newly released drugs can overwhelm even the most studious physician. Pharmacists can be very helpful on advising both physicians and patients on the advantages and disadvantages of specific preparations, dose adjustments, drug-on-drug and drug-disease interactions, and side effects. Pharmacy consultation and review is generally available for care in the hospital and mandated for care in the nursing homes. Pharmacists should package all medications in suitable containers that bear adequate instructions written in a type size that older people can read, and they should explain verbally how to take the medicine.

Some pharmacists provide written information to older people when prescriptions are filled. It is likely that these developments will increase with advances in computer technology.

Pain

Unrelieved pain is one of the most common complaints among older people. Between 25 and 50 percent of elderly people have significant pain. Among people living in nursing homes, the proportion may be between 45 and 80 percent. Pain causes depression, decreased socializaion, sleep disturbances, impaired walking, increased usage of health services, and increased medical costs. Although less thoroughly explored, pain may also affect specific arthritis complaints, balance and gait disturbances, falls, lack of progress with rehabilitation, taking too many medications, cognitive dysfunction, and malnutrition. Moreover, pain and its management carry significant implications for quality of life, especially with regard to people with terminal illness and people who live in nursing homes.

Causes of Pain   The most common cause of pain appears to be arthritis and other muscle and bone conditions. Malignancy is also a common cause. One-third of people with active cancer and two-thirds with advanced cancer suffer significant pain. Shingles (herpes zoster), poor circulation, and inflammatory disease involving the blood vessels are some other specific pain syndromes that are known to affect older people in disproportionate numbers.

Theories that view pain as a simple sensation have long been abandoned, and pain is now recognized as a very complex sensory experience modified by a person's memory, expectations, and emotions. A number of anatomical and biochemical findings support what is known as the "gate control" theory of pain. This theory postulates that sensory information can be inhibited in the spinal cord. Although it seems to apply to pain in the body, the theory may not apply to pain that originates within the central nervous system. Two types of sensory information are relayed from the spinal cord to the brain. A fast track relays information directly to the brain about the location and quality of the pain, such as sharp, severe, and sudden. A slow track relating to the emotional qualities of pain is thought to produce such descriptors as "burning," "frightening," or "cruel." There is also a neural system to inhibit pain that influences pain transmission at the spinal cord level. This system, which descends from the midbrain to the spinal cord, appears to be very important in modulation of pain sensation.

The extremely complicated interaction of these systems may explain the diverse nature of pain perception and responses to various treatments such as opiates (narcotics), antidepressants, transcutaneous nerve stimulation therapy, acupuncture, and placebo effects.

Pain is usually characterized as acute or chronic. Acute pain, defined by its distinct onset and relatively short duration, usually occurs with some additional symptoms within the nervous system: fast heart rate, sweating, or a sudden elevation in blood pressure. Such symptoms imply the existence of an endangering injury. Chronic pain, which usually has a duration of more than three months, ordinarily does not occur with such neurologic symptoms and is often strong or intensely felt out of proportion to any indications of immediate danger. Chronic pain occurs with long-standing functional and psychological impairment.

Pain is such an individual experience that it usually requires a multidimensional approach to its assessment. To ensure an accurate assessment, physical, functional, and psychological evaluations should be combined, beginning with a thorough interview and physical exam. The interview generally establishes the presence of any medical conditions and provides a description of the experience of pain. Factors that worsen or relieve the pain are explored, including any physical or social limitations. For a person with chronic pain, sudden changes in the character of the pain may indicate deterioration in the condition or a new injury. These need careful evaluation. In addition, many different pain-producing conditions may coexist in any given person, especially in the context of malignancy. Each condition may require a different treatment approach.

Older people may underreport symptoms because they think the pain is caused by aging and progression of their disease. People who have cancer may not report pain because they are afraid of what the pain may mean or they may feel that it cannot be relieved. Elderly people often have multiple illnesses, and care must be taken to avoid attributing acute pain too quickly to some preexisting illness. What makes finding the cause even more challenging is that chronic pain is often variable, and that both the character and intensity of pain may fluctuate.

Functional impairment is an important guide for pain management in older people. Impairment in advanced activities of daily living such as psychosocial functions (social role, hobbies, recreation, etc.) may correlate with the presence and severity of pain. The information gained from the interview and physical examination can be useful in assessing the person's functional capacities.

The Evaluation of Pain

Figure 47. Pain-Intensity Scale

PAIN DESCRIPTOR SCALE

VISUAL ANALOGUE SCALE

0 No Pain

1 Mild

├────────────────┤
No pain   Worst pain

2 Distressing

3 Severe

Make a mark on the line
for the severity of your pain.

4 Horrible

5 Excruciating

Source: Ferrell BA. Pain management in elderly patients. *Journal of the American Geriatrics Society.* 1991;39:67.
Reprinted with permission.

A psychologic assessment is also conducted as part of the evaluation. Most people with chronic pain have significant symptoms of depression or anxiety and may benefit dramatically from psychologic or psychiatric intervention. Various pain assessment scales have been developed to help both doctors and researchers more accurately measure and document pain experiences (see Figure 47).

Records such as a pain diary provide the physician with a description of the person's individual pain experience and can be particularly useful in determining pain management. In people with cognitive impairment, body language such as facial grimaces and agitation may be important behavioral cues indicative of pain. Specific pain-rating scales such as numerical or verbal descriptor scales quantify the intensity of the person's pain and assess pain at a particular moment—for example, in response to therapy.

General Pain Management

In the past 15 to 20 years, pain management has become very sophisticated, with specialized pain centers, multidisciplinary teams, and the development of high-technology pain management applications. Pain management may involve special problems for older people, but very few studies describe management techniques specifically for elderly individuals. For the most part, pain management strategies have been based upon studies of younger people and people with pain caused by malignancy.

Initially, the control of most acute pain relies on the treatment of the underlying disease and on short-term administration of pain relievers. Chronic pain, however, usually requires a multidimensional approach consisting of various behavioral and coping strategies as well as pain relievers and other drugs.

Drug treatment alone is usually not effective in chronic pain management. A combination of drug and nondrug techniques usually results in more effective pain control, with less reliance on medications that can produce major side effects in elderly people. The possible side effects of many pain-relieving drugs cannot be overstated. In general, people with pain caused by malignancy respond well to the constant administration of opiate (narcotic) pain relievers. The long-term use of these analgesics (pain relievers) remains controversial in the management of chronic pain not due to malignancy. Analgesics should be reserved for more severe pain that is unrelieved by other approaches. It should also be remembered that pain caused by nerve irritation, such as that resulting from shingles (herpes zoster), diabetes mellitus, and stroke, may respond to antidepressants or anticonvulsant medications.

Pain-Relieving Drugs in Older People

Oral or injectable pain-relieving medicines, the most common treatments for pain, fall into two broad categories: nonsteroidal anti-inflammatory drugs (NSAIDs) and narcotics. NSAIDs affect pain indirectly by blocking a class of compounds called prostaglandins that appear to be mediators in the pain process. They provide specific relief for inflammatory conditions that stimulate pain. These drugs have a pain-relieving effect that is characterized by a ceiling effect; that is, a level at which increasing the dose does not result in increased pain relief. Often working well individually or in combination with narcotic analgesics, NSAIDs may be especially helpful in managing cancer pain affecting the bone. They are not generally habit-forming. However, NSAIDs have been associated with a variety of adverse effects in older people, including stomach irritation, ulcer disease, kidney problems, and the tendency to cause bleeding. Although they are usually the safest form of pain relief for mild to moderate pain, experts have begun to question their overall safety among frail, older people.

Narcotic analgesic medications act on the nervous system to decrease the perception of pain. Some of these drugs—morphine, for example—may also have anesthetic properties and are used in providing anesthesia for surgery. With no absolute upper limit of dose, narcotics have been shown to relieve many types of pain, although they appear to be much less effective in managing chronic pain due to nerve irritation, compared with managing pain from other causes. Short-term studies of pain after surgery and for cancer have shown that compared with younger people, the elderly are more sensitive to the pain-relieving properties of these drugs.

Narcotics may produce such side effects as memory disturbances, constipation, and habitual use among elderly people. Suppression of breathing does not seem to occur if the drugs are carefully increased in dose until the pain is relieved. As with most psychoactive drugs, narcotics may produce inconsistent and variable effects. However, when they are administered appropriately, the effects of narcotics remain the best understood and the most predictable. Morphine remains the standard by which all other pain relievers are compared and is the drug of choice for severe pain. The reluctance of physicians to prescribe morphine has been overly influenced by recent political and social pressure generated by the reaction to illegal drug use. One study of over 12,000 medical records found only 4 cases of narcotic dependency produced medically. Psychologic dependence does not come from the use of morphine and other narcotics that are used to relieve pain. It appears that once the pain goes away, the narcotics are no longer desired.

Such side effects of narcotics as constipation and nausea do not wear off with time, and along with other symptoms may make the overall management of pain more difficult. Because of this, it is important to begin a bowel regimen at the same time the older person is started on these narcotics; such a regimen should include increasing fluids and the use of special lubricating agents and other medications.

Antidepressants, antiepileptics (drugs that are used to control seizures), and some sedatives are sometimes used to help control certain types of chronic pain. For example, the treatment of underlying depression or mood disorders with antidepressants may enhance other pain management strategies. In addition to reducing anxiety, stress, and tension, these drugs may also help the person have a good night's sleep. Chronic pain is an exhausting experience, and most people cope better if they have adequate sleep.

Although older people are more sensitive to the pain-relieving capacity of pain relievers (and their side effects), the doses and incremental increases remain the physician's decision. In the final analysis, the best advice is, "start low and go slow."

Patient-controlled analgesia (PCA) has proven to be an effective strategy in pain management. In this approach the person sets her own dose of medication; this often balances the person's pain tolerance and the side effects more effectively. Although PCA is often used with continuous intravenous infusions of pain relievers, the concept remains valid for other pain management strategies.

Advances in pain management strategies that do not include drugs have been strongly advocated for pain relief. These techniques include transcutaneous electrical nerve stimulation (TENS), physical therapy, biofeedback, hypnosis, and distractive techniques. In individual circumstances each of these techniques can be quite effective.

Non-pharmacologic Pain Management

Transcutaneous electrical nerve stimulation has been used for a variety of older people's chronic pain conditions, such as painful nerves caused by diabetes, shoulder pain or bursitis, and for fractured ribs. Although the overall effectiveness of TENS is in doubt, some people who receive it experience relief of their symptoms. Its effectiveness often wears off after a few months, although some people have had years of pain relief. Care must be taken to avoid skin irritation and possible burns from the electrodes, especially when treating people with memory problems. (Chapter 8 has additional information about TENS units and other modalities.)

Physical methods such as heat, cold, and massage can be helpful in managing musculoskeletal pain. Many of these measures relax tense muscles and prove soothing for a variety of complaints. They can be managed by older people, thus giving them and their families a sense of control over the symptoms and the treatment. However, caution must be exercised with the prolonged use of heat or cold in older people, to avoid burns and other skin injury.

Biofeedback, relaxation, and hypnosis are some of the maneuvers that may be effective in controlling pain, although they are not as useful in people with cognitive impairment. These approaches require the skills of a trained psychologist or therapist.

Perception of pain may be decreased by a variety of distractions. Many people find comfort in music, meditation, or prayer. In general, as much involvement in activities, exercise, and recreation as the person can tolerate should be encouraged, since inactivity and immobility may contribute to depression and enhanced pain. Humor therapy also has a significant role in pain relief.

Sleep Problems

Disturbed sleep at night, sleepiness during the daytime, or both, are common complaints among older people. They are also important symptoms of the psychiatric disorders that may occur in late life, especially depression and dementing illness. Complaints of disturbed sleep are especially common among community-living elderly people who live alone, are unemployed, depressed, or bereaved. The use of sleeping medications increases steadily with advancing age, as does the likelihood of many types of sleep-related behavioral disturbances such as wandering at night, confusion, and agitated behavior. These disturbances may frustrate caregivers and may trigger a family's decision to institutionalize an older relative. Sedating medications are commonly prescribed for elderly people in the nursing home setting.

The Causes of Sleeping Difficulties

Sleeping states and sleep schedule change with age, which reflects both the aging process and the impact of any existing physical and psychiatric disorders. There are two very different states of sleep: nonrapid eye movement (NREM) sleep and rapid eye movement (REM) sleep. NREM sleep represents a quiescent brain whereas REM sleep represents an activated brain. During REM sleep, the heart rate, breathing rate, and blood pressure tend to increase compared to these values during NREM sleep. REM sleep is governed by activity in cells of one part of the brain; NREM sleep is influenced by activity in two other brain areas. The most important age-related changes in sleep include a decreased continuity of sleep with an increase in the number of arousals during sleep; a tendency for the major period of sleep to occur earlier in the night; a tendency for REM sleep also to occur earlier in the night; a decrease or a loss of the very deepest parts of NREM sleep; increased napping during the day; and a tendency to spend more time in bed. While this last tendency may be a response to poor sleep, it only seems to perpetuate the problem and make sleep quality worse. Other important age-associated changes in sleep include a decrease in the amount of growth hormone secreted and alterations in the sleep-associated secretion of other hormones.

Studies of sleep in healthy elderly people have also noted gender-related differences: Elderly men show poorer sleep maintenance than women. Paradoxically, older women are more likely than men to complain of sleep problems and to receive sleeping pills, possibly because they are more sensitive to sleep quality and sleep losses than older men. This may be especially true for the mood-disrupting effects of sleep loss.

Depression and dementing illness such as Alzheimer's disease produce characteristic changes in the way we sleep. The changes of sleep that occur with depression include a shortened time between the onset of sleep and REM sleep, various brain wave changes, and early morning awakening. Over half of people with depression experience some improvement in their symptoms after a night of sleep, but over 80 percent of these people relapse if they remain untreated after one night of sleep deprivation. Sleep in patients with Alzheimer's disease gets worse as the dementia progresses and is characterized by a more variable sleep-wake pattern, decreased eye movements in the REM stage, a normal or increased interval from the beginning of sleep to the development of REM sleep, and increased breathing problems occurring during sleep.

The body's internal clocks are called circadian rhythms, and they exert powerful effects on the regulation of sleep, particularly the temperature rhythm. The body temperature cycle is generally an accepted marker for the biological clock that seems to drive the daily cycles in REM sleep, alertness, and vigilance. Most likely, REM sleep is near the lowest level of daily temperature rhythm.

Human temperature rhythms tend to flatten out and shorten with age, and this range reduction seems to result from an increase in the daily low point. These changes influence older people's preference for earlier bedtimes and wake-up times. Sleep disturbances such as insomnia show a blunting in the body's sleep temperature rhythm.

Lifestyle changes also contribute to sleep problems that occur in old age. For example, the fact that many older people spend increased time in bed may reflect a feeling that they have little reason to get up; their opportunities for social and physical activity may be diminished. Among institutionalized older people, environmental factors such as temperature, noise, and lighting undoubtedly provide important and perhaps deleterious changes in the time cues for the regulation of sleep and wakefulness.

How Common Are Sleep Problems? As many as 30 percent of people over the age of 60 suffer from and complain of poor sleep quality on a regular basis. Interestingly, only about 1.6 percent of those over the age of 65 complain of getting too much sleep. Significant depression is much higher in people of any age who have sleeping difficulty (see Chapter 15 for more on depression). Between 20 and 25 percent of older people living in the community regularly use some form of sleeping pills. Older people frequently complain that their sleep is not refreshing and they have difficulty in maintaining sleep. Younger people are more likely to complain of difficulty in getting to sleep. As already noted, older people may also report trouble in maintaining alertness during the day, which may reflect the need for more sleep.

Sleep-related behavioral disturbances such as agitation at night, night-walking, shouting, and urinary incontinence are also important issues. The widespread prescriptions of sedative medications in nursing homes probably reflect, in part, the clinical importance of these sleep disturbances and behavioral problems. About 30 percent of the nursing home inhabitants receive medication for sleep on a regular basis.

Snoring has received the most attention among sleep behaviors. Habitual, severe snoring occurs in about 10 percent of men and about 3.5 percent of women ages 40 to 67. It seems more common in men with high blood pressure and in men with heart disease or stroke. Severe snoring is likely to reflect complete closing of the airway during sleep leading to a condition of impaired breathing called sleep apnea. Several studies have shown that sleep-disordered breathing increases with advancing age, but more commonly in men than in women. In one large community-based study, the prevalence of sleep-disordered breathing was about 25 percent. In addition, the prevalence rates were higher in men than in women, and were higher in nursing home residents and in hospitalized individuals than those who lived in the community.

Sleep disturbance is also a major debilitating reaction to bereavement and frequently persists following spousal bereavement. The importance of this sleep disturbance in late-life bereavement can be significant. It may lead not only to depression but also to self-medication with alcohol and sleeping pills.

Classification of Sleep Disorders

The two major categories of sleep disorders are the insomnias—disorders in getting to sleep and maintaining sleep—and the hypersomnias—disorders of excessive daytime sleepiness. About 40 percent of people with persistent insomnia and about 50 percent of people with hypersomnia are related to psychiatric disease.

The key symptoms are complaints of insomnia, nonrefreshing sleep, excessive daytime sleepiness, a shift in the timing of the sleep period, frequent periods of sleep and wakefulness during the day, and changes in mood, performance, and alertness as a result of these sleep changes.

Evaluation of Sleep Disorders

The person who is having sleeping problems should discuss with a physician how long these problems have been present and any likely contributing factors. Temporary disturbances lasting two to three weeks are usually determined by the specifics of the particular situation. More persistent problems, those lasting more than a month, indicate more serious, underlying medical or psychiatric conditions and require a more detailed evaluation. The person's sleep partner (if any) is usually eager to share information concerning the sleeping problem. Additionally, the person or the partner or other caregiver can keep a sleep log over a two-week period to determine the quality of sleep during the 24-hour day. The usefulness of the sleep log is improved if the information includes schedules of sleep and naps as well as social activities, information about meals, medications, and exercise. After reviewing this information a physician may recommend, among other things, an adjustment in drug use, both prescription and self-medications (alcohol and caffeine, for instance). Factors contributing to sleep disturbances in older people and possible additional problems are shown in Tables 48 and 49. Sometimes an evaluation in a sleep laboratory is recommended if the person has heavy snoring, excessive daytime sleepiness, severe muscle jerks at night, or restlessness of the legs during sleep. A sleep laboratory study can also be done if an initial attempt to treat the problem fails.

Treatment for Sleep Problems

Most older people should realize that some sleep disturbance, particularly mild insomnia, may be an unavoidable consequence of aging. The reinforcement of a regular sleep-wake schedule, together with limiting the time in bed to no more than seven or eight hours nightly, is important to counteract the age-related tendency to replace a consolidated period of sleep with a more scattered sleep-wake cycle.

Practically speaking, the older person with insomnia should be encouraged to maintain control of the sleep schedule by going to

Table 48. Factors Contributing to Sleep Disturbances in Older People

- Age-dependent decreases in the ability to sleep ("sleep decay")
- Sleep-disordered breathing (sleep apnea) and jerking of the legs
- Excess napping
- Psychiatric disorders
- Medical disorders
- A tendency to spend excessive time in bed
- Sedating medications taken during the daytime
- Inadequate lighting (too dark by day or too light at night) and excessive heat or noise
- Loneliness, inactivity, and boredom

bed only when sleepy, by getting up at the same time each morning, by reducing the time for naps to no more than 30 to 45 minutes a day, and by limiting the nightly time in bed to seven hours. In addition, the person should avoid using the bedroom for activities that are not conducive to sleep. This will serve to keep the bed as a powerful stimulus to sleep. When a person is encouraged to follow such suggestions he has an increased sense of control over the schedule and stimuli for sleep, which diminishes the need for sleeping pills. Other facets of the initial treatment approach involve reducing the amount of nicotine, alcohol, or caffeine; avoiding fluids just before bed (to lessen the need to urinate in the middle of the night); the timing of physical activity, meals, medications, and sleep periods (including naps); and removing depressant or stimulant drugs.

Regular exercise, particularly if it leads to improved fitness, may improve the quality and depth of sleep in late life. Also, a behavioral technique called sleep restriction therapy may be particularly useful among older people with insomnia. In this treatment, the

Table 49. Causes of Sleep Disturbances in Older People

- Irregular sleep-wake scheduling

- Evening self-medication, especially nicotine, alcohol, or caffeinated beverages

- Use of the bed for activities other than sleep

- Dependency on sleeping pills

- Other medication effects

- Sleeping at an earlier time in the 24-hour day

- Heavy snoring or obstructive breathing during sleep

- Feelings of restlessness in the legs

- Psychiatric disorders

- Medical disorders such as congestive heart failure or esophageal reflux person is taught to spend less time in bed at night in order to create a modest sleep deficit, which then reduces sleep fragmentation.

The cause of the sleep disorder must be determined if at all possible before an older person uses sleeping pills. Most experts on sleep disorders agree that there is a role for sleeping pills in a situation that is temporary or for persistent insomnia that is related to nonpsychotic psychiatric disorders. Before prescribing sleeping pills, a doctor should alert the patient to the effects the pills will have on thinking, breathing, alertness, and performance, among other factors.

Surprisingly few studies have provided information about the use of sleeping pills in very old people with dementia or related mental conditions. The normal classes of sleeping pills such as the benzodiazepines do not offer a useful long-term strategy for successful management of sleeping problems in older people. This is especially true for older people with dementing illness. For the nondemented person with severe insomnia who cannot function without sleep-promoting medication, the use of a low-dose sedating antidepressant may be a useful alternative. Antidepressants retain their sedating effects for a longer time than benzodiazepines but without incurring the development of tolerance, daytime symptoms, or withdrawal symptoms. These medications may have other effects, however, such as causing drops in blood pressure when a person is standing, and this must be taken into consideration. Frequently, people with sleep disorders have depressive symptoms that may benefit from the use of these antidepressant compounds. For people with major depressions, tricyclic antidepressants usually prolong the time between onset of sleep and REM sleep and suppress REM sleep to an appropriate 8 to 10 percent of total sleep. In short, some antidepressant medications seem to restore the sleep to a pattern closer to that seen in younger people.

Diphenhydramine, another medication, has long been used to promote sleep in older people, but its effectiveness is not as clear as that of other compounds and its usefulness in older people may be limited. If it is determined that muscle jerks at night (myoclonus) are a major cause of the person's insomnia, then a benzodiazepine may be helpful. Although the cause of nocturnal leg jerks is unknown, these medications seem to keep the person from waking up during the jerks, allowing normal sleep. Generally, in this condition it is important to use the benzodiazepines with the shortest elimination half-life.

The only reliable way to determine that the sleep disturbance is due to disordered breathing (sleep apnea) is for the person to participate in a sleep laboratory. There are many causes of this sleep apnea and an important element may be closing of the upper airway muscles leading to blockage and breathing difficulty. Whether this disorder requires treatment and what the treatment should be depends upon complex considerations. Interventions range from such behavioral changes as weight loss and reduction of alcohol consumption to significant surgical procedures involving the nasal passages, back of the mouth, and throat.

The Outlook for People with Sleeping Problems

While physicians generally assume that sleep disturbance in late life tends to be chronic and intermittent, there is little information to guide them in this assumption. It seems reasonable to assume that a sleep disturbance will most likely occur in relation to medical and psychiatric conditions that then are seen as part of the cause of the complaint. One major aspect of sleep duration in late life is in its relationship to death. For example, men who report fewer than four hours of sleep per night have about three times higher the likelihood of dying within six years compared with those who sleep seven to eight hours per night.

Walking Problems, Immobility, and Falls

Mobility refers to a person's ability to physically maneuver through the environment. Personal mobility depends upon being able to move from one surface to another and to propel oneself either by walking or by wheelchair. Immobility, therefore, is defined as having a problem in one or more of these areas. Falls are unintentional changes in position that result in hitting the ground. Generally, an event is not called a fall if a person faints or is overcome by a hazard, such as being hit by a car. Falls and immobility are related because immobility can lead to falls, which, in turn, may further reduce mobility. Because walking difficulties and falls often share the same causes and risk factors, let us consider them together.

Prevalence of Walking Problems, Falls, and Fall Injuries

Many older people have difficulty in walking and transferring from one place to another. (See Chapter 8 for more information.) If one defines a walking problem as significant slowing or an abnormal walking pattern, then gait disorders affect 15 to 20 percent of older people. About 20 percent of people who are over age 75 require help from someone to get out of a chair. Thirty percent of this group of people also have difficulty climbing stairs. In addition, 40 percent of people older than 75 are unable to walk for half a mile, and slightly less than 10 percent cannot walk across a room without the help of another person. Because the ability to move through the environment is essential for daily functioning, walking problems are partially responsible for the functional decline in activities of daily living that commonly occurs with aging. Severe immobility, defined as being unable to get out of a chair or a bed, can lead to other complications such as pressure ulcers, contractures of the joints, and urinary incontinence.

Each year, one-third of older people living in the community who are 75 and older fall. Of these one-half fall repeatedly. In nursing homes, the fall rate is estimated at one to two falls per person per year. The chance of falling increases with age.

In this country, the sixth leading cause of death in people over age 65 is accidents. The majority of these accidents are from falls. Broken bones and soft tissue injuries such as bruises and scrapes account for most of the nonfatal injuries related to falls. About 5 percent of falls in older people result in a fracture; 1 percent result in a hip fracture. In addition, 5 to 10 percent of falls cause restrictions in activity or result in a serious injury, such as a major bruise, joint dislocation, or sprain, requiring medical care. Although it is uncommon, a collection of blood between the brain and the skull, called a subdural hematoma, is a potentially devastating fall-related injury. Unfortunately, injuries other than hip fractures have not been studied thoroughly enough to provide accurate estimates of how often they occur, what lasting effects they cause, and what costs they incur.

Another disability caused by falls is the fear of falling again. This leads to self-imposed restriction of activity. Between 10 and 25 percent of people who have fallen admit to avoiding activities such as shopping or housekeeping because of their fears of falls or injury. Family members and other caregivers may also discourage activity. These physical and psychological consequences of falls and immobility contribute to the functional decline in many elderly people.

The causes and risk factors for falls and immobility can be understood by considering the various components that are necessary for us to remain stable while on our feet. Being stable requires the highly coordinated input and response of the several body systems: nervous, musculoskeletal, cardiovascular, respiratory, and others. Falls and immobility result either from a single disease that impairs a major component of stability or, more commonly, from the accumulated effect of multiple diseases superimposed on each other and on age-related changes. Some of the important age-related changes in balance include increased swaying from side to side and slowed responses to changes in position. The changes in walking that occur with age include a decreased step length, decreased walking speed, and increased time spent on both feet. These changes have very little significance until diseases and disorders become superimposed on them.

The Causes of Walking Problems and Falls

Various diseases can interfere with a person's balance, impair the gait, or promote falls and often affect the neurologic and musculoskeletal systems, including stroke, Parkinson's disease, severe arthritis in the neck, vitamin B_{12} deficiency, and problems with the lower back. Gait abnormalities are common and can involve difficulty in starting to walk, a stooped-over posture, variability in the steps, staggering, decreased height of the steps resulting in a shuffling kind of gait, and inability to walk in a straight line. People with these difficulties are usually able to keep from falling forward but may topple backward very easily.

Falls Caused by Single Conditions

Probably the most common cause of walking difficulty related to spinal cord disease in the older age group is cervical spondylosis, or degeneration of the cervical spine (the section of the spine located in the neck). Factors that predispose people to this condition include congenital narrowing of the spinal canal in the neck, trauma, bony growths that narrow the canal, and specific forms of arthritis such as rheumatoid arthritis. Numbness and tingling of the fingers and clumsiness with fine-motor tasks such as buttoning clothing are early symptoms. As the condition progresses, there may be mild weakness in the legs and difficulty in feeling vibration in the feet. The walking problems probably result from a combination of changes in muscle strength, coordination, and difficulty in telling one's position in space (the medical term for this is proprioception). While the degenerative changes of the cervical spine may be seen on X rays of the neck, additional studies, such as computed tomography (CT) or magnetic resonance imaging (MRI), may be needed to demonstrate that the spinal cord is pinched in the neck.

There are other spinal canal conditions that cause walking difficulty. Narrowing of the spinal canal in the low back can occur with neck disease or it can occur independently. Most people with this condition (over 90 percent) feel a sense of pain, numbness, or weakness in the buttocks, thighs, or legs on standing or walking or sometimes with exercise. Usually these symptoms go away when the person sits down or lies down. The majority of people with this condition also have low back pain. A physical examination may show a change in neurologic reflexes in the ankle and knee and mild muscle weakness, particularly in the legs. Because serious diseases such as cancer can also produce neck and back problems, the older person with any change in walking ability should be evaluated carefully by a physician.

Sometimes blood vessel disease in the brain causes problems with walking. This is more common among people with high blood pressure; walking difficulty may result from changes in small blood vessels or even from small strokes.

Severe musculoskeletal problems can also result in instability, difficulty in walking, and falling. Severe arthritis of the hips or knees can compromise walking as a result of pain, muscle weakness, or loss of joint flexibility.

Falling can also be a sign of a sudden illness such as pneumonia, urinary tract infection, or congestive heart failure. About 5 percent of the time, falls are signals of these significant underlying diseases.

Falls Due to Multiple Conditions

The majority of falls have several causes and result from the accumulated effect of multiple impairments of sensory, neurologic, and musculoskeletal components.

Diseases and disabilities in the eyes, ears, and balance control systems can increase the risk of falling and instability. Changes in the eyes that occur with age include slow adaptation to the dark and difficulty in accommodating to distances. Age-related diseases such as cataracts, macular degeneration, and glaucoma are also common. Visual orientation in space (and with movement) may be more relevant to falling than visual acuity—the ability to read letters along a line as in a standard vision test. Changes in the ear are common among older people and can create a sense of motion (vertigo), dizziness in response to head movements, and decreased stability in the dark. Factors that predispose to inner-ear disease include past exposure to certain antibiotics; present use of aspirin, tobacco, alcohol, and other drugs; head trauma; and previous ear infections or ear surgery. In addition, diseases that affect the balance system in the ear such as Ménière's disease are more common in older people.

The proprioceptive system orients people in space during changes in body position or when other senses are impaired. The system is made up of the joints in the neck, hips, knees, and feet, special receptors located in other joints, and other connections within the brain and nervous system. When an older person has difficulty maintaining balance as the body changes position, this is most likely due to malfunction of the nerve endings in the legs and feet. This condition is seen with diseases such as diabetes mellitus and vitamin B_{12} deficiency, both of which are more common in elderly people. As mentioned earlier, severe neck disease can also result in proprioceptive abnormalities. People with such abnormalities may complain of dizziness, a sense of motion, or unsteadiness when they turn their head. A common symptom is the inability to feel vibration in the legs and feet.

Because the central nervous system handles all of this sensory information, it is not surprising that central nervous system disorders including dementing illness, contribute to instability, immobility, and falling. Dementing illness increases the risk of falling even among people without a specific gait problem.

The movement aspect of the balance system involves the nervous system, muscles, joints, and bones. Disease or disabilities that affect any of these components such as arthritis, muscle weakness, or foot problems can result in an increased risk of imbalance and falling. Calluses, bunions, toe deformities, and deformed toenails, for example, may impair spatial orientation or cause limping or stumbling.

A sudden drop in blood pressure may act in concert with other conditions to cause falls and difficulty walking, but it is sometimes severe enough by itself to cause a person to fall. Medications, dehydration, and changes in the blood vessels and nervous system can all be culprits. People who feel dizzy, faint, or experience a fall within an hour after eating may have these symptoms because of a drop in blood pressure that occurs after meals.

Medications are significant as potential, and correctable, contributors to balance problems and falling. Any medication that affects the nervous system can increase the risk of falling and injury, such as sedatives, drugs given for anxiety, antidepressants, diuretics, heart medications, drugs for arthritis, and pain relievers. The greater the total number of medications a person receives, the greater the risk of falling.

Sedatives increase a person's chance of falling by 28 times. Dementing illness makes a person 5 times more likely to fall compared with people without dementing illness; leg problems make a person about 4 times more likely to fall. Among people living in nursing homes, weakness of the hip muscles, poor balance, and taking more than four medications are each independently predictive of falling during a year. All people who have three or more of these risk factors are highly likely to fall in the course of a year.

How the Environment Influences Falls

Over 75 percent of falls by elderly people occur at home. Tripping over objects or on stairs or steps is the most common cause. Environmental factors not only increase the chance of falling but they may also impair mobility. Low soft chairs, low toilet seats, a lack of things to hold on to, and poor access to light switches or dim lighting are just a few examples of environmental impediments.

Most falls occur during ordinary actions such as walking or changing position. Only about 5 to 10 percent of falls by people living in the community occur during clearly hazardous activities such as climbing a ladder or standing on a chair. The more active the person is the greater the risk of falling.

The ideal goal is to minimize the risk of falling while maximizing the person's mobility and independence. The best assessment and treatment plan will incorporate the preferences of the person, the family, the caregiver, and the physician.

Preventing Falls

Falling and immobility can be minimized in many ways; regular exercise is certainly a good strategy for reducing the likelihood of falling. However, once a fall or balance problem has occurred, it is important to review any previous falls and other risk factors and evaluate the person's balance and gait. Once any balance and gait problems have been identified, treatment solutions should include medical, rehabilitative, and environmental components. Medical and surgical interventions are aimed at eliminating or reducing the impairments; rehabilitative interventions are designed to help people compensate or adapt to impairments; and environmental interventions are directed at decreasing the impact of the impairments (see Chapter 8 for rehabilitation options).

The first step in evaluating ways to reduce falling is understanding its origin. A basic checklist that includes sensory, neurologic, musculoskeletal, and systemic diseases is useful (see Table 50). A careful review of medications is also an important part of this evaluation.

As indicated in Table 50, the results of the evaluation help determine the range of possible medical, rehabilitative, and environmental interventions. For example, people with impaired vision should see their opthalmologist for a change in their glasses, or if necessary, for evaluation of cataracts. They should also be advised to maximize the lighting inside their home to avoid falls due to poorly visualized obstacles.

Proprioceptive contributors to balance problems can often be detected by checking the range of movement in the neck. A physician can check for various disease states such as vitamin B_{12} deficiency. If a condition is uncovered, rehabilitative and environmental interventions include balance exercises, using appropriate walking aids, and wearing appropriate footwear. Firm shoes register a much better sensation of spatial relations to the feet than does walking barefoot or using slippers. Walking on thick carpets or uneven surfaces can also cause problems. People with proprioceptive difficulty should be careful in the dark because they tend to rely so much on their vision to maintain their balance.

Table 50. Possible Interventions for Fall Risk Factors

RISK FACTORS	POSSIBLE INTERVENTIONS
VISION	
Medical	Eyeglasses; cataract extraction
Rehabilitative	Balance and gait training; low-vision aids
Environmental	Good lighting; home safety assessment; architectural design that minimizes distortions and illusions
HEARING	
Medical	Earwax removal; hearing evaluation
Rehabilitative	Training in hearing aid use
Environmental	Decrease of background noise
INNER-EAR DYSFUNCTION	
Medical	Avoidance of certain drugs
Rehabilitative	Special exercises
Environmental	Good lighting (increased reliance on visual input); home safety assessment
NECK AND NERVE PROBLEMS	
Medical	Diagnosis and treatment of specific diseases such as spinal cord compression, vitamin B_{12} deficiency
Rehabilitative	Balance exercises; appropriate walking aid
Environmental	Good lighting (increased reliance on visual input); good footwear; home safety assessment
CENTRAL NERVOUS SYSTEM DISEASES	
Medical	Diagnosis and treatment of specific diseases such as Parkinson's disease
Rehabilitative	Physical therapy; balance and gait training; appropriate walking aid
Environmental	Home safety assessment; appropriate adaptation (e.g., high, firm chairs, raised toilet seats, grab bars in bathroom)
DEMENTIA	
Medical	Avoidance of sedating drugs
Rehabilitative	Supervised exercise and ambulation
Environmental	Safe, structured, supervised environment

Musculoskeletal evaluation is an important part of the assessment. In individual circumstances, any of a number of interven-

RISK FACTORS	POSSIBLE INTERVENTIONS
MUSCULOSKELETAL PROBLEMS, INCLUDING HIP AND KNEE WEAKNESS, ANKLE WEAKNESS, FOOT PROBLEMS	
Medical	Diagnosis and treatment of specific diseases
Rehabilitative	Balance and gait training; muscle-strengthening exercises; back exercises; correct walking aid; correct footwear; good foot care (e.g., nails, calluses, bunions)
Environmental	Home safety assessment; appropriate adaptations
POSTURAL HYPOTENSION	
Medical	Diagnosis and treatment of specific diseases; avoidance of offending drugs; careful medication review; rehydration; identification of precipitating situations (e.g., meals)
Rehabilitative	Reconditioning exercises; graded pressure stockings
Environmental	Elevation of head of bed
DEPRESSION	
Medical	Review medication regimen
MEDICATIONS, ESPECIALLY SEDATIVES, PHENOTHIAZINES, ANTIDEPRESSANTS	
Medical	Determination of lowest effective dose of essential medication; readjustment and discontinuation when possible; selection of shorter-acting medications
ACUTE ILLNESS; NEW OR INCREASED MEDICATIONS	
Medical	Diagnosis and treatment of specific diseases; starting of medications at low dose and increasing slowly
Environmental	Increased supervision during illnesses or with new medications

Source: Adapted from Tinetti ME, Speechley M. Prevention of falls among the elderly. *New England Journal of Medicine.* 1989;320:1056. Reprinted with permission.

tions can be helpful. Examples of these include relief of pain, muscle strengthening, range-of-motion exercises, balance and gait training, back exercises, correct footwear, good foot care, and appropriate walking aids.

For people with a sudden drop in blood pressure on standing, the specific causes must be addressed. In addition to these, the therapy can involve eliminating or providing substitutions for any offending medications. Other useful steps include ensuring adequate intake of fluids, liberalizing salt intake, and flexing the ankles, wrists, and hands just before getting up. Elevating the head of the bed can also be useful. For people with a fall in blood pressure after meals, smaller meals and consuming judicious amounts of caffeine may sometimes help.

Evaluating Balance and Gait There are also several simple, practical, less expensive techniques to evaluate balance and gait. The simplest part of a physician's or caregiver's evaluation involves watching the person get up from a chair, walk a few steps, turn around, walk back to the chair, and sit down again. Difficulty or unsteadiness in any of these actions requires further evaluation. If stair climbing is a regular part of the person's daily activities, it, too, should be evaluated.

Assessment of the home is very important because most falls occur there. An environmental checklist that outlines the types of hazards to look for is shown in Table 51. To some extent, what actually constitutes an environmental hazard depends upon the person's problems. By helping to involve the person in the identification of hazards and developing a plan of care, home care can be improved significantly.

People who live in nursing homes are generally more frail than people who live in the community. More subtle hazards can affect them such as ill-fitting shoes, pants that are too long, or slippery floors. In certain circumstances, the objects used to improve safety may actually increase the risk of injury. For example, bed rails can be climbed over, walking aids can be tripped over, and restraints can be entangling.

Finally, in addition to identifying the predisposing factors, balance and gait problems, environmental hazards, and other factors, there should be a review of any previous falls. A knowledge of such things as newly prescribed medications, any new illness, recurring dizziness, or other symptoms may help to explain why a fall occurred and to prevent others. For example, if the fall occurred during a worsening of congestive heart failure, then closer observation and evaluation of the person would be warranted if the heart failure recurred or if the person had another fall.

The person's activity at the time of the fall should also be considered. If the person was not doing something considered hazard-

Table 51. Strategies for Reducing Environmental Fall Hazards

ENVIRONMENTAL FACTOR	STRATEGIES
Lighting	Nonglare and without shadows; switches accessible to room entrances; night-light in bedroom, hall, bathroom
Floor surfaces	Throw rugs with nonskid backing; carpet edges tacked down; carpets with shallow pile; nonskid wax on floors; cords out of walking path; small objects (e.g., clothes, shoes) off floor
Stairs	Good lighting with switches at top and bottom; securely fastened bilateral handrails that stand out from wall; top and bottom stair marked with bright, contrasting tape; risers no more than 6 inches; steps in good repair; nothing stored on steps
Kitchen	Items stored so that reaching up and bending over not necessary; secure stepstool available if climbing necessary; firm, nonmovable table
Bathroom	Grab bars for tub or shower and toilet; nonskid decals or rubber mat in tub or shower; shower chair with handheld shower; nonskid rugs; raised toilet seat; locks removed to ensure access
Outdoors	Attention to cracks in pavement, holes in lawn, and rocks, tools, and other tripping hazards; walkways well lit and free of ice and wet leaves; stairs and steps as above
Institution	All the above; bed at proper height (not too high or low); no spills on floor; appropriate use of walking aids and wheelchairs
Footwear	Firm, nonskid, nonfriction soles; low heels (unless accustomed to high heels); no walking in stocking feet or loose slippers

Source: Adapted from Tinetti ME, Speechley M. Prevention of falls among the elderly. *New England Journal of Medicine.* 1989;320:1058. Reprinted with permission.

ous, as is most often the case, the preventive emphasis should be on improving the safety and effectiveness of the activity, on balance and gait training, and on improving the safety of the environment in which the activity occurred.

RESOURCES

While this list represents a comprehensive guide to organizations that address the clinical care needs of older people, it is not a resource of all social service agencies and organizations that assist older citizens. If you have questions that do not specifically relate to one of the following organizations, please contact your state Administration on Aging. These state agencies can provide information on local services and to other local agencies. Their telephone numbers are available in your phone directory.

General Aging

Administration on Aging
330 Independence Ave., SW
Washington, DC 20201
(202) 619–0724

Aging Network Services
4400 East-West Hwy.
Bethesda, MD 20814
(301) 657–4329

American Association of Homes for the Aging
901 E St., NW
Washington, DC 20004–2242
(202) 783–2242

American Association of Retired Persons
601 E St., NW
Washington, DC 20049
(202) 434–2277

American Geriatrics Society
770 Lexington Ave., Suite 300
New York, NY 10021
(212) 308–1414

American Red Cross
18th and D St., NW
Washington, DC 20006
(202) 737–8300

American Society on Aging
833 Market St.
San Francisco, CA 94103
(415) 882–2910

Children of Aging Parents
1609 Woodbourne Rd.
Levittown, PA 19057
(215) 945–6900

Disabled American Veterans
807 Maine Ave., SW
Washington, DC 20024
(202) 554–3501

Eldercare Locator
(800) 677–1116

Legal Services for the Elderly
130 West 42d St., 17th Floor
New York, NY 10036
(212) 391–0120

National Aging Resource Center on Elder Abuse
c/o American Public Welfare Association
810 First St., NE, Suite 500
Washington, DC 20002–4205
(202) 682–2470

National AIDS Clearinghouse
PO Box 6003
Rockville, MD 20849–6003

National Alliance for Senior Citizens
1700 18th St., NW
Washington, DC 20009
(202) 986–0117

National Association for Hispanic Elderly
Asociacion Nacional Pro Personas Mayores
3325 Wilshire Blvd.
Los Angeles, CA 90010–1724
(213) 487–1922

National Association for Home Care
519 C St., NE
Washington, DC 20002
(202) 547–7424

National Association of Area Agencies on Aging
1112 16th St., NW
Washington, DC 20036
(202) 296–8130

National Caucus and Center on Black Aged, Inc.
1424 K St., NW
Washington, DC 20005
(202) 637–8400

National Citizens's Coalition for Nursing Home Reform
1424 16th St., NW, Suite 202
Washington, DC 20036
(202) 332-2275

National Council of Senior
    Citizens
1331 F St., NW
Washington, DC 20004
(202) 347–8800

National Council on Patient
    Information and Education
666 11th St., NW, Suite 810
Washington, DC 20001

National Council on the Aging
409 3d St., SW
Washington, DC 20024
(202) 479–1200

National Hospice Organization
1901 North Moore St., Suite 901
Arlington, VA 22209
(703) 243–5900

National Indian Council on Aging
City Centre, Suite 510W
6400 Uptown Blvd.
Albuquerque, NM 87110
(505) 888–3302

National Institute on Aging
    Information Center
PO Box 8057
Gaithersburg, MD 20857
(800) 222–2225

National Pacific/Asian Resource
    Center on Aging
Melbourne Tower, Suite 914
1511 Third Ave.
Seattle, WA 98101
(206) 624–1221

National Rehabilitation
    Information Center
8455 Colesville Road, Suite 935
Silver Spring, MD 20910–3319
(800) 227–0216

National Senior Citizens Law
    Center
1815 H St., NW, Suite 700
Washington, DC 20006
(202) 887–5280

National Shut-In Society, Inc.
1925 North Lynn St., Suite 500
Rosslyn, VA 22209
(703) 516–6770

United Seniors Health
    Cooperative
1331 H St., NW
Washington, DC 20005
(202) 393–6222

Resources on Specific Health Problems

MEMORY AND THINKING PROBLEMS

Alzheimer's Association
919 North Michigan
Chicago, IL 60611
(800) 272–3900

Alzheimer's Disease Education
    and Referral Center
PO Box 8250
Silver Spring, MD 20907–8250
(800) 438–4380

NEUROLOGIC PROBLEMS

American Academy of Neurology
2221 University Ave., SE
Minneapolis, MN 55414
(612) 623–8115

American Parkinson's Disease
    Association
60 Bay St., Suite 401
Staten Island, NY 10301
(800) 223–2732

Epilepsy Foundation of America
4351 Garden City Dr.
Landover, MD 20785
(800) 332–1000

Huntington's Disease Society of
    America
140 West 22d St., 6th Floor
New York, NY 10011–2420
(800) 345–4372

National Institute of Neurological
    Disorders and Stroke
31 Center Dr., MSC 2540
Bethesda, MD 20892–2540
(800) 352–9424

United Parkinson's Foundation
833 West Washington Blvd.
Chicago, IL 60607
(312) 733–1893

PSYCHOLOGICAL PROBLEMS

National Alliance for the
    Mentally Ill
2101 Wilson Blvd., Suite 302
Arlington, VA 22201
(800) 950–6264

National Mental Health
    Association
Information Center
1021 Prince St.
Alexandria, VA 22314–2971

SKIN PROBLEMS

American Academy of
    Dermatology
PO Box 4014
Schaumberg, IL 60168–4014
(708) 330–9830

American Academy of Facial
    Plastic and Reconstructive
    Surgery
1110 Vermont Ave., NW, Suite 220
Washington, DC 20005–3522
(800) 332–FACE

The Skin Cancer Foundation
P.O. Box 561
New York, NY 10056

JOINT, MUSCLE, AND BONE PROBLEMS

American Academy of Orthopedic
  Surgeons
6300 North River Rd.
Rosemont, IL 60018

American Podiatric Medical Assoc.
9312 Old Georgetown Rd.
Bethesda, MD 20814
(800) FOOT–CARE

Arthritis Foundation
1314 Spring St.
Atlanta, GA 30309
(800) 283–7800

Lupus Foundation of America
4 Research Pl., Suite 180
Rockville, MD 20850–3226
(800) 558–0121

National Arthritis and Musculoskeletal and Skin Diseases
  Information Clearing House
Box AMS
9000 Rockville Pike
Bethesda, MD 20892
(301) 495–4484

National Osteoporosis Foundation
1150 17th St., NW, Suite 500
Washington, DC 20036

HEAD AND NECK PROBLEMS

American Academy of
  Otolaryngology—Head and
  Neck Surgery, Inc.
1 Prince St.
Alexandria, VA 22314
(703) 836–4444

HEART AND CIRCULATION PROBLEMS

AHA's Stroke Connection
(800) 553–6321

American Association of
  Cardiovascular and Pulmonary
  Rehabilitation
7611 Elmwood Ave., Suite 201
Middleton, WI 53562
(608) 831–6989

American Heart Association
7272 Greenville Ave.
Dallas, TX 75231–4596
(800) AHA–USA1

Courage Stroke Network
3915 Golden Valley Rd.
Golden Vally, MN 55422
(612) 588–0811

National Heart, Lung and Blood
  Institute
PO Box 30105
Bethesda, MD 20824–0105
(301) 251–1222

National Institute of Neurological
  Disorders and Stroke
31 Center Dr., MSC 2540
Bethesda, MD 20892–2540
(800) 352–9424

National Stroke Association
300 East Hampden Ave.
Englewood, CO 80110–2654
(303) 762–9922

DIABETES

American Diabetes Association
1660 Duke St.
Alexandria, VA 22314
(800) DIABETES

National Diabetes Information
  Clearinghouse
1 Information Way
Bethesda, MD 20892–3560

LUNG AND BREATHING PROBLEMS

American Association of
  Cardiovascular and Pulmonary
  Rehabilitation
7611 Elmwood Ave., Suite 201
Middleton, WI 53562
(608) 831–6989

American Lung Association
1740 Broadway
New York, NY 10019–4374
(212) 315–8700

National Heart, Lung and Blood
  Institute
PO Box 30105
Bethesda, MD 20824–0105
(301) 251–1222

DIGESTIVE PROBLEMS

American Liver Foundation
1425 Pomptom Ave.
Cedar Grove, NJ 07009
(201) 256–2550

National Digestive Disease
  Information Clearinghouse
2 Information Way
Bethesda, MD 20892–2480

United Ostomy Association
36 Executive Park, Suite 120
Irvine, CA 92714
(714) 660–8624

NUTRITIONAL CONCERNS

Food and Nutrition Information
    Center
10301 Baltimore Blvd.
Room 304
Dept. of Agriculture, NALB
Beltsville, MD 20705–2351

National Association of Meal
    Programs
101 North Alfred St.
Alexandria, VA 22314
(703) 548–5558

URINARY PROBLEMS

HIP (Help for Incontinent People)
PO Box 544
Union, SC 29379
(800) BLADDER

National Kidney and Urologic
    Diseases Information
    Clearinghouse
3 Information Way
Bethesda, MD 20892–3560

National Kidney Foundation
30 East 33d St.
New York, NY 10016
(800) 622–9010

The Simon Foundation for
    Continence
PO Box 835
Wilmette, IL 60091
(800) 237–SIMON

SEXUALITY AND SEXUAL CONCERNS

American College of Obstetricians
    and Gynecologists
409 12th St., SW
Washington, DC 20024
(202) 347–1140

Hysterectomy Educational
    Resources and Services
    Foundation
422 Bryn Mawr Ave.
Bala Cynwyd, PA 19004

SIGHT PROBLEMS

American Academy of
    Opthalmology
PO Box 7424
San Francisco, CA 94120–7424
(415) 561–8500

American Foundation for the Blind
15 West 16th St.
New York, NY 10011
(800) 232–5463

American Optometric Association
243 North Lindbergh Blvd.
St. Louis, MO 63141–7881
(314) 991–4100

Better Vision Institute
1800 North Kent St., Suite 904
Rosslyn, VA 22209
(800) 424–8422

Foundation for Glaucoma
    Research
490 Post St., Suite 830
San Francisco, CA 94102
(800) 826–6693

National Eye Institute
Information Office
Building 31, Room 6A32
Bethesda, MD 20892
(301) 496–5248

National Society to Prevent
    Blindness
500 East Remington Rd.
Schaumberg, IL 60173
(800) 331–2020

HEARING PROBLEMS

American Tinnitus Association
PO Box 5
Portland, OR 97207
(503) 248–9985

Better Hearing Institute
PO Box 1840
Washington, DC 20013
(800) EARWELL

International Hearing Society
20361 Middlebelt Rd.
Livonia, MI 48152
(810) 478–2610

National Institute on Deafness and
    Other Communication
    Disorders
Information Office
Building 31, Room 3C35
9000 Rockville Pike
Bethesda, MD 20892
(301) 496–7243

Self Help for Hard of Hearing
    People
7910 Woodmont Ave., Suite 1200
Bethesda, MD 20814
(301) 657–2248

CANCER

American Cancer Society, Inc.
National Headquarters
1599 Clifton Rd., NE
Atlanta, GA 30329
(800) 227–2345

National Cancer Institute
Cancer Information Service
9000 Rockville Pike
Bethesda, MD 20892
(800) 422–6237

INDEX